Fertility Counseling: Clinical Guide

Fertility Counseling: Clinical Guide

2nd Edition

Edited by
Sharon N. Covington
Shady Grove Fertility, Rockville, MD

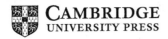

CAMBRIDGE
UNIVERSITY PRESS

CAMBRIDGE
UNIVERSITY PRESS

University Printing House, Cambridge CB2 8BS, United Kingdom

One Liberty Plaza, 20th Floor, New York, NY 10006, USA

477 Williamstown Road, Port Melbourne, VIC 3207, Australia

314–321, 3rd Floor, Plot 3, Splendor Forum, Jasola District Centre,
New Delhi – 110025, India

103 Penang Road, #05–06/07, Visioncrest Commercial, Singapore 238467

Cambridge University Press is part of the University of Cambridge.

It furthers the University's mission by disseminating knowledge in the pursuit of
education, learning, and research at the highest international levels of excellence.

www.cambridge.org
Information on this title: www.cambridge.org/9781009014298
DOI: 10.1017/9781009030151

First published 2015
This second edition published 2023

A catalogue record for this publication is available from the British Library.

Library of Congress Cataloging-in-Publication Data
Names: Covington, Sharon N, editor.
Title: Fertility counseling : clinical guide / edited by Sharon N Covington.
Description: Second edition. | Cambridge, United Kingdom ; New York, NY :
Cambridge University Press, 2022. | Includes bibliographical references and
index.
Identifiers: LCCN 2022020589 (print) | LCCN 2022020590 (ebook) | ISBN
9781009014298 (paperback) | ISBN 9781009030151 (ebook)
Subjects: MESH: Infertility – psychology | Reproductive Techniques, Assisted –
psychology | Counseling
Classification: LCC RC889 (print) | LCC RC889 (ebook) | NLM WP 570 | DDC
616.6/92–dc23/eng/20220624
LC record available at https://lccn.loc.gov/2022020589
LC ebook record available at https://lccn.loc.gov/2022020590

ISBN 978-1-009-01429-8 Paperback

....

My passion for the field of fertility counseling derives from what family means to me –

the family created with the love and unwavering support from my dear husband of over 50 years, Barry T. Covington, and the energy, enthusiasm, common values and bond shared with the children we were blessed with and their growing families:

Michelle Covington Harmon, her husband Scott and their children Sean, Michaela and Liam;

Brendan Truitt Covington, his wife Darlene and their children Luke and Elaina;

Laura Covington MacNevin, her husband Tom and their daughter Margaret

Family is more than just a word . . . it is something that exists within your heart.

Contents

V Special Topics in Fertility Counseling

VI Practice Issues

Online resources and tools for fertility counseling practice are available at www.cambridge.org/coving ton-clinical-guide
Password: ClinicalGuide2023

Preface

Fertility Counseling: Clinical Guide Volume

The formulation of the second edition of *Fertility Counseling* occurred during the time of COVID-19. As the world changed dramatically and instantly, so did we. Our mental health services were never more important. My dear friend and colleague Linda Applegarth and I were teaching a year-long training program, The Fertility Counseling Postgraduate Course, via live video conference to an international group of clinicians eager to learn this field. When COVID-19 hit in March 2020, and despite the worldwide shut down, we were able to continue our course without missing a beat. Hearing the stories of what mental health professionals from India, the Philippines, Mexico, Greece, Australia, the Middle East, Africa (to name a few countries), as well as across the US and Canada, were experiencing in their work and personal lives was both heartbreaking and awe-inspiring.

In teaching this course and listening to my students over the last five years, the vision for a second edition was realized: a two-volume approach consisting of a clinical guide and an in-depth exploration of the concepts presented through case studies. In class, I often use the analogy that we will be building a house over the year. As it relates to this edition, the foundation starts with a thorough understanding of the medical and psychosocial issues of infertility and theoretical context of reproductive psychology. The framing of the house includes the therapeutic approaches to providing fertility counseling – individual, couple and group therapy, and supporting methods pertaining to sexual therapy, the intersection of psychiatric disorders with infertility, and the use of spirituality in treatment. Then we explore the rooms – counseling gamete/embryo donors and recipients, gestational surrogate participants, as well as issues related to disclosure and family life after donor conception. Understanding the needs of all our patients, including diverse groups who may or may not be infertile and, yet, often feel marginalized, is imperative – LGBQ+,

transgender people requesting fertility preservation and/or family building assistance, patients of races or cultures different from their healthcare professionals, and the often-overlooked experience of men in treatment. Additional issues to consider, such as reproductive loss, trauma and resiliency, can "shake or shape" the structure of treatment for both patients and fertility counselors. Pregnancy and postpartum adjustment can present new challenges for our patients as well as unanticipated conflict when the fertility counselor becomes pregnant. Last, the roof of the house pertains to issues in clinical practice that help hold the structure together and protect it: legal framework, practice management and competency including telemental health which has shifted the way most fertility counselors practice, and the ever-changing complexities in reproductive medicine that continue to present ethical challenges for all clinicians. Having a strong ethical platform to address these issues provides both a roof and a foundation in fertility counseling.

With the encouragement of my long-time, wonderfully supportive editor at Cambridge, Nick Dunton, who recently retired, the scope of the second edition expanded to twenty-seven chapters in each volume – fifty-four chapters in all, a calculation I failed to make when first committing to the revision! In considering the necessary updates and additions, I thought about feedback from readers, changes in reproductive medical care over recent years, and how terminology in this field continues to evolve and change, reflecting today's culture. What is accepted today may be considered antiquated or inappropriate tomorrow. The most prominent example, "anonymous" has been eliminated from our reference since anonymity no longer exists as a result of direct-to-consumer DNA testing.

I am honored to have had an esteemed group of clinicians, researchers, academics, advocates, and colleagues write chapters in these volumes – forty-eight contributors in all. Many are cherished friends as well as pioneers in the field of fertility counseling, while others are talented young practitioners whom I got to know as students in my course. While the list is too long to mention each by name, I hope all know how much I appreciate their support and admire their work and dedication to this field. I am so grateful for these authors' enthusiasm, support, shared vision and willingness to commit to this project during the demands presented by COVID-19. Thank you all!

Sharon Covington
December 2021

Contributors

G. David Adamson, MD
Director, Equal3, A Professional Corporation, Cupertino, CA;
CEO, ARC® Fertility; Cupertino, CA;
Clinical Professor, ACF, Stanford University, Stanford, CA; and Associate Clinical Professor, University of California San Francisco, CA, US

Linda Applegarth, EdD
Clinical Associate Professor of Psychology, Departments of Obstetrics & Gynecology, Reproductive Medicine, and Psychiatry
The Ronald O. Perelman/Claudia Cohen Center for Reproductive Medicine
Weill Medical College of Cornell University
New York, New York

Lauren Magalnick Berman, PhD
Licensed Psychologist,
Fertility Psychology Center of Atlanta, LLC,
Atlanta, GA, US

Kate Bourne, BSW
Private Practice, Melbourne, AU

Laura Covington, PhD
Clinical Social Worker,
Shady Grove Fertility and Covington & Hafkin and Associates
Washington, DC, US

Sharon N. Covington, MSW
Director of Psychological Support Services, Shady Grove Fertility, Rockville, MD and
Assistant Clinical Professor, Department of Obstetrics and Gynecology, Georgetown University School of Medicine, Washington, DC, US

Marilyn Crawshaw, PhD, CQSW
Department of Social Policy & Social Work, University of York, York, UK

Teni Davoudian, PhD
Assistant Professor of Psychiatry, Director of Psychological Services at Division of Reproductive Endocrinology, Oregon Health & Science University, Portland, OR, US

Eileen Dombo, MSW, PhD
Associate Professor and Assistant Dean & PhD Program Chairperson, The National Catholic School of Social Service, The Catholic University of America, Washington, DC, US

Carrie Eichberg, PsyD
Licensed Psychologist, Boise, ID, US

Jane Ellis, BA, CQSW
Donor Conception Network, London, UK

Megan Flood, MA, MSW
Licensed Independent Clinical Social Worker, Washington, DC, US

Trudie Gerrits, PhD
Associate Professor, Medical Anthropologist, University of Amsterdam,
Amsterdam Institute of Social Science Research, The Netherlands

Elaine Gordon, PhD
Clinical Psychologist, Independent Private Practice, Santa Monica, CA, US

Maya Grobel, MSW
Licensed Clinical Social Worker, Private Practice, CEO of EM•POWER donation LLC,
Los Angeles, CA, US

Kimberly Grocher, PhD
Clinical Social Worker, Independent Practice, NY and FL
Lecturer, School of Social Work, Columbia University;
Lecturer of Social Work in Psychiatry, Weill Cornell

Medical College; Adjunct Professor, Graduate School of Social Services, Fordham University, NY, US

Sarah R. Holley, PhD
Professor, Clinical Psychology, San Francisco State University, and HS Assistant Clinical Professor, Department of Psychiatry and Behavioral Sciences, University of California, San Francisco, CA, US

Astrid Indekeu, PhD
Licensed psychologist, sexologist, private practice, Hasselt, Belgium, Fellow at Centre for Sociological Research, KU Leuven, Leuven, Belgium

Janet Jaffe, PhD
Co-founder and Co-director of the Center for Reproductive Psychology, San Diego, CA, US

Jamie Joseph, PhD
Licensed Psychologist, Independent Practice
Coral Springs, FL, US

Laura Josephs, PhD
Clinical Assistant Professor of Psychology
The Ronald O. Perelman/ Claudia Cohen Center for Reproductive Medicine Weill Medical College of Cornell University New York, NY, USA

Erika Kelley, PhD
Clinical Psychologist, Department of Obstetrics and Gynecology, University Hospitals Cleveland Medical Center; Assistant Professor, Departments of Reproductive Biology and Urology, Case Western Reserve University School of Medicine, Cleveland, OH, USA

Sheryl Kingsberg, PhD
Clinical Psychologist and Chief, Division of Behavioral Medicine, Department of Obstetrics and Gynecology, University Hospitals Cleveland Medical Center; Professor, Departments of Reproductive Biology, Psychiatry and Urology, Case Western Reserve University School of Medicine, Cleveland, OH, US

Susan Klock, PhD
Professor, Departments of Obstetrics and Gynecology and Psychiatry, Northwestern University Feinberg School of Medicine, Chicago, IL, US

Kristy Koser, PhD
Licensed Professional Clinical Counselor, Aporia Counseling & Psychotherapy, PLLC
Berlin, OH, US

Irving Leon, PhD
Adjunct Associate Professor of Obstetrics and Gynecology, Michigan Medicine,
Ann Arbor, MI, US

Rayna D. Markin, PhD
Associate Professor in Counseling, Villanova University; Licensed Psychologist, Attune Philadelphia Therapy Group,
Philadelphia, PA, US

Molly Moravek, MD, MPH
Associate Professor and Director, Fertility Preservation Program, Division of Reproductive Endocrinology and Infertility, Department of Obstetrics and Gynecology, Department of Urology, University of Michigan, Ann Arbor, MI, US

Jeanne O'Brien, MD
Reproductive Endocrinologist and Chairperson, Ethics Committee,
Shady Grove Fertility, Rockville, MD, US

Lauri A. Pasch, PhD
Professor, Department of Psychiatry and Behavioral Sciences
University of California, San Francisco CA, US

Brennan Peterson, PhD
Professor, Chapman University
Departments of Marriage and Family Therapy & Psychology
Crean College of Health and Behavioral Sciences
Orange, CA USA

William Petok, PhD
Licensed Psychologist, Independent Practice,
Baltimore, MD, USA

Rachel Rabinor, MSW
Licensed Clinical Social Worker, Certified in Perinatal Mental Health
Independent Practice, San Diego, CA, US

Trystan Reese
CEO, Collaborative Consulting, Portland, OR, US

Mary Riddle, PhD
Associate Teaching Professor of Psychology, Department of Psychology,
The Pennsylvania State University,
University Park, PA, US

Patricia Sachs, MSW
Licensed Clinical Social Worker,
Shady Grove Fertility and Covington & Hafkin and Associates
Rockville, MD, US

Tara Simpson, PsyD
Licensed Psychologist,
Shady Grove Fertility and Covington & Hafkin and Associates
Rockville, MD, US

Margaret Swain, RN, JD
Attorney in Private Practice,
Baltimore, MD, US

Carol Toll, MSW
Licensed Clinical Social Worker,

Shady Grove Fertility and Covington & Hafkin and Associates
Rockville, MD, US

Uschi Van den Broeck, PhD
Clinical Psychologist and Family Therapist,
University Hospitals Leuven, Gasthuisberg,
Leuven University Fertility Center (LUFC), Leuven, Belgium

Katherine Williams, MD
Clinical Professor of Psychiatry, Stanford University School of Medicine
and Director of the Women's Wellness Clinic, Stanford, CA, US

Landon Zaki, PsyD, PMH-C
Licensed Psychologist
Bloom Therapy
San Francisco, CA USA

Julianne E. Zweifel, PhD
Department of Obstetrics & Gynecology
University of Wisconsin School of Medicine & Public Health,
Madison, WI, US

Collaborative Reproductive Healthcare Model
A Patient-Centered Approach to Medical and Psychosocial Care

Sharon N. Covington and G. David Adamson

Introduction

There is nothing "typical" about the average patient who seeks fertility treatment today. Rapid advancement in technology and changes in societal views of reproductive rights have created choices and options for family building few could have imagined one generation ago. Heterosexual/opposite-sex couples, while still the norm, are being joined by a diverse group of adults who also long for children. Same-sex couples, transgender individuals, single men and women, older people beyond normal reproductive capacity, and those facing life-threatening medical circumstances or serious genetic conditions, have access to reproductive techniques that will allow them to have a child or children. In addition, are those who present wanting to preserve fertility options for the future through cryopreservation of their gametes, or even family members requesting sperm retrieval posthumously after a sudden, tragic death.

This chapter will lay the foundation for subsequent chapters in this book regarding the medical and psychosocial assessment and treatment of individuals and couples needing reproductive medical assistance. Optimal patient care involves the collaboration of numerous healthcare professionals (doctors, nurses, laboratory scientists, paraprofessionals, administrative staff, as well as mental health professionals) working together to provide reproductive medical services. Over the years, there has been a dramatic shift in the recognition of the psychological consequences of infertility and the role fertility counselors play as an integrated part of the treatment team. There is international consensus that the complex psychosocial issues of infertility patients' experience cannot be separated from the extraordinary reproductive technologies physicians use to treat these problems (i.e., "You can't separate what is being done to your body, from how you feel about what is being done to your body"), which necessitates a collaborative approach to care.

The addenda referred to in this chapter are available for download at www.cambridge.org/covington-clinical-guide

The American Society for Reproductive Medicine (ASRM) and the European Society for Human Reproduction and Embryology (ESHRE), as well as numerous other professional organizations and governmental policies, recognize this multidisciplinary method [1,2]. In addition, there is recognition that, for patients seeking medically assisted reproduction (MAR), "optimal care" requires attention to patients' psychological well-being as well as the quality of their interactions with staff, clinicians and other personnel during treatment [3]. Negative intrapersonal psychological reactions to treatment and difficulties in interactions with others during treatment can create a psychological burden for patients, affecting compliance and their ability to make decisions about continuing with treatment. Thus, "best practice" in reproductive healthcare will include ways to minimize patients' emotional and psychological distress, while providing effective clinical care in a positive environment.

As clinicians and colleagues, the authors have spent their careers advocating for the medical and psychosocial integrative care proposed by Covington with the "collaborative reproductive healthcare model" [4] and by other authors as "patient-centered care" [5] or "integrated approach" [6]. This model has a biopsychosocial approach in which the diagnosis and treatment of impaired reproduction are considered in terms of a variety of aspects impacting an individual's/couple's experience with infertility: physiological, psychosocial, interpersonal, familial, spiritual, cultural and societal. A patient's overall health, functional status, emotional well-being, quality of life and resiliency are influential factors in how s/he can navigate the condition. This approach emphasizes the importance of healthcare professionals and patients as collaborators in diagnosis, treatment and health maintenance to achieve optimum results. This collaborative model integrates the best medical and psychosocial patient care, and is responsive to patient values and needs. The approach in this chapter will be to present this model through a medical and psychosocial overview of the evaluation and treatment of infertility.

Overview of Infertility

In our modern world, most people think that getting pregnant is easy. They think this because a combination of sociologically driven delayed parenting, effective contraception and societal silence regarding infertility creates the perfect storm for disbelief when pregnancy does not occur almost immediately when they "try to get pregnant." Everyone is different, so some couples are highly fertile, others less so but still normal, some have sufficiently impaired fertility that they can be considered subfertile (although there is no agreed definition for this term) and some do not get pregnant within one year of having regular unprotected intercourse and, by the World Health Organization (WHO) definition, are considered infertile [7–9]. Since almost half of couples with no identifiable fertility problem will get pregnant in the second year of trying without any medical intervention, these couples often need and/or receive very little diagnosis and treatment [10]. Couples who fail to get pregnant after five years can be considered sterile, although very rarely pregnancies will occur without medical intervention even in these couples [11].

Importantly, in 2017 the International Glossary on Infertility and Fertility Care, led by the International Committee Monitoring Assisted Reproductive Technologies (ICMART) in partnership with most of the leading reproductive medicine societies in the world, recognized infertility also when due to an impairment of a person's capacity to reproduce either as an individual or with his/her partner, and confirmed again that infertility is a disease which generates disability as an impairment of function [8]. The WHO also published an Infertility Fact Sheet in 2020 that stated, "A wide variety of people, including heterosexual couples, same-sex partners, older persons, individuals who are not in sexual relationships and those with certain medical conditions, such as some HIV sero-discordant couples and cancer survivors, may require infertility management and fertility care services."

Infertility is now defined by the WHO, the American Medical Association and all the major reproductive medicine societies in the world as a "disease." Primary infertility means that the patient has never been pregnant. A woman experiencing infertility after having ever been pregnant, regardless of the outcome of that pregnancy, has secondary infertility. Recurrent miscarriage, historically defined as three spontaneous pregnancy losses, but now defined as the spontaneous loss of two or more clinical pregnancies and usually investigated at that time, is not considered to be infertility, but is a different disease classification [8] (please see the Glossary at the end of this book for other definitions of infertility and fertility care described in this chapter).

It is very difficult to determine the prevalence of infertility. However, studies that have been done suggest that about 7–9% of couples are infertile at any given time [12,13]. Traditionally, the causes of infertility in younger patients (<35) are ovulation problems in about 15% of cases, tubal/pelvic pathology in 35%, male factor in 35%, unexplained in 10% and other causes in the remaining 5% of cases (Figure 1.1). However, over the past two decades, as women and men have delayed attempts at pregnancy, ovulation and hormonal problems, along with decreased egg quality, affect about 40% of the couples, pelvic problems occur in about 30%, cervical/combined factor (e.g., vaginal/cervical abnormalities and failure to have sex) in about 5% and primarily male factor in about 25%. In addition, reduced sperm quality may affect an additional 25% of couples in which a female factor is the primary cause. Some, but not all, studies suggest that decreased ovarian reserve associated with the older age of women

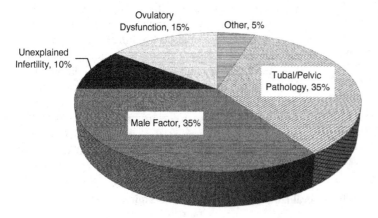

Figure 1.1 Causes of infertility in couples.

attempting pregnancy is much more common in developed countries and pelvic factors, such as fallopian tube adhesions and occlusion, are more common in lower-to-middle income countries.

In developed countries a very common cause of difficulty getting pregnant is advanced age. The increased educational and economic opportunities for women have, understandably, resulted in many women delaying childbearing to pursue other life goals and interests. However, the female reproductive system has not changed. A baby girl is born with about 700,000 to one million eggs, the number of which continues to decrease over time. At puberty there are approximately 350,000–500,000 eggs

(Figure 1.2) [14]. Women's fertility is at its peak from about age 23–31, and then begins to decrease because of a declining number of eggs and reduced percentage of eggs with a normal number of chromosomes (fewer euploid, i.e., normal number of chromosomes in the eggs and more aneuploid, i.e., abnormal number of chromosomes in the eggs). This results in a decreased pregnancy rate of approximately 3% per year from age 31–34, and 8% per year to age 39, so that at age 39 the average woman has about half the chance of getting pregnant than she did at age 31. From age 39–42 the chance of pregnancy is reduced about half again (Figure 1.3) [15]. Therefore, the chance that a woman in her mid-twenties will get pregnant is about 30% on the first

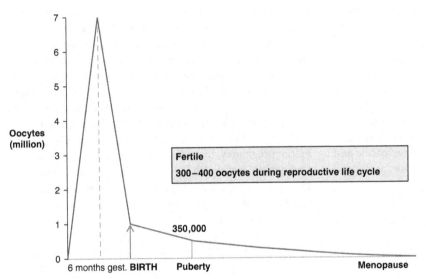

Figure 1.2 Oocyte numbers over a lifetime (adapted from [14]).

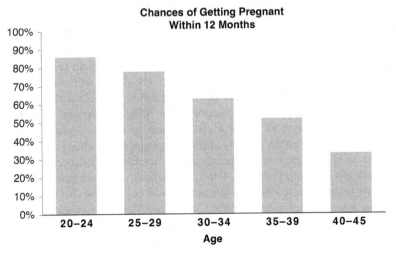

Figure 1.3 A woman's chance of getting pregnant by age (adapted from [15]).

cycle without contraception, dropping gradually to about 10% on her sixth cycle and 3–5% by the twelfth cycle. Each of these numbers is approximately half as high for a 39-year-old woman and one-quarter as high for a 42-year-old woman [16]. While there is a wide range of ovarian reserve in women at any given age, age remains the most important predictor of the ability to get pregnant and deliver a healthy baby [17].

Male fertility is less well understood. Fertility decreases with age in men, but much less than in women, with a man in his fifties having about 70% the capability of creating a pregnancy that he had in his twenties. Additionally, rates of autism, schizophrenia and bipolar disorders and other problems may be higher in children born to older fathers [18]. Most of the time, when sperm quality is poor, a cause cannot be found. Situations that can cause male infertility include prior testicular surgery for cancer, chemotherapy or radiation treatment for cancer, serious testicular injury, undescended testicle(s), mumps after childhood, social and prescription drugs that interfere with spermatogenesis, sexually transmitted infections, obstruction of the vas deferens duct that transports sperm from the testicles to the penis, complications of hernia operations, exposure to environmental toxicants, possibly large varicocele and testicular exposure to high temperatures for prolonged periods of time.

General lifestyle and other factors can affect fertility. The commonest of these in developed and even many developing countries (now designated lower-to-middle income countries or LMIC) is obesity, which reduces fecundity through hormonal and ovulatory dysfunction in women and can also affect male sperm quality [19,20]. Excessive exercise and/or decreased weight for women can reduce fertility also. Other factors can include excessive use of alcohol, smoking, social drugs, certain prescription medications, exposure to environmental toxicants, radiation exposure, or excessive heat for men. It is important to emphasize good health habits with respect to diet, exercise and sleep. All reproductive-age women would benefit from taking a supplemental multivitamin, iron, folate, vitamin D and calcium [21].

Generally, women who are younger than 35 and don't get pregnant after one year of unprotected intercourse should seek professional assistance from their gynecologist or a reproductive endocrinologist. Because of the reduction in fertility that occurs with age, women aged 35–40 should see a physician after about 6 months of no contraception, and women 40 or older after 3 months. Of course, if a couple has a history of an issue that might contribute to fertility problems, they should see a fertility specialist when they start attempting or, even better, when they decide that they will want to have a family. Examples of such problems are prior chemotherapy or radiation, irregular menstrual cycles, known hormonal problems, history of pelvic surgery, endometriosis, ruptured appendix or surgery on the cervix and, for the male, history of penile, testicular or hernia operations, or exposure to heat, environmental toxicants, chemotherapy, radiation or other drugs that can affect sperm production.

The goal of fertility treatment is to optimize the number of healthy eggs that can potentially be fertilized in any given cycle and result in implantation of embryo and birth of a healthy singleton baby. Treatment of patients with low ovarian reserve can be done by using oral or injectable medications that increase the number of eggs ovulated. However, the quality of the eggs is not changed by these medications. Additionally, the risk of miscarriage and of having a baby with a birth defect increases with age. Fertility treatment can be used to overcome some, but not all, of these problems. Modern testing can help to identify babies with problems during pregnancy, and sometimes with in vitro fertilization (IVF) even before pregnancy, by testing embryos using preimplantation genetic testing (PGT), a rapidly evolving technology that raises important biological, societal, ethical and counseling issues that require expert interpretation and support (see Chapter 27 for further discussion).

When patients present to the physician with infertility, it is important to recognize the reason the patient is there. It is not to diagnose, not to treat, but rather to intervene to obtain the desired outcome – a healthy singleton baby. The barriers to achieving this patient goal are several: medical conditions in the female and/or male, the patient's age, financial barriers and psychological stress. Based on numerous clinicians' experience, approximately 50–60% of patients seen in a tertiary care center will have a baby [22]. About 10% will decide not to pursue treatment because the prognosis is very poor, while about 30% will not achieve their goal because of financial and/or psychological barriers: 10% financial reasons alone, 10% psychological reasons alone and 10% a combination of the two. Additionally, even the patients who do get pregnant will often experience significant financial and/or emotional challenges during their treatment. If the physician is to optimize intervention, these issues must be actively addressed. These challenges are even more severe in LMIC, where financial ruin and societal isolation are more common.

Reproduction: Physiology and Pathophysiology

For pregnancy to occur, a healthy egg must be released from the ovary (ovulation) and be fertilized by a healthy sperm. Sperm are deposited at the cervix and make their way up through the endocervical canal and uterus to meet the egg, which has been picked up by a normally functioning fallopian tube from the ovarian surface or pelvis. The uterus must be functional and the endometrial lining must be able to respond to the estrogen and progesterone hormones secreted by the ovary so that the endometrium is prepared for implantation of the blastocyst. The blastocyst results from the fertilization of the egg and its development into a zygote and then an embryo and then the blastocyst by day 5 after fertilization (Figure 1.4).

The process of ovulation begins with the pulsatile release of gonadotropin releasing hormone (GnRH) from the hypothalamus at the base of the brain. This pulsatile release can be affected by weight, stress and other factors. The frequency of pulses changes during the menstrual cycle to cause the production of follicle stimulating hormone (FSH) by the pituitary gland, causing the follicles in the ovary to develop. The ovary must have follicles (the number of which become reduced with age) containing cells that make estrogen in the follicular phase (the first half of the menstrual cycle leading up to ovulation). During the follicular phase, approximately 10–20 follicles begin to grow, but eventually one exerts dominance over the others through a process of natural selection (the best one grows and the others stop growing). The rapidly increasing estrogen level from the cells in this enlarging follicle stimulates the release of luteinizing hormone (LH) by the pituitary gland, which causes the egg in the follicle to mature and to be released from the follicle (ovulation).

The egg is released into the pelvis and is picked up by the fallopian tube. The egg only lives about 12–24 hours, so it is important for sperm to be present when the egg is ovulated. The sperm, which have swum up from the cervix, fertilize the egg in the fallopian tube. Sperm will live 2–4 days in the female reproductive tract. The fertilized egg is called a zygote. The cells divide and at 3 days, the eight cells are called an embryo. The embryo continues to grow in the fallopian tube and enters the uterus at 5–6 days, comprises about 150–250 cells, and is called a blastocyst. The blastocyst floats in the uterus for about a day before implanting in the endometrium. The endometrium has been stimulated to grow by the estrogen from the follicle.

After ovulation, the follicle collapses on itself and becomes more vascularized and is called a corpus luteum ("body yellow"). This structure then makes progesterone under the influence of LH and some FSH that is produced by the pituitary gland. The progesterone is essential for the endometrium to develop properly so that implantation of the blastocyst can occur. If implantation and pregnancy occur, the trophoblast (early placenta) secretes human chorionic gonadotropin (hCG) which is the hormone tested for to detect pregnancy. The hCG stimulates the corpus luteum to continue producing progesterone until the placenta takes over with progesterone production at approximately 8–10 weeks of pregnancy. Progesterone is necessary to maintain the developing pregnancy.

Understanding the physiology of reproduction, it is no wonder there may be many things that impede,

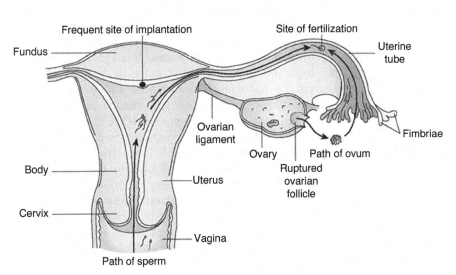

Figure 1.4 Female reproductive anatomy and physiology.

diminish or get in the way of fertilization and implantation. While there are many specific causes of infertility, the general categories are simple:

1. *Female factors:*
   a. Egg and hormonal factors: decreased ovarian reserve based on age or other factors; ovulation abnormalities from hypothalamic/pituitary gland dysfunction, polycystic ovarian syndrome (PCOS – diagnosed by the presence of two or three of the following symptoms/signs: (1) irregular ovulation; (2) clinical or biochemical hyperandrogenism; or (3) antral follicle count equal to or greater than 20 in either ovary, or ovarian volume equal to or greater than 10 ml in either ovary), or abnormal weight; hormonal problems such as thyroid disease, hyperprolactinemia or renal gland disease; and endometrium problems affecting implantation.
   b. Pelvic/anatomic factors: uterine problems such as fibroids, adenomyosis, polyps, adhesions or congenital abnormalities; tubal problems such as adhesions, internal fibrosis or obstruction; pelvic peritoneal problems such as endometriosis or adhesions; cervical or vaginal abnormalities preventing deposition of sperm at the cervix and/or access of sperm into the uterus and fallopian tubes [23].
2. *Male factor:* azoospermia, oligospermia, decreased motility or morphology; genetic disorders (e.g., Klinefelter's); erectile dysfunction (ED), ejaculatory dysfunction or other problems affecting the delivery of sperm to the cervix at the appropriate time [24].
3. *Combined factor:* having intercourse at the wrong time with respect to timing of fertilization; using lubricants that harm sperm.
4. *Unexplained:* in about 10–20% of cases, a definitive cause of infertility is not identifiable and the diagnosis is "unexplained infertility." However, this diagnosis is commonly thought to represent an undiagnosable egg or sperm problem.

Evaluation of Infertility: Collaborative Care

Medical Management

Initial assessment of infertility includes a history and physical examination of both male and female partners [25]. The female history involves asking about menstrual history, prior pregnancies and attempts at prior pregnancy, fatigue, constipation and other symptoms of thyroid disease, breast secretions, acne and hirsutism. Use of exogenous hormones such as estrogen found in soy-based products and alternative medicine such as herbs or other supplements are potentially important because these bioactive compounds can interfere with the patient's own hormones. History of issues affecting pelvic factor, such as prior abdominal/pelvic operations, sexually transmitted infections (STI) and pelvic pain with menses, intercourse or bowel/bladder function, is also significant. Male factor should be assessed by history of prior pregnancies created and/or exposure to pregnancy, sexually transmitted infections, urethritis, prostatitis, reproductive injuries, accidents, operations or diseases, undescended testicle(s), environmental toxicants, excessive heat, erectile dysfunction, obesity, genetic causes, hormonal abnormalities and other reproductive problems [26]. Combined factor history includes cervical operations, frequency and timing of intercourse and use of lubricants. General questions regarding weight, diet, exercise, sleep, smoking, alcohol or drug use, exogenous hormones, alternative medicines, other medications, general health and prior fertility testing and treatment are important for both female and male patients.

Female Testing

Physical examination includes general health, height and weight, blood pressure and respiratory rate. Visual examination of the external genitalia, vagina and cervix should be performed followed by bimanual examination of the uterus, ovaries and rectovaginal area. The thyroid should be examined, along with the breasts for galactorrhea (nipple secretions) and the skin for acne or hirsutism (abnormal facial hair, periareolar hair).

Initial testing for causes of infertility is fairly simple. Table 1.1 lists common blood work used to test for ovarian reserve and the normal levels [27]. In addition, hyperandrogenemia (increased male hormone levels) can be tested with testosterone and possibly other androgenic hormone levels in selected situations. The clomiphene citrate challenge test (CCCT) is a more sensitive test of ovarian reserve than cycle day 3 FSH alone and is occasionally helpful. Karyotype (chromosome testing) is occasionally indicated to rule out genetic problems. Endometrial biopsy to date the endometrial development is a traditional test that has been shown not to be helpful and is no longer performed. Newer tests such as the endometrial receptivity assay are sometimes performed but are yet to be validated to improve live birth rates.

Table 1.1 Ovarian reserve testing [27]

Blood levels

Anti-mullerian hormone (AMH: normal ~ > 1 ng/ml);
follicle stimulating hormone (FSH: normal ~ <10 miU/ml)
Estradiol (E2: normal ~ < 80 pg/ml)
Thyroid stimulating hormone (TSH: normal < 2.5 miU/l);
prolactin levels (PRL: normal ~ 25 ng/ml).

Ultrasound

Antral follicle count (AFC: normal ~> 7)

Pelvic factor is usually assessed initially with ultrasound to obtain information about the uterus (e.g., uterine myomas, which are benign muscle tumors of the uterine wall), congenital abnormalities (septate uterus may be associated with infertility, single and double uterine abnormalities with pregnancy complications) and endometrial thickness and characteristics; the ovaries (size, antral follicle count, ovarian cysts); the fallopian tubes (hydrosalpinx or complete distal obstruction of the fallopian tube), paratubal cysts and possibly endometriosis (only endometriomas which are ovarian cysts of endometriosis and deeply infiltrative endometriosis can be seen on ultrasound). A saline infusion sonogram (SIS, also known as a sonohysterogram or SHG) provides additional sensitivity (ability to detect a real abnormality) to identify intrauterine polyps, myomas or adhesions. After an ultrasound, the most common test of the pelvic organs is a hysterosalpingogram (HSG). The HSG is a radiological procedure that is better at documenting whether the uterine cavity is normal shape and whether the fallopian tubes are open and/or have intratubal damage or peritubal adhesions. Very occasionally magnetic resonance imaging (MRI) or computerized tomography (CT) may be used to help define abnormalities of the uterus or ovaries or other pelvic masses. Surgical procedures that can be used to further diagnose and then to treat problems that have been identified by imaging technology include hysteroscopy (passing a small telescope through the cervix to look into the uterine cavity) and laparoscopy (passing a small telescope through a sub-umbilical incision into the abdomino-pelvic cavity to look at the internal organs) with hydrotubation (injection of colored fluid through the fallopian tubes to check for patency), which are minor surgical procedures that usually require anesthesia.

Male Testing

Male testing is almost always initiated with a semen analysis to measure volume of semen, pH, liquefaction, count, motility and morphology. Normal parameters by the World Health Organization Standard (6th edition) count are volume is 1.4 ml or more, count 16 million/ml or higher, total motility 42% or more, progressive motility 30% or more and strict morphology 4% or higher [28]. Morphology is especially difficult to assess and many men have slightly decreased morphology. Antisperm antibody and other male tests rarely add additional useful information except perhaps for men with prior vasectomy considering reversal [29].

Tests for combined factor generally involve sexually transmitted infection testing for HIV 1 and 2, HTLV (human T lymphotropic virus) I and II for men, hepatitis B and C, syphilis, chlamydia and gonorrhea. The traditional test for combined factor, the postcoital test, has been shown not to be helpful and is no longer performed [30].

General/systemic tests for hematology (blood, spleen), biochemistry (liver, kidneys, parathyroid), and blood sugar (pancreas) are generally indicated if not done within the past 1 to 2 years. Obese patients or those with family history of diabetes mellitus should be tested with fasting blood sugar (normal <100 mg/dl) and HgA1c (a measure of glucose metabolism, normally less than 5.7%).

Genetics testing has become much more common in the last several years. This can include preconception testing to identity single gene defects or translocations that can increase risk of morbidity and mortality and preimplantation genetic testing during IVF cycles to identify normal and abnormal embryos, the latter having decreased chance of pregnancy and a higher chance of poor maternal and fetal outcomes [31].

The purpose of testing is not to do tests or, in fact, to simply make a diagnosis. The purpose of testing is to determine the prognosis for the patient given the test results, and how that prognosis can be improved by: intervention with lifestyle or other general/systemic changes; hormonal treatment of specific ovulation or other hormone problems; controlled ovarian stimulation to increase the number of eggs ovulated in a given month; surgical intervention to improve the pelvic organs; male factor treatment with drugs or surgery; or combined factor treatment to get more, better sperm closer to the egg(s) at the right time. All diagnostic tests and medical or surgical interventions should be focused on improving the patient's quality of life by better disease management and, specifically, meeting the desired wish of delivering a healthy singleton baby.

At this planning visit, their physician may explain to a couple that infertility represents the fifth highest burden of disease globally in reproductive-age individuals, and that learning one is infertile often carries an emotional impact equivalent to that of a diagnosis of HIV or cancer [32]. Additionally, this is a condition that often must be dealt with by the couple alone because it is generally not discussed socially, even while there can be significant pressures from other family members to have children. Infertility is often the first major challenge a young couple face together, so it is important to communicate clearly to each other how they feel and what they want to do. The husband/partner can be educated about the fact the woman (or female partner receiving treatment in a same-sex relationship) almost always experiences much more pressure and emotional stress, and so the partner must support her personally and socially; and she needs to express appreciation for these efforts, even though they cannot completely resolve her emotional burdens. The importance of obtaining the best available evidence, asking questions and making logical decisions can be emphasized. The value of emotional support through good nutrition, sleep and exercise as well as meditation, prayer, yoga, acupuncture, mindfulness, or other mind–body exercises and support groups is emphasized. The important role of individual, couple and/or group counseling during treatment is explained. They are provided with written materials on the medical and emotional aspects of infertility, support resources and information, and the psychological services available at the clinic (see Addendums for examples of support resource materials).

Psychosocial Management

Despite the media attention often given to infertility, few people ever anticipate they will have problems getting pregnant or carrying a baby. There is mounting evidence that men and women frequently underestimate their reproductive time clock as well as lifestyle issues that can affect childbearing (e.g., smoking, body weight, alcohol, drug and caffeine consumption), and it is suggested that people should be encouraged to think about parenthood goals in a similar way as one does other important life goals, like education and careers [3]. In addition, advances in technology in cryopreservation of oocytes have opened a new area of counseling for women needing to preserve their fertility due to a medical problem, usually cancer treatment, or by choice to use in the future (see [33], pp. 212–235 on fertility preservation counseling). Hence, mental health professionals (MHP) in all types of practice settings can play an important role in helping

their clients understand and consider preconception issues, fertility awareness and reproductive options.

The intention and planning of family creation is something that takes place psychologically long before it ever occurs physically. Individuals and couples begin thinking about having a child and being a parent often while still children themselves, as the imaginary journey towards parenthood begins. The longer one walks down this path, the stronger the attachment to the "wished-for" baby. If difficulties occur along the road, assistance may be needed to achieve the dream of a child. These difficulties may be caused by medical or genetic issues, which result in infertility, or by other life circumstance, such as not finding a partner or sexual orientation, whereby people are technically not "infertile" but nonetheless need medical assistance (now described as "fertility care") to have a child. No matter what the path is that has brought an individual or couple to seek MAR, every person brings a history that will impact how he or she experiences impaired reproduction (see Chapter 2 on reproductive psychology).

Psychosocial Context

Reproduction is a basic human need, influenced by strong psychological, cultural and social drives. Griel and colleagues [34] describe infertility as a "socially constructed reality" rather than purely a medical condition with psychological consequences. Individuals and couples must embrace the role of parenthood as a desired social role or they would not seek medical assistance. For couples, it is a condition that affects them both, no matter who is identified as impaired, and is most evident as a state of "absence" (i.e., no child) rather than disease or symptoms. In addition, there are strong sociocultural influences in both developed and LMI countries that shape how an individual or couple experience infertility. In pronatalist cultures, childlessness is surrounded by shame and stigma, while in developed societies, not having a child may be viewed as a voluntary, viable choice. Griel et al. state, "The experience of infertility is shaped by the social context ... [and] best understood as ... a process whereby individuals come to define their ability to have children as a problem, to define the nature of that problem, and to construct an appropriate course of action" ([34], p. 141).

In a controversial revision of Maslow's hierarchy of needs theory, Kenrick and colleagues [35] renovated the pyramid by replacing "self-actualization" and putting "parenting" at the top, reflecting new findings from the fields of neuroscience, developmental and evolutionary psychology. They contend that reproduction is not just about producing children, but also raising and parenting them so they, in turn, will reproduce. Therefore, all the effort that goes into parenting (e.g., caring, feeding, nurturing, educating children) is based in deep-rooted psychological urges that are a hallmark of being human and are passed down from generation to generation.

Thus, parenthood is not only a desired social role, but also a biologically driven need, creating the "perfect storm" for psychological distress when thwarted. It is well established in the literature (and throughout this text) that infertility is an inherently stressful experience that creates great emotional turbulence in the individual and/or couple the longer it goes on. So, whether by impairment or circumstance, patients presenting for MAR will need psychological support and assistance throughout the treatment process. While most couples presenting to clinics are emotionally well-adjusted and not fundamentally different from others, they are more likely to experience distress over time, affecting self-esteem and life satisfaction, because of infertility [34].

Men and women will experience infertility differently in both the way they feel and the way they cope. Most studies indicate that women experience greater infertility-related stress, reporting more symptoms of depression and anxiety than men. Men also experience infertility stress, but with less emotional affect and more indirectly, through the effect it has on their partner and concern about her [34]. The emotional context changes when infertility is gender-specific (i.e., female factor or male factor), with the diagnosed individual within a couple having a more negative response typically reflecting negative feelings surrounding diminished self-esteem, self-image and body-image [36]. Consequently, shame may become a defining force as an individual feels there is something inherently wrong or defective about themself. Feelings of grief and loss, well documented throughout the literature, are the emotional response and continue when treatment is unsuccessful and, finally, when moving on to third party reproduction.

Regarding coping strategies, women display higher levels of seeking social support (e.g., talking to friends and family), avoidant behavior of painful situations (e.g., baby showers, pregnant friends) and information-seeking. Men tend to use distancing from the pain of infertility and problem-solving [37]. Similar dynamics may occur in same-sex relationships. These different partner/gender-related coping strategies may give rise to additional stress within a couple's relationship, as women seek more ways to obtain emotional support, while men attempt to problem-solve and, when not effective, distance themselves out of

frustration. This dynamic can be played out further in their sexual relationship, which is explained in the adage: "Women need to feel loved (i.e., emotionally supported, feeling truly understood) in order to have sex, and men need to have sex (i.e., take action, physical response) in order to feel loved." Thus, infertility can have a powerful effect on a couple's sexual relationship, not only due to the repeated, time-sensitive, performance demands of procreation, but also because of the differences in the ways men and women cope with distress (see also Chapter 4 on couples and Chapter 6 on sexual therapy).

Assessment

Infertility is not experienced in a vacuum and needs to be understood within the context of the history a patient brings to it. Just as physicians would not begin to treat a patient without comprehensive history-taking and doing a thorough medical examination, fertility counselors also must take a similar approach. Tools are available to help gather information, as well as self-administered interventions for patients in need of additional emotional support.

There are several self-report, standard screening tools for depression and anxiety which are easily administered, readily available on the Internet, and in numerous languages. The Patient Health Questionnaire (PHQ-9) screens for the presence and severity of depression and takes less than 3 minutes to complete. The Generalized Anxiety Disorder (GAD-7) can be used for screening and severity measuring of anxiety. Research has shown that psychological distress is common during infertility treatment, yet most patients are not screened for, nor receive referrals to, mental health services [38]. It is also important for all healthcare professionals to routinely assess fertility patients' coping and distress as part of standard care (not in response to someone "falling apart") and provide support resources. All patients bring a psychosocial history into their reproductive experience, which has a profound effect on how they feel and deal with it. The psychological side effects of medications used during treatment, and considerations for patients with a psychiatric history and on psychotropic medication, can impact treatment as well as interactions with the treatment team (see Chapter 7 on the intersect between psychiatric disorders and infertility).

Besides standard instruments used in the screening of depression and anxiety, several infertility-specific screening tools have been developed that help clinicians identify how patients are doing and their level of distress. These tools are validated, self-administered instruments, quick to take, and can be easily interpreted by clinicians. FertiQoL can be completed online by patients (http://sites.cardiff.ac.uk/fertiqol/download), is currently available in 46 languages, and takes about 10–15 minutes to complete [39]. It assesses the impact of fertility problems and its treatment on a patient's quality of life along domains of personal, social and relational life. SCREENIVF has been found to be highly predictive of those at risk for treatment distress, which helps in directing patients towards additional psychological support [40]. The Fertility Problem Inventory (FPI) is another validated tool that measures an individual's infertility-related stress as well as the impact on a couple's relationship [41]. Any of these screening tools will help the fertility counselor in the assessment of a patient's current functioning and need for support as treatment progresses.

Anticipation, Prevention and Support

For patients entering treatment, it may feel like embarking on a journey and entering a strange land where you don't speak the language or know the terrain you must travel. In this sense, fertility counselors, along with other members of the treatment team, will serve as guides. Metaphors like this abound that relate to the struggles and issues faced by patients, from the "emotional rollercoaster" of treatment cycles, "road maps" of where one has been and is going, and "bridges" that need to be crossed to reach a goal or connect to divergent paths or views. Since both words and visualizations are used, metaphors can be a powerful tool to open ways of thinking, evoke emotions, help understanding and change perspective with infertility patients.

Preparatory counseling is seen as both helpful and a valuable service for new patients entering treatment [42]. Patients need to anticipate what is ahead and should be provided with information and reading materials which are racially and culturally sensitive to the diversity of patients entering a practice. Materials regarding medical conditions, treatment options, the emotional experience of infertility, support services and resources should be available in printed versions to share during a counseling session, as an electronic file that can be emailed to patients prior to meeting, and on the clinic website. These educational materials and resources become the fertility counselor's "tools of the trade" and having them readily available and organized is important. Being able to anticipate what is ahead emotionally, where and how difficulties may arise and what strategies might help, can prevent more serious problems. Helping patients understand that "an ounce of prevention is worth

a pound of cure" may help them be more adaptive and resilient to the distress of infertility.

Support becomes a pivotal piece of care for all members of the treatment team. Patient-centered care is supportive and focuses on positive communication with staff – empathy, respect, sensitivity, trustworthiness and responsiveness. As all MHPs know, these interactions are the basis of forming a therapeutic relationship in counseling. While individual and couple counseling should be easily accessible for patients, the reality is that only a small minority will follow on their own and those given a referral for counseling during a "crisis" often deem it as another example of their inadequacy [38,43] (see also Chapters 3 and 4 on individual and couple fertility counseling).

Research has shown that the most effective psychosocial intervention is group counseling along with psychoeducation, normalizing the emotional response to infertility, teaching effective coping strategies and educating patients on various aspects related to treatment and family building [43]. These groups can consist of periodic (weekly/monthly), open-ended gatherings which are more emotion-focused on dealing with treatments (e.g., general infertility, recipients of donor gametes, intended parents or gestational surrogates, secondary infertility, etc.), skill-building (e.g., mind–body techniques, cognitive–behavioral strategies, etc.), or specific topics providing more psychoeducation (e.g., adoption discussion, disclosure assistance, etc.), yet all will be offering patient support [44]. Patient organizations, such as Resolve, continue to provide support, advocacy and information, while the Internet has dramatically changed the way patients access information, seek support (chat rooms, blogs, social media, etc.) and obtain education [45]. Furthermore, during COVID-19, virtual support groups via telehealth have provided a life-line to isolated fertility patients (see Chapter 5 on group counseling).

Spirituality is another form of support, often overlooked by clinicians, which should be considered by fertility counselors (see Chapter 8 on spirituality). Religion and spirituality usually occur within a cultural context of the patient going through treatment and may provide important information about how infertility is perceived. Patients with a strong spiritual foundation utilize this belief system to cope with the sense of loss of control, to help in decision-making and to find meaning and purpose from the experience. While many clinicians, both medical and psychological, are uncomfortable with addressing religion and spirituality, research continues to show this is a neglected area that fertility patients wish was discussed [46].

The importance of delivering all reproductive medical services, including fertility counseling, in a racially, culturally and LGBTQ+ sensitive approach, is imperative. Dramatic shifts in recent years in the awareness of how services have been directed, most often in a heteronormative, racially and culturally color-blind way, have frequently created greater distress in patients seeking fertility care (see Chapters 16, 17, and 18 for a deeper discussion on these issues related to fertility counseling with diverse populations). Similar issues can also be experienced by men going though fertility treatment, who may feel marginalized or left out of discussions with healthcare professionals, as much of treatment focuses on the female partner (see Chapter 15 on the male experience). Fertility counselors must be attuned to the unique health needs as well as disparities existing for all patients needing and seeking reproductive medical care.

Treatment of Infertility: Collaborative Care

Medical Intervention

There are multiple potential medical interventions for infertility, but they can, generally, be grouped into three categories: observation, standard/conventional treatment and in vitro fertilization (IVF). While recurrent miscarriage is not strictly a category of infertility, the management during treatment will also be addressed. A fourth category of medical intervention, third party reproduction (donor sperm, donor egg, gestational surrogate), is not technically a treatment for infertility and will be discussed in the next section.

Lifestyle Choices to Optimize Pregnancy

Patients can optimize their chance for pregnancy by healthy lifestyle choices [21]. People attempting pregnancy should get 8 hours of sleep, eat a healthy, balanced diet, get a moderate amount of exercise and maintain normal weight [19]. Studies show that women with a body mass index (BMI) of greater than approximately 30 begin to have decreased pregnancy rates. Women with a BMI less than about 19 can also experience ovulation disorders and less chance of pregnancy. Women should not do more than about 2 hours of aerobic exercise per week, but there are no limits on non-aerobic exercise such as weights, yoga, walking and swimming. Smoking significantly reduces fertility and should be avoided [21]. Men should avoid exercise that might cause significant increase in testicular heat, for example, long bicycle rides or excessive use of hot tubs or saunas, as well as excessive heat from laptop computers, the proverbial tight underwear, or other sources of heat. For women, alcohol should be avoided or at least limited to small amounts in the follicular phase before ovulation, although there are no good studies on how much, if any, alcohol is entirely safe. Men may have small amounts of alcohol, less than two standard drinks of beer or wine or other alcohol per day although, again, there are no studies that prove any specific amount is entirely safe. Two to five cups of coffee or similar amount of caffeine per day from other sources is acceptable for women or men. Similarly, drug and medication use should be limited to that which is absolutely necessary. Any questions should be directed to the patient's personal physician. Social drugs, toxicants such as pesticides, paint sprays, hair/cosmetic sprays, industrial chemicals and radiation should be avoided. Prenatal vitamins with calcium, iron and folate for the woman and a male multi-vitamin with antioxidant are recommended. Appropriate tests and vaccinations for rubella, chicken pox, whooping cough, Zika and COVID-19 and other diseases should be obtained according to Centers for Disease Control (CDC) recommendations [47,48].

Observation Only Without Treatment

Observation alone is sometimes appropriate in young women with a short duration of infertility and no obvious causes of infertility after at least an initial history, physical examination and simple testing that show normal menstrual function, normal sperm and appropriately timed intercourse. Usually not more than 3–6 months of observation alone is indicated. Intercourse should occur every 2 days plus or minus half a day (i.e., every 1.5 to 2.5 days, or every 1 to 3 days at the outside). Intercourse should begin not later than 16 days before the expected menses based on the woman's shortest cycle in the past 6 months (i.e., if the shortest cycle in the past 6 months is 26 days, intercourse should start on day 26–16 = Cycle Day (CD) 10 where CD 1 = the first day of the last menstrual period) [21]. Basal body temperature charting can occasionally be used retrospectively to confirm ovulation and urinary LH sticks (ovulation predictor kits) can be used to help time intercourse, but intercourse should begin several days before an expected rise. Assessing cervical mucus for viscosity can be informative but generally not sufficiently so to be the primary method of timing intercourse [21]. Pre-Seed, canola oil or mineral oil can be used as a lubricant but other lubricants should be avoided because they may reduce sperm function. Position of intercourse does not matter, and the woman can remain supine after intercourse for 10 or so minutes if she chooses, although the potential benefit of this is unproven.

While mind–body/integrative care programs, yoga, acupuncture and other holistic approaches likely can improve the patient's sense of well-being and enhance their ability to comply with and manage their fertility care, thus boosting their chances to take home a baby, there is no credible evidence that these alternative medicine approaches will intrinsically increase biologic pregnancy rates. Herbal medicines and other alternative ingestions can reduce pregnancy rates if they contain bioactive ingredients that interfere with normal ovulation or controlled ovarian stimulation (COS).

Standard Fertility Treatment

After undergoing the tests noted above to assess sperm, eggs, uterus and combined factors, specific problems should be treated. Thyroid disease should be managed with thyroid supplement or appropriate treatment of hyperthyroidism. Hyperprolactinemia can be treated with bromocryptine or cabergoline after pituitary assessment for markedly elevated prolactin levels that can be associated with pituitary adenoma. Hyperandrogenism can be treated with dexamethasone or other appropriate medications. Insulin resistance can be treated with weight loss/metformin/insulin or other appropriate medications.

After testing and management of general lifestyle factors and general health conditions, treatment of specific fertility problems usually involves the use of hormones and/or minor or major surgery for the female, treatment of the male with hormones or minor surgery, or treatment of both with intrauterine insemination (IUI), IVF or use of donor sperm, eggs or gestational carrier (now commonly called surrogate). The goal of treatment is to increase the chance of pregnancy in each menstrual cycle by bringing more egg(s) together with more sperm in the best possible pelvic environment at the right time.

Female Factor

See Figure 1.5. Oligo-ovulation can be treated with clomiphene citrate (Clomid or Serophene) usually starting with a dose of 50 mg per day cycle day 5 through 9 and increased

Figure 1.5 Female factor algorithm.

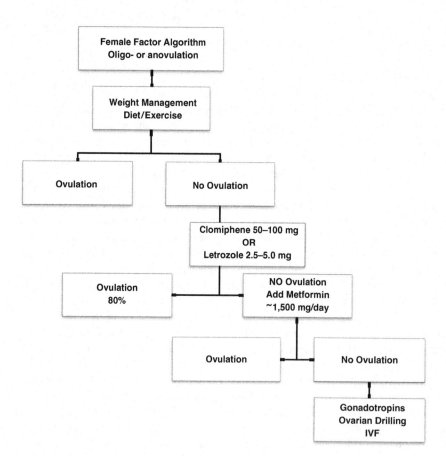

as necessary [50]. Empiric ovarian stimulation (OS) is usually performed with clomiphene 100 mg for 5 days starting on cycle day 3, 4 or 5, with similar pregnancy rates regardless of start day. Letrozole 2.5 to 5 mg per day can be used if clomiphene is not successful or in place of clomiphene if patients experience side effects from clomiphene. Letrozole is likely superior to clomiphene in PCOS patients and should be the first line of treatment [51]. Metformin can be considered as first-line treatment in selected patients [52]. OS should be monitored with ultrasound on approximately cycle day 11 to assess response to treatment with at least one or two maturing follicles (~ >15 mm) but not an excessive number that could lead to increased risk of multiple pregnancy (< 4 mature follicles) [53]. The risk of twin pregnancy with clomiphene is approximately 8% and triplets 0.5%. Other side effects of clomiphene include thinning of the endometrium, headaches, hot flashes, vaginal dryness, mood changes, breast tenderness and occasionally photophobia or other eye symptoms. The cause of the latter is unknown, but thought possibly to be vascular in nature, and is sufficient to merit discontinuation of clomiphene use. Ovarian hyperstimulation syndrome (OHSS) with ovarian cysts is very rare with clomiphene.

Cancer, such as breast, ovarian and endometrial, is more common in women with infertility. The evidence does not support a relationship between fertility drugs and an increase in these cancers, though more studies are needed. However, there may be a small increase in the slower-growing, less-invasive borderline tumors in women treated with clomiphene [53].

Type 1 amenorrhea, which is very uncommon, can be treated with very low dose gonadotropins. Patients undergoing any type of gonadotropin treatment must be carefully monitored with ultrasound to follow the follicle number and size, and usually also with blood estradiol levels [54–56]. (OHSS) affects 1–3% of women treated with gonadotropins and occurs following administration of hCG (see the "IVF" section for more details.) More importantly, while gonadotropins can be very effective, they also carry the risk of twins and even triplets and higher order multiples [57]. Such pregnancies have much higher risks of a baby with a serious medical problem and of maternal pregnancy complications. Prematurity, which occurs much more frequently in multiple pregnancy, is the major, but not only, cause of these problems. Today, there are very few patients who benefit from gonadotropins that are used outside of Type1 amenorrhea or in IVF cycles. The increased pregnancy rates, decreased risks, shorter time to pregnancy and increased cost-effectiveness of IVF almost always

make it a better treatment choice than gonadotropins and IUI [57–59].

Some patients have lesions in their uterus that reduce or prevent the chance of pregnancy. Intrauterine polyps, which result from excessive growth of the endometrium from estrogen stimulation, can be identified by ultrasound and treated by hysteroscopy. Hysteroscopy involves passing a small telescope through the cervix, usually as an office procedure or a short, outpatient procedure with intravenous sedation and monitored anesthesia care, and then using scissors or forceps to remove the polyp. A dilatation and curettage (D&C) is often done at the same time. Myomas, also called fibroids, result from excessive growth of a single cell in the muscle wall of the uterus. Myomas can occur in any number, location and size in the uterus: pedunculated (on a stalk outside the uterus), subserous (just under the outer layer of the uterus), intramural (in the wall of the uterus), submucous (protruding into the uterine cavity) and intracavitary (almost completely into the uterine cavity). Myomas that distort the uterine cavity reduce pregnancy rates and should be removed before fertility treatment. Large and/or multiple intramural myomas may reduce IVF pregnancy rates and removal should be considered before IVF. Myomas that cause pain or abnormal bleeding should also be removed. Intrauterine myomectomy can be accomplished with a hot electrosurgical loop resection or sometimes scissors and forceps. Intrauterine scarring or adhesions can also be diagnosed and cut or removed at hysteroscopy. Such adhesions are not common and usually result from complications of a pregnancy associated with trauma to the endometrium and infection. Severe adhesions are called Asherman's syndrome.

Some patients have an abnormally developed uterus. Most congenital abnormalities do not reduce pregnancy rates but may be associated with increased complications of pregnancy because the uterine cavity is either too small or abnormally shaped, leading to problems with the functioning of the placenta during pregnancy and/or premature labor. However, a relatively common abnormality called a septate uterus – in which there is a fibrous septum in the middle of the uterus – is possibly associated with increased miscarriage rates and should be removed before attempting pregnancy. This is easily done by resection with scissors during a hysteroscopy. After some, usually more extensive, hysteroscopic procedures, the patient has a balloon catheter left in the cavity for a few days, antibiotics and/or estrogen hormones to help the endometrium regrow and reduce the risk of adhesions forming inside the uterus.

Other uterus, fallopian tube or pelvic problems can reduce pregnancy rates and can be treated by laparoscopy or laparotomy. Both operations require general anesthesia. Laparoscopy involves passing a small telescope into the abdomino-pelvic cavity through the umbilicus (i.e., "belly button"). Laparotomy usually involves a small "bikini" incision. If a very small abdominal incision is made, this is called a mini laparotomy. Myomas that distort the uterine cavity, but cannot be removed by hysteroscopy, can be removed at laparoscopy or laparotomy [60]. Adhesions around the uterus, ovaries or fallopian tubes can usually be removed at operative laparoscopy. Different energy sources such as electrosurgery, laser or scissors can be used depending on surgeon preference, with no difference in effectiveness. Blocked fallopian tubes can be repaired, although if damage is severe and the tube is blocked at its distal end near the ovary (hydrosalpinx), then pregnancy rates are still very low afterwards (10–20%) and ectopic pregnancy risk is high, so IVF is more appropriate. Very badly damaged tubes with hydrosalpinges should be removed because their presence reduces IVF pregnancy rates [61]. Endometriosis is a common disease of the pelvis that can result in different types of inflammatory lesions on the pelvic peritoneum, adhesions around the uterus, tubes and ovaries, cysts in the ovaries (endometriomas), invasion into the uterine wall (different than adenomyosis) and deep endometriosis (DE), especially in the pelvic

cul de sacs and between the rectum and the vagina. Surgical treatment of endometriosis increases pregnancy rates and reduces commonly associated pain symptoms [62–64]. Some women who have had bilateral tubal sterilization may benefit more from tubal reversal (microreanastomosis) than from IVF [61].

Male Factor

See Figure 1.6. Male factor problems also need attention. Healthy lifestyle behaviors are usually the most important. Some men may benefit from clomiphene citrate 25 mg per day continuously, or treatment of chronic prostatitis or other infections. Surgical treatment of varicocele, which is a varicose vein of the testicular vein, may be indicated if the man has pain symptoms associated with the varicocele and/or it is very large. The role of varicocele in infertility and its treatment has been controversial for decades. Current recommendations are to offer varicocelectomy to the male partner when all of the following are present: a varicocele is palpable, the couple has documented infertility, the female has normal fertility or potentially correctable infertility and the male has one of more abnormal semen analyses or sperm function test results [29,65]. Other serious anatomic abnormalities are rare but should be treated. Men with obstructive azoospermia may benefit from testicular or epididymal biopsy and cryopreservation of sperm or, for men with a vasectomy, a surgical reconnection of the vas deferens

Figure 1.6 Male factor algorithm.

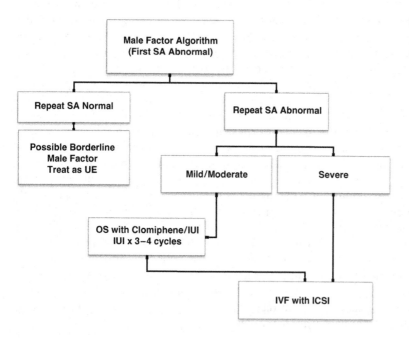

(vasovasostomy) [66]. Male fertility decreases slightly with age and the risk of having a baby with a problem, especially autism-related disorders, increases very slightly. Genetic tests have identified over 100 genes related to autism and other disorders, as well as epigenetic associations, but there are no known specific diagnostic tests or treatment to make accurate predictions or remedy these conditions. Combined factors can be treated with sperm washing and intrauterine insemination [67]. This procedure enables more motile sperm with normal shape to be placed closer to the egg(s) at the right time in the cycle when ovulation is occurring. Depending on the clinical situation, this can increase the pregnancy rate only a small amount to up to two to three times. It can also be used when intercourse is difficult for psychological reasons in the male or female. Of course, such situations should also be addressed with counseling to identify and treat underlying psychological issues.

Unexplained Infertility

See Figure 1.7. Up to 10–20% of couples have unexplained infertility, the diagnosis typically being made after the basic evaluation fails to reveal an obvious abnormality [68]. It is not recommended to perform IUI in natural cycles for the treatment of unexplained infertility. It is less effective than OS with IUI and likely no more effective than expectant management. It is not recommended to use either clomiphene citrate or letrozole with timed intercourse, as both are no more effective than expectant

management. It is not recommended to use gonadotropins with timed intercourse because there is either no difference in pregnancy outcomes compared to OS with oral agents or higher pregnancy rates are associated with a higher risk of multiple-gestation pregnancy. There is strong evidence that clomiphene citrate with IUI is superior to expectant management and natural-cycle IUI for the outcome of live-birth rate in couples with unexplained infertility and is recommended. Multiple gestation pregnancy rate with clomiphene citrate with IUI treatment ranges from 0 to 12.5%. Clomiphene and letrozole have similar outcomes and both are superior to expectant management and natural-cycle IUI. Of note, letrozole is not FDA approved for treatment of unexplained infertility but is considered an effective and well tolerated option. It is not recommended to use letrozole or clomiphene citrate plus conventional-dose gonadotropins with IUI, because improved pregnancy rates over OS-IUI with oral medications are also associated with an increased risk of multiple-gestation pregnancy. It is not recommended to use low-dose or conventional dose gonadotropins with IUI in the treatment of unexplained infertility, as both are more complex and expensive, and likely no more effective than OS with oral medications with IUI. Higher pregnancy rates are associated with higher multiple rates. A single IUI can be performed between 0 and 36 hours relative to hCG injection in OS with IUI treatments. Overall, it is recommended that couples with unexplained infertility initially undergo

Figure 1.7 Unexplained infertility algorithm.

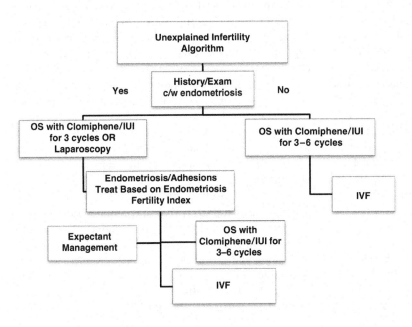

a course (typically three or four cycles) of OS and IUI with oral agents. For those unsuccessful with OS and IUI treatments with oral agents, IVF is recommended rather than OS and IUI with gonadotropins. In recent years, excellent studies confirm that IVF is more cost-effective than gonadotropins and IUI, and so it is usually the most appropriate treatment after failed clomiphene and/or IUI [57–59]. Laparoscopy may be indicated in younger patients with clinical suspicion of endometriosis or adhesions, short duration of infertility, other fertility factors reasonably within normal limits, and who are prepared to attempt with conventional treatment for at least 9 to 12 months after surgery if the prognosis remains favorable.

Recurrent Miscarriage

Recurrent miscarriage or recurrent pregnancy loss (RPL) is often the most difficult clinical situation for both patients and physicians to manage. This is so because of the emotional trauma associated with miscarriage and our inability to identify the reason for pregnancy loss in 50–75% of patients [69,70]. It is important to counsel patients that, even with three or more prior pregnancy losses, the chances for a successful live birth are 50–60%, depending on maternal age and parity, even with no treatment. Most pregnancy losses are sporadic and caused by random genetic factors that increase with age. It is appropriate to investigate RPL after two consecutive clinical pregnancy losses. Assessment of RPL focuses on screening for genetic factors and anti-phospholipid syndrome, assessment of uterine anatomy, hormonal and metabolic status and lifestyle factors. Investigation may include karyotype screening of potential parents, screening for anticardiolipin antibodies, lupus anti-coagulant, and anti-beta 2, glycoprotein I, sonohysterogram, hysterosalpingogram and/or hysteroscopy, thyroid and prolactin screening and karyotyping of products of conception with the second or additional miscarriages. Identified problems should be treated when possible. Women with persistent, moderate to high levels of circulating antiphospholipid antibodies can be treated with a combination of prophylactic doses of unfractionated heparin and low-dose aspirin. Psychological counseling and support are especially important for couples with RPL (see Chapter 22 on RPL counseling).

In Vitro Fertilization (IVF)

Generally, after diagnostic tests are done, systemic problems addressed and specific causes of infertility identified and treated, standard treatment is performed for 3 to 6 months, if there are no identifiable issues that suggest only IVF can solve the medical problem. Issues that usually should result in immediate referral to IVF include advanced maternal age (approximately 38 and older), diminished ovarian reserve, significant tubal damage, two or more ectopic pregnancies, moderate to severe male factor, severe endometriosis, failed prior treatments and/or prolonged infertility. If 3 to 6 months of standard treatments do not result in an ongoing pregnancy, most patients are candidates for IVF, although laparoscopy may be indicated for some. Occasionally, in younger patients or those with miscarriages, standard treatment can effectively be used for a longer period of time. IVF can be a successful treatment for most, but not all, patients. IVF does not improve uterine factor and cannot change egg quality. All patients considering IVF need to be thoroughly counseled regarding IVF. Issues about which the patients need to be made aware and decisions they need to make are discussed below.

An IVF cycle sometimes consists of suppressing the ovaries with oral contraceptives for three weeks so that all the eggs start maturing at about the same time when ovarian stimulation begins. Different types of ovarian suppression and stimulation cycles include long luteal suppression with the gonadotropin releasing hormone (GnRH) agonist leuprolide acetate (Lupron), leuprolide acetate flare cycles and GnRH antagonist cycles with cetrorelix (Cetrotide) or ganirelix (Antagon). No studies show any protocols are superior to long luteal suppression protocols with GnRH agonist. A study comparing estradiol priming antagonist, antagonist +/oral contraceptive pill priming, long luteal protocol, leuprolide acetate stop protocol, and flare showed no difference changing stimulation protocol on repeat conventional ovarian stimulation cycles [71]. There are no studies that demonstrate any specific protocol will increase pregnancy rates in poor responders. In patients who are classified as poor responders and pursuing IVF, strong consideration should be given to a mild ovarian-stimulation protocol (low-dose gonadotropins with or without oral agents) due to lower costs and comparable low pregnancy rates compared with traditional IVF stimulation protocols [72].

Injectable fertility medications can be human menopausal gonadotropins (HMG) that contain both FSH and LH and are sold as Repronex or Menopur. Follitropins are recombinant FSH, sold as Follistim and Gonal F. The scheduling and protocols for monitoring these subcutaneous injections are complex and need to be explained in detail and specific written instructions given to patients. Ovarian cancer risk is of historical concern but reasonably good data conclude there is likely very little risk of ovarian carcinoma and/or very few patients are ever affected [53]. Additional medications such as dexamethasone, bromocryptine and/or growth hormone may occasionally be used in selected patients. However, these and other "add-ons," including preimplantation genetic testing, endometrial receptivity assay (ERA) and immunological treatments add cost to IVF cycles, often without any evidence of increased pregnancy rates, and so should be avoided unless there are sound clinical indications [73,74].

The goal of fertility treatment is to optimize the number of healthy eggs that can potentially be fertilized in any given cycle and result in implantation of embryos and birth of a healthy singleton baby. It is not possible to know with certainty how any woman will respond to ovarian stimulation medications until they are used. There is a risk of either not responding much at all with very little or no benefit from the ovarian stimulation, or the risk of responding too much, with the risk of large ovarian cysts, pelvic pain and/or OHSS. The potentially significant medical risks of OHSS include pelvic discomfort from large ovaries, nausea, vomiting, accumulation of fluid in the peritoneal, pleural and/or pericardial sac resulting in a distended abdomen, difficulty breathing and/or cardiac problems. Significant fluid imbalance in the body can result in a very high concentration of red blood cells in the vascular system, cause blood clots, kidney and/or liver failure or affect other vital organs. Hospitalization is needed in about 1 in 300 patients and in the rarest of cases, death can occur. If pregnant, a second wave of OHSS can occur, and complications can be more severe with multiple pregnancy [75]. Minor side effects include inflammation and bruising at the injection site.

Use of these fertility medications does increase pregnancy rates but does not reduce miscarriage rates, the risk of pregnancy complications, or birth defects/abnormal babies. Women experiencing infertility generally have approximately 1.5 to 2 times the risk of perinatal complications regardless of whether they use fertility drugs or the method of getting pregnant. Approximately 10–15% of cycles are cancelled before egg retrieval because of low response to gonadotropins or hyperstimulation/OHSS.

After ovarian stimulation, which lasts about 8 to 12 days on average, human chorionic gonadotropin (hCG) is used to trigger final maturation of the eggs. Trade names for these drugs are Novarel, Ovidrel and Pregnyl. Leuprolide acetate (Lupron) trigger can be used in antagonist cycles to avoid OHSS. Sometimes double triggers are used. It is essential to time carefully this injection with respect to time of egg retrieval procedure, the usual interval being about 35–36 hours. Trigger medications and protocols have become much more complex in the past several years, yet their relative effectiveness is still being assessed [76].

The egg retrieval procedure involves monitored anesthesia care with conscious sedation performed in a procedure room or surgery center. A small needle is passed through the posterior vaginal wall into the ovary using transvaginal ultrasound guidance. Each follicle is entered and the follicular fluid is aspirated into a small test tube, which is passed to an embryologist who looks at the fluid under a microscope to identify and separate any eggs into a separate small dish. The procedure takes approximately 15 to 30 minutes. The patient goes home about an hour after the procedure. The risks of the procedure include anesthetic complications, drug reactions, breathing or heart problems, neurologic problems, bleeding, infection, or blood clots. However, the procedure is, overall, very safe. Rarely, no eggs are retrieved or the eggs that are found are not viable. This happens about 3% of the time, usually in older patients. Additionally, on average only approximately two-thirds of the eggs retrieved will be of appropriate maturity to be fertilized. Furthermore, even eggs that have normal maturity do not all have normal chromosomes. At age 35 less than half of the eggs have normal chromosomes and at age 40 the percentage of normal eggs is approximately 10–20%.

While eggs are being retrieved from the patient, her partner will provide a sperm specimen by masturbation. The sperm specimen will then be prepared in the embryology laboratory for insemination of the partner's eggs. In situations in which the male has erectile dysfunction or any other type of problem that might make it difficult or uncertain that he can collect sperm on the day of egg retrieval, it can be arranged for the male to come in the day before to the laboratory and collect a specimen that will be kept overnight and used for insemination the next day. Alternatively, the male can collect a specimen days or weeks in advance and have it frozen in the laboratory and stored until the day of egg retrieval. In very selected cases of men with very poor sperm quality or other obstructive ejaculatory duct problems, sperm can be obtained surgically from the testicle or epididymis by a urologist using procedures called testicular sperm extraction (TESA) or microsurgical epididymal sperm aspiration (MESA) at the same time as the female partner is having eggs retrieved. However, if the male partner is sterile or the female patient has a same-sex partner or is single, donor sperm will be used for fertilization of the eggs.

Eggs can be fertilized by standard fertilization in which case about 50,000 to 100,000 sperm are placed around the eggs. In cases in which there is concern about the sperm quality, or occasionally for other reasons, intracytoplasmic sperm injection (ICSI) or injection of one sperm into one egg can be performed. This procedure is done in approximately 70% of cycles in the US. ICSI increases the chances that at least some eggs will be fertilized, but ICSI does not increase the fertilization rate if the sperm function normally. Unfortunately, some men have normal semen analysis but their sperm do not function normally, and thus ICSI can be helpful for them. Approximately 70–90% of normal-appearing eggs will fertilize. In cases in which it is not clear if ICSI is needed, the eggs can be split into both types of fertilization if sufficient mature eggs are retrieved. Eggs are checked one day after fertilization to see if normal fertilization has occurred, called the 2 pronuclear (2 PN) stage.

Embryos can be cultured to day 3 at which time they are at a cleavage stage or approximately 8-cell stage. On day 3, embryos are graded by the number of cells and the appearance of those cells. Embryos can also be grown from day 3 to day 5 or 6 in culture, at which time they are a 150–250-cell blastocyst [77]. The probability a blastocyst will implant and result in a baby is about 1.3 to 1.4 times higher than a cleavage stage or day 3 embryo. However, only about 50% of the embryos grow in culture from day 3 to day 5. Most, but not necessarily all, of the embryos that fail to grow are abnormal. Therefore, patients who choose to continue with culture to blastocyst stage will have fewer blastocysts to choose from than day 3 cleavage stage embryos, and some patients, especially older patients, might have no blastocysts to transfer. Additionally, there are some concerns that embryos remaining in culture might experience "imprinting" problems where the expression of genes is influenced, and some studies suggest that babies born after culturing to blastocyst may have more abnormalities. However, the vast majority of babies born from blastocysts are healthy and the pregnancy rate for each blastocyst transferred is significantly higher than for a day 3 embryo. There are clinical reasons to transfer on either day 3 or day 5, and these must be discussed and decided upon with each patient individually. There is no convincing evidence that cumulative live birth rates are increased by growing day 3 embryos to blastocysts and transferring them on day 5. Non-invasive systems to assess embryo growth using time-lapse imaging and artificial intelligence are in clinical use and may improve our ability to select better embryos for transfer. Most transfers are now done at the blastocyst stage unless there are only a few poor-quality embryos on day 3.

Preimplantation genetic testing (PGT) can be done to identify selected known genetic problems in the patient and/or her partner: PGT-M for monogenic disorders, PGT-A for aneuploidy and PGT-SR for structural rearrangements [31]. Approximately three to seven cells are removed from the cells that will make the placenta and sent to the laboratory for analysis. PGT-M and PGT-SR are 95% to over 99% accurate. PGT-A is less accurate because of sampling and platform errors, mosaicism and self-correction of embryos. It appears to be helpful for advanced maternal age patients with numerous embryos but its optimal application is still being studied.

Multiple pregnancy is the major complication of IVF and results from many factors. Approximately 70% of infertile patients say they would like twins. Nevertheless, twins have approximately 1.2 to 2 times the risk of serious, permanent physical and/or mental abnormalities or death. The risk of serious pregnancy complications for the mother is also increased about twice as much. Therefore, it is important to have as a goal the birth of a healthy singleton baby and patients need to be carefully counseled about the risks. The best way to ensure this is to perform elective single embryo transfer (eSET). eSET can be performed with either a day 3 cleavage stage embryo or day 5 blastocyst. For patients in their late thirties, it can be appropriate to transfer two day 3 embryos, but the risk of twins is too high to transfer more than one blastocyst in most patients unless the patient is in her forties. Only one known-euploid embryo (from PGT-A) should ever be transferred. Each patient will have the number to transfer finalized after the number and quality of the embryos are determined during the cycle [78].

Assisted hatching is a technique that involves making a small hole in the embryo cell wall with a laser beam on day 3 if the patient meets certain criteria, namely age 38 or more, prior failed IVF cycle(s), cryopreserved/thawed embryos, or thickened outer cell wall (zona pellucida) [79]. Reasonably good studies suggest an increase in pregnancy rates as a result of assisted hatching. The procedure may be associated with a small increase in identical twin pregnancies, which are associated with a lower chance of a healthy baby.

The embryo transfer procedure is done under abdominal ultrasound guidance and is painless. Sometimes the procedure just takes a few minutes and sometimes it can take longer because of difficulty passing the catheter through the endocervical canal into the uterus. Patients are usually asked to limit their activities significantly for the day following embryo or blastocyst transfer, primarily for emotional reasons because it has been claimed, but not proven, that this will increase pregnancy rates. No anesthesia is required for the embryo transfer.

It is necessary to provide progesterone or other hormonal support to the endometrium in the luteal phase because the ovary has been suppressed by the GnRH agonist or antagonist. Progesterone can be given intramuscularly in the buttock, which has been proven effective for over 50 years, yet can be painful. Vaginal suppositories or capsules can be used instead and are not associated with pain but are found to be messy by some patients and have been shown to be equivalent, but not superior to, intramuscular progesterone. Progesterone taken for a short period of time generally does not have serious side effects, but some patients do experience nausea, constipation, breast enlargement and tenderness, headache, fluid retention and depression.

Approximately 10 to 14 days after the embryo transfer a serum pregnancy test is done to determine if the embryo(s) has implanted and is developing. It is best not to be overly active during these two weeks because the ovaries are usually enlarged from the gonadotropin drugs and a high degree of activity will potentially increase pelvic discomfort and risk ovarian cyst leakage and pain or ovarian torsion.

Approximately two-thirds of patients who have a positive pregnancy test following IVF will deliver a baby. The proportion who will miscarry in the first trimester, or lose a baby in the second or third trimester, ranges from about 15% for patients around age 25 to 75% for a woman age 45. About half the pregnancy losses will occur in the first two weeks after the first positive pregnancy test and most of the remaining losses will occur before 12 weeks of pregnancy. After 12 weeks of pregnancy only about 5% of pregnancies will be lost. Ectopic or tubal pregnancy occurs in about 2–4% of patients and must be carefully diagnosed and managed with either methotrexate injections or surgery. The vast majority of IVF babies are healthy, but the risk of an abnormal baby is about 1.2 to 1.6 times higher than the general population. The risk increases for all women who have a multiple pregnancy and for all women who are older. Tests, most but not all of which are non-invasive, can be performed to help assess the baby during the first and second trimester. Cell-free DNA blood tests, quadruple testing, chorionic villus sampling (CVS), amniocentesis, and ultrasound testing are the types of tests that are generally discussed with and performed by the patient's obstetrician.

Induced fetal reduction, also known as pregnancy reduction, is a difficult topic to discuss because of the emotional and ethical/societal aspects associated with it. It should not be considered a backup for replacing too many embryos and is uncommonly performed. Nevertheless, it is a relatively easy, safe and effective procedure that can significantly reduce the risk of multiple pregnancy, especially high order (triplet or more) pregnancy, and increase the probability of a healthy mother and baby. The risk of losing the entire pregnancy because of the procedure is approximately 5% but the improvement in pregnancy and fetal outcome is greater than that, especially for triplet or higher order pregnancies.

It is possible to cryopreserve by vitrification (an ultra-fast freezing process) any viable embryos or blastocysts that were not transferred in the fresh cycle. Pregnancy rates in frozen/thaw embryo transfer cycles (FET) following vitrification are similar to fresh transfer and appear to be as safe with respect to good outcomes with healthy babies. A much higher proportion of cycles are now having all embryos frozen ("freeze-all") because PGT is performed and time is needed for analysis; for embryo banking to get multiple good embryos before beginning transfers; because of less-than-optimal endometrium for implantation; to reduce the risk of OHSS; or for fertility preservation and later use. Embryos or blastocysts have been kept frozen and successfully thawed for 10–20 years or more. It is important to discuss the eventual need to use the embryos or blastocysts to attempt a pregnancy or to dispose of them in the future if they are not needed. Disposition options include transfer into the patient's uterus, donation to research, donation to another patient or discarding.

Either natural FET cycles or medicated FET cycles can be used to transfer thawed embryos. The natural cycle requires no medications but more monitoring than the medicated cycle and has a higher chance of being cancelled because the time of ovulation cannot be adequately determined or the endometrial lining does not seem adequate. The medicated cycle does require medications but is more predictable. Both types of cycles have similar financial cost and pregnancy rates.

Live birth rates per cycle start for both fresh transfer cycles and FET should be discussed with the patients. Future treatments depending on whether the cycle goes well or poorly and whether the patient is pregnant or not should be discussed before the cycle starts. The health of babies born from IVF should be discussed. Many studies have concluded that babies born after IVF and ICSI have a slightly higher (approximately 1.2 to 1.6 times) risk of being abnormal. It is not entirely clear, but most experts think this is primarily due to the patient population being treated, that is infertile patients, who will have slightly higher reproductive risks and slightly fewer good outcomes than patients with no reproductive problems who get pregnant without difficulty. It is not thought that the IVF procedure itself creates much risk, although there may be some small risk that could come from handling eggs and sperm and from culturing embryos outside the body. The risk of abnormal babies with ICSI appears to be slightly higher than that with conventional or standard IVF fertilization, and is likely related to the population of patients needing ICSI to get pregnant. A condition called hypospadias, in which the urethral opening on the penis is on the underside of the penis, may occur slightly more often. The major risk from IVF is having multiple pregnancy, which increases the risk of having a baby with a problem about 1.2 to 2.0 times from 2.5% to 4% for major problems or death. However, it is important to note that the great majority of IVF and ICSI babies are healthy.

The average number of IVF cycles done by patients in the US is approximately two. Many patients will do three or four fresh cycles, but few do more than that. Patients should know that fewer than half of all patients get pregnant on their first cycle. However, even on the sixth or seventh cycle the pregnancy rate is about half as high as it is on the first cycle in populations of patients who have continued to undergo IVF cycles for that long. Most patients find that frozen/thaw cycles are much less demanding and cost much less so that they can do more of them, although there are still emotional costs associated with doing multiple cycles and patients do drop out of treatment for both financial and/or emotional reasons [3]. Besides further IVF cycles, the patient needs to be informed about other options including donor egg and/or sperm, donor embryo, adoption or child-free living.

Patients need to know that, while concerns have been expressed about long-term risks of IVF treatment associated with ovarian stimulation or egg retrieval and anesthesia, there are no confirmed known longer-term risks. Additionally, there are benefits from pregnancy, including reduced risk of breast, ovarian and other cancers. Patients should be informed about additional sources of information including the American Society for Reproductive Medicine (ASRM) website (www.asrm.org), the European Society of Human Reproduction and Embryology (ESHRE) website (www.eshre.org), the ASRM patient website (www.reproductivefacts.org), the

Society for Assisted Reproductive Technology (SART) website (www.sart.org), the Centers for Disease Control site for ART results (www.cdc.gov), RESOLVE (www.resolve.org), FIGO (https://endometriosis.org/) and other legitimate fertility websites.

Psychosocial Intervention

Therapeutic Approaches

The longer patients pursue treatment, the more difficult it becomes. Each cycle or new approach to treatment comes on the heels of failure, which takes an emotional toll. The fertility counselor can offer a safe haven to process feelings of anxiety, sadness and loss as well as assist with coping strategies to deal with the next cycle of treatment. As has been noted, individual, couple and group fertility counseling (Chapters 3–5) provide treatment modalities for not only processing the myriad of feelings related to infertility (grief, loss, shame, guilt, etc.), but also help in developing effective coping strategies that facilitate resiliency and healing from the life-altering experience. The repeated experience of reproductive loss is traumatic and navigating this "battlefield" during therapy creates challenges for both the patient and the fertility counsellor. The impact of reproductive trauma on the therapeutic relationship is discussed further in Chapter 20.

An overlooked aspect of the therapeutic relationship is when the fertility counselor (or other reproductive medical professional) becomes pregnant. The therapeutic alliance is altered and intense feelings for the patient and reactions in the clinician may be triggered. The self-disclosure of the pregnancy unfolds transference/countertransference dynamics which can feel like "walking a tightrope." Chapter 24, on the pregnant fertility counselor, delves into an important topic that has not previously been addressed in the literature.

During the COVID-19 pandemic, all MHPs had to rapidly change the way they delivered care, from in-person sessions to virtual meetings via telehealth platforms. Fertility counselors continued to provide crucial support to patients who were suddenly cut-off from their medical professionals and treatment, at the same time ensuring services were delivered competently, legally and ethically. The dramatic switch to telemental health because of the pandemic has established a "new normal" in the way we are able to deliver fertility counseling services, especially to patients living remotely and in underserved areas of the world. Chapter 25 on telemental health in fertility counseling presents a model for how this can be done competently in both fertility counseling and third-party assessments.

Processing Trauma and Promoting Resiliency

Trauma, a profound emotional response to a distressing event or experience, is a layered part of the infertility journey. The loss of a much-desired pregnancy and longed for baby is one of the most difficult, traumatic reproductive experiences for patients as well as their caregivers. Even more difficult is when a patient/couple is faced with the onerous decision to terminate a much-wanted pregnancy due to fetal anomaly or to reduce a multiple pregnancy. The empathic assistance, support, understanding and direction of a fertility counselor can be a lifeline for patients and is discussed further in Chapter 21 on pregnancy loss as well as Chapter 22 on recurrent pregnancy loss counseling.

Resiliency refers to the concept of an individual's ability to adapt to adversity and cope flexibly with life's challenges, thus reflecting how one copes with stress and one's emotional hardiness. It is seen as a process and not a character trait, and thus is not a personality characteristic one is born with but rather can be a learned behavioral adaptation to a distressful event or significant trauma. Resilience has been studied extensively in the literature with regard to loss and potential trauma [80] and more limitedly, in relation to the distress of infertility [81]. What is important for fertility counselors to understand (and is addressed further in Chapters 2, 19, and 20 of this book) is that the trauma of infertility can also lead to positive changes referred to as posttraumatic growth (PTG). Individuals and couples have the opportunity to learn new skills in communication, coping, and resiliency that will help in the future when faced with other life difficulties [82].

Drawing from this research, fertility counselors should consider ways to enhance resiliency as indicated by Table 1.2. Having programs that teach cognitive–behavioral techniques (e.g., cognitive restructuring, positive thinking, etc.) ideally in a group setting, which allows for social connections, is essential. Clinics should also have tools available to help with times known to be especially stressful for patients, specifically the two-week waiting period after treatment and before getting pregnancy results. The Positive Reappraisal Coping Inventory (PRCI) is a low-cost, easy to administer, self-help intervention that increases positive affect during the two-week waiting period, helps in coping during early pregnancy for RPL patients, as well as dealing with uncertainty in

Table 1.2 Promoting resiliency during infertility

Emphasize behavioral skills which enhance resiliency:
- Learn relaxation techniques
- Teach cognitive re-appraisal
- Identify active coping strategies
- Practice health-enhancing behaviors
- Promote optimism and acceptance
- Encourage social connections and sharing of feelings.
- Increase self-esteem, self-acceptance, and self-adequacy.
- Identify spiritual resources and "the bigger picture" beyond oneself.
- Find a positive meaning and purpose to the experience of infertility.

other stressful situations [83]. Chapter 19 provides a deeper discussion on resiliency and adaptation in responding to reproductive loss.

Integrative/complementary care programs, specifically for fertility patients, are becoming increasingly popular, offering classes in yoga, breathing, graduated relaxation, meditation, mindfulness, guided imagery and nutrition counseling, as well as offering acupuncture services. Helping patients develop active coping skills, such as self-care or breaking problems down into manageable pieces, and drawing upon spirituality has been shown to be effective in building resiliency. Rebuilding self-esteem and being able to find meaning in the infertility experience, with both thought and action, is also an important part of the counseling process. In sum, incorporating cognitive–behavioral skills, active coping, spirituality and finding ways to put meaning and purpose to the adversity enhances resiliency. Many such programs can be found digitally in apps that are mobile-friendly and have proliferated because of COVID-19.

Third Party Reproduction: Collaborative Care

More than other aspects of infertility care, third party reproduction requires the coordinated, collaborative approach of numerous professionals (i.e., medical, psychological, legal, and donor/gestational surrogacy agencies) together with multiple participants (intended parents, gamete donors/surrogates and their partners) to help in family building. Terminology is changing, reflecting the realities of donor-conceived people's consumer groups, social media and most notably direct-to-consumer DNA testing eliminating the possibility of anonymity between gamete donors and recipients. Thus, anonymous donation is now referred to as nonidentified (deidentified/unknown) and known as directed donation, terms that will be used throughout this text. The complexities related to the end of anonymity, DNA testing and the linking of gamete donors and their offspring are discussed further in Chapter 13.

Medical Issues

Sperm donation has been performed since biblical times. Until the past century, this involved sperm deposition with intercourse, and until the last few decades fresh sperm placed around the cervix (cap insemination) or into the uterus after sperm washing (IUI). However, improvements in sperm freezing technology and concerns over sexually transmitted infections, particularly HIV, have resulted in almost all inseminations now being done with cryopreserved sperm from screened individuals. This procedure was for many years called artificial insemination or AI, but now is called partner or husband insemination (HI) or donor insemination (DI). Donor insemination has most commonly been used for heterosexual couples with severe male factor infertility. However, since IVF became more available in the mid-1980s, and especially ICSI in the early 1990s, severe male factor can be treated by IVF/ICSI. That technology development, along with other societal changes, has resulted in a more common use of donor sperm being with single women and LGBTQ+ people who wish to have children. The use of donor sperm and donor eggs is regulated by the Food and Drug Administration (FDA) and requires sexually transmitted infection and other screening of both nonidentified and directed donors. The intended recipients receive donor sperm specimens from regulated sperm banks and choose the donor based on physical characteristics and qualities they value and desire. Further, at the request of intended parents, offspring and in some cases national legislation, sperm banks have initiated an "identity-released" donor program where sperm donors agree to allow the release of personal information and even contact with donor-conceived children when they reach the age of 18. Given developments in genetics and social media it is no longer possible to ensure "anonymity," a situation that must be carefully discussed with all parties involved in third party reproduction. Directed sperm donors can still be used, but this is less commonly done and more often carried out in a non-medical environment.

Egg donation is a recent development since IVF became more available in the mid-1980s. From a medical perspective, the process of egg donation is more involved than sperm donation. Different characteristics of egg donors, the basis on which they can be chosen, characteristics of different agencies, ASRM and ESHRE guidelines, the process of assessing donors by patients and the important characteristics for the patient and her husband need to be discussed with patients [84].

Egg donor screening involves a detailed history, family history, physical examination and specific gynecologic examination, in particular for antral follicle count, anti-mullerian hormone (AMH) and follicle stimulating hormone (FSH) and estradiol (E2) levels, general hematology and biochemistry tests, genetic testing and screening, sexually transmitted infection screening and testing, drug and nicotine screening and testing, psychological screening and counseling, and an explanation of management of the egg donor during fresh donation cycles.

Legal issues, including consent forms, control and management of the eggs and embryos, split donor cycles, reciprocal IVF cycles, requirements for establishing parenthood, potential changes in law over time and situations and issues to be considered and avoided need to be discussed with the intended parents. Psychological issues such as deidentified versus directed donors, legal issues surrounding anonymity, the potential for telling the child and other family members about egg donation and reproductive choices the couple would face over the child's lifetime should be addressed by both the physician and the fertility counselor. Also, discussion of financial issues including the cost of egg donation, insurance and payment options need to be addressed.

Recipients need to understand medical management during the cycle, including the fact the egg donor is also a patient, the screening and timeline for the donor, medical management of the donor and other aspects of the relationship with the donor. Medical management of the female recipient, who will undergo what amounts to a medicated cycle preparing her uterus ready to receive an embryo, is important to understand. Options such as freezing all the embryos for later transfer and the obtaining of cryopreserved eggs from an egg bank are also possible options for consideration. The male role involves screening and the provision of the sperm.

Egg donation, in many countries, is generally nonidentified now and so issues of anonymity and disclosure must be discussed and resolved before starting a cycle. As noted, anonymity is impossible to guarantee given developments in genetics and social media. When directed egg donors are involved, the nature of the ongoing relationship needs to be determined and finalized to the extent possible. The medical process for egg donors is the same as for IVF patients, with careful coordination of the cycle with the female recipient and sperm from her male partner.

Other options that are performed much less commonly but that are appropriate for some patients are embryo donation and gestational carrier or surrogacy. *Embryo donation* is an excellent option, but the problem is that not many people decide to donate embryos. This occurs because embryos are generally donated by patients who have had successful IVF treatment, in which case they have children from the cohort of embryos that are frozen and so often consider the embryos to be siblings of their living children, making embryo donation more psychologically difficult. Chapter 11 describes the intricacies involved in counseling embryo donors and recipients.

Gestational surrogacy (GS), also referred to as gestational carrier (GC), is an option for patients who don't have a uterus because of developmental or disease problems, or who have a non-functional uterus, history of pregnancy losses or underlying medical condition that makes pregnancy risky. Same sex male couples and single males also need surrogates. GSs may be recruited or be a relative or friend of the intended parent(s) (IPs). All the considerations of egg donation apply, plus the added issues of pregnancy in another person and longer-term relationship issues, all of which need to be discussed, agreed upon and finalized in writing before undertaking a GS cycle. Psychological assessment and counseling for all parties involved in third party reproduction – intended parents, donors and GS participants – should be mandatory. Chapter 12 focuses on special considerations in counseling and assessment in GS arrangements (see [33], pp. 122–135 on gestational carrier participant screenings).

Psychosocial Issues

When patients move on to third party reproduction, they do so either out of an experience of loss and often repeated treatment failure, or because life circumstance necessitates the need for reproductive assistance. Whatever the reason, there is a common thread to the experience because using a donor or GS correlates with "loss," be it genetic connection or biological connection by carrying a pregnancy and giving birth, which must be grieved. For couples who have exhausted all treatment options for a genetically or biologically shared baby, third-party assistance is their last, best hope.

For LGBTQ+ couples or single individuals, these treatments offer hope for the family of their dreams, yet also the realization that it will not happen without

the assistance of another person or people, whether directed or nonidentified ([33], pp. 166–179 for more information on fertility counseling with single women and men). More recently, transgender people (those individuals whose gender identity does not align with that assigned to them at birth) are seeking care in ART programs to preserve their fertility or grow their families, described further in Chapter 17. Because of the multifaceted issues (medical, psychological, legal, ethical, social, etc.) involved in third-party reproduction, the ASRM, ESHRE and numerous other regional and legislative organizations recommend that all participants receive counseling and psychological education before undergoing treatment. Today, as many as five individuals may come together in these arrangements – intended parent 1 and 2 (heterosexual or same sex couple), a sperm donor, ovum donor and a woman (or transmale) who will carry the pregnancy – which generates a complex psychosocial situation to manoeuvre during the counseling process.

Third-party counseling, psychoeducation and assessment is a fundamental component of the work fertility counselors do, and is a multifaceted, nuanced process. Section III of this text explores what is involved in the psychoeducation, screening and preparation of gamete recipients (Chapter 9) and donors (Chapter 10) in nonidentified arrangements. Counseling directed or known participants in third-party reproduction presents more complex psychosocial issues, whether the parties are family members/friends or recruited as in GS, and involves careful coordination with all involved (see [33], pp. 136–149 for more details on counseling known participants). Helping patients understand long-range issues to consider, including disclosure to their children, is an important part of recipient/intended parent counseling now and in the future, and is addressed throughout this section.

Decision-making in Infertility: Collaborative Care

Reviewing Family Building Options

Throughout the treatment process and during times of decision-making, it can be helpful to reconsider all family building options. To review, couples wishing to get pregnant have, in general, six potential options from which to choose, although not all options apply to all patients. These options begin with no specific fertility treatment but an approach in which patients optimize their chance for pregnancy by healthy lifestyle choices with respect to sleep, diet, exercise, alcohol, drug and medication use, along with prenatal vitamins with calcium, iron and folate for the woman and a male multi-vitamin with antioxidant. Timing of intercourse every 1 to 3 days and the potential use of urinary LH test kits to confirm ovulation may be helpful. Basal body temperature recording and mucus testing are not generally helpful but might be used in selected couples.

A second option is standard fertility diagnosis and treatment. Patients undergo diagnostic tests for hormonal/ovarian reserve, pelvic, male, combined and systemic factors that affect fertility. After testing, treatment can involve management of identifiable problems of the female by use of hormones, minor or major surgery; treatment of the male; the use of intrauterine insemination and/or management of general health conditions. The goal of treatment is to increase the chance of pregnancy in each menstrual cycle by bringing more egg(s) together with more sperm in the best possible pelvic environment at the right time.

A third option is IVF, the treatment with the highest chances for pregnancy for almost all infertility patients regardless of the cause of their infertility. However, it is more involved for the patient and more expensive, so it is not always the best choice for a given patient. With IVF, ICSI is the single most effective treatment for male factor infertility of almost any severity. However, IVF does not improve egg quality and does not treat problems with the uterus.

A fourth option is egg donation, sperm donation or gestational surrogacy that can be used in situations in which the egg and/or sperm number and/or quality is very low or unavailable from a partner, or the uterus is absent or severely abnormal. Another person can provide eggs, sperm or a uterus (gestational surrogate), as third-party collaborators. The major barriers to third-party reproduction are personal values, psychological considerations for the patient and financial cost. The cost of an egg donation cycle is approximately $35,000 to $65,000 although the chances for a baby are 65–75%. Sperm donation is cheaper at generally less than $1,000 per cycle but pregnancy rates are approximately 10–20% per cycle. GS costs are approximately $85, 000–$150,000 or more.

A fifth option is adoption or foster care. Adoption can be a very successful way for patients to have a family, while foster care can provide an opportunity to care and parent both in the short- and long-term. Public adoption can take a long time and is often more available to younger patients. Private or international adoption is often chosen by patients but is quite involved and can be expensive, costs varying depending on many factors between approximately $25,000 to $75,000. Adoption specialists, including agencies and attorneys, are available to educate and guide about the process and various options. However, it is concerning to note that the number of children (particularly infants) available for adoption nationally and internationally has decreased dramatically in recent years, making this family building option much more difficult ([33], pp. 197–211 has more information on counseling fertility patients considering adoption).

A sixth option is child-free living. Child-free living, which means a conscious decision not to have children or, in some cases, to continue with the number of children already born but not attempt to have more, is a very reasonable choice for many people. While children are wonderful and may be critical to many people's life goals, not everyone has to be a parent, and certainly not if they choose not to be. Child-free living has some economic, time, happiness and lifestyle advantages that balance off some of the benefits of having children. Thus, this is a choice all patients should at least consider before pursuing fertility diagnosis and treatment.

Cost–benefit Analysis

With so many options, all very different, making decisions can be difficult for patients. A framework for this that can be helpful is performing cost–benefit analysis of the different treatment options.

The **benefit** of any treatment choice is equal to the value of that choice to the patient/couple, multiplied by the probability of a successful outcome, which is a healthy baby. The outcomes are potentially different with the different options: her or his own biologic child, a child resulting from involvement of a donor, an adopted child, or no child at all. The value of each outcome to patients is unique to the intended parent(s) and can only be determined by them, not the physician. The physician's role is to provide patients with information and guidance to help them make the best reproductive decision for themselves. The probability of a healthy baby is a prognosis that can be approximately estimated by the physician by applying the best available evidence in the literature to the patient's unique clinical situation. Interpreting the literature can be a difficult exercise given the plethora of studies, many of them not well designed and/or with other biasing factors. Utilizing national and/or professional guidelines is generally the best approach [86]. SART has a predictive model (https://w3.abdn.ac.uk/clsm/SARTIVF/tool/ivf1), as do some free phone apps based on algorithms, one free one being *FertilityNow*. Patients also need to be directed to legitimate sources of information so that they do not waste time, money and emotional energy pursing inappropriate tests and treatments (e.g., www .reproductivefacts.org). Together, the patient and physician can determine the level of benefit for the different options and start to prioritize approaches to treatment. For any treatment option to be appropriate it must, therefore, have both reasonable value to the patient and reasonable chance of occurring if treatment is undertaken.

The benefits of any treatment must be balanced by the costs. There are four types of **costs**. The first cost is **financial ($)**. Financial cost is important because approximately two-thirds of patients whose treatment doesn't result in a baby and are not successful because they must drop out due to financial barriers. This occurs because some infertility treatments are expensive, but more so because many insurance plans do not provide much infertility coverage. To manage this problem, many fertility clinics have financial counselors who will ascertain as best they can the insurance coverage the patient has, and explain to them other financial packages, plans and financing to help deal with the financial challenges many patients face with fertility treatments.

The second cost is **time (T)**. A patient's fertility becomes reduced over time and is often much reduced even when the patient is first seen because of her age and duration attempting pregnancy. Therefore, the time treatment takes is an important consideration in making choices.

The third cost is the **potential health risks of diagnosis and treatment (Rx)**. Fertility treatment is generally safe. The biggest risk, by far, is the risk of success, that is, a pregnancy confers more risk on the woman than any of the tests or treatments that are generally undertaken in fertility management. However, risks can be increased significantly if the patient has an underlying medical condition such as obesity, has a multiple pregnancy, or has complications from fertility drug use, such as OHSS, or from a surgical procedure. Long-term risks are thought not to occur, or to be very minor, or to occur in a very small proportion of patients treated.

The fourth and often biggest cost is emotional or **psychological (Ψ)**. Patients with infertility can suffer emotional stress equivalent to those of other diagnoses such as HIV and cancer. Infertility can profoundly affect a woman's sense of personhood, marital relationship, sexual and reproductive self, family place and responsibility and social worth. Women are almost always more severely affected than men. Strategies to deal with this situation include having frank communication and agreement with the partner, having strong partner understanding and support, obtaining accurate information about infertility and fertility treatment, asking questions of the physician, and undertaking resiliency activities such as yoga, prayer, meditation, self-help groups, professional counseling or other integrative care programs. For a choice to be a good choice, a depiction of a cost–benefit analysis might look like this:

$$\text{Benefit} > \text{Cost}$$
$$\text{OR}$$
$$\text{Value} \times \text{Probability of Success} > \$ + T + Rx + \Psi$$

After obtaining the appropriate diagnostic tests, couples who are aware of the value to them and prognosis of the different choices, and know the costs, can prioritize the choices and initiate treatment. The process of assessment of costs and benefits should be continuously carried out, and a formal reassessment with the physician performed at least every 3 months because the infertility situation changes over time. In this way optimal management of the patient's infertility can occur, and the maximum chance for pregnancy and a healthy baby can be achieved.

Stopping Treatment

When treatment has been successful, patients transition away from the reproductive medical practice, ideally, towards normalcy in pregnancy, birth and parenthood. While the pregnancy after infertility is at greater risk prenatal and postpartum, most patients navigate the process without significant difficulties [87]. For those where treatment is not successful, they will need to decide if they will remain childless (or with secondary infertility, without more children) or will seek parenthood through adoption. Ending treatment and moving on in either direction will require a process of grief and mourning made more difficult due to the invisible nature of this profound loss – the death of the dream child.

Postpartum and Family Life after Treatment

Successful fertility treatments present a new set of biopsychosocial stressors. Pregnancy and postpartum often involve marked life changes, and, for the carrying parent, unprecedented hormonal fluctuations. The peri- and postnatal period is recognized as a window of vulnerability for the development or exacerbation of psychopathology. All parents, regardless of their ethnicity, socioeconomic status, relationship status, and reproductive history, are susceptible to perinatal mood and anxiety disorders (PMADs) and should be educated about and assessed for PMADs. Chapter 23 explores pregnancy and postpartum adjustment as well as issues to consider in PMADs after fertility treatment.

Adjustment to parenthood and family life after assisted reproduction is usually not on the radar of many patients using assisted reproduction. Years of energy focused on trying to have a child present new challenges when pregnancy is achieved and a baby is born. Parents must adjust beliefs about genetic relationships, what it means to be a family, and develop a healthy process of ways to honestly tell the story of how they became a family ([33], pp. 252–264 also offers a framework for helping parents talk to donor-conceived children). Chapter 14 presents an in-depth discussion on family life after donor conception, and the importance of ongoing professional and peer support.

Exit Counseling

Patients who are not successful with treatment will make the decision to end trying to have a child either consciously or unconsciously. At times a "default" decision is made when patients stop treatment, deciding they need a break (often due to the psychological stress of treatment or financial burdens) yet never to return, or to defer decision-making on alternative family building. The avoidant behavior extends over time and becomes an unconscious choice to remain childless, adding to a sense of being "unresolved." For others, the emotional journey of disengagement from treatment is a conscious, emotionally charged process in decision-making. Based on a longitudinal study of infertile couples, Daniluk [88] identified four stages in the transition to childless after infertility, along a continuum of themes including: "hitting the wall," "reworking the past," "turning toward the future" and "renewal and regeneration." Each of these stages involves approximately a 10-month period, thus taking about 3.5 years to fruition, a reference point that is often very useful for patients to understand. For fertility counselors, helping patients make a conscious decision to end treatment without success may also involve assisting the physician to give their patients permission to stop [89].

A conscious decision to end treatment without having a baby is difficult and may necessitate help in fertility counseling to say a "formal" goodbye. Grieving is the hardest work one ever does in life and is made more difficult when the loss is elusive, amorphous and invisible, as with the death of a dream baby. Normal mourning rituals often don't feel appropriate and patients may struggle with how to recognize their loss in a meaningful way. One powerful therapeutic tool is to task patients to write a letter of goodbye to their dream child: visualizing and naming the child; discussing how wanted s/he was and why; what were their hopes, plans, and wishes for the child; and why they must say goodbye. It is an extraordinarily emotional undertaking where patients need the time, space and emotional energy to build up to the task.

Another aspect of exit counseling for all patients, whether pregnant or not, is to address the consequences that protracted infertility can have on an individual and/or couple's relationship. Most notable is a couple's sexual relationship, which is discussed in detail in Chapters 4 and 6. Also significant are single women who may have struggled through years of treatment and faced decisions along the way they wouldn't have imagined at the start: creating embryos with donor egg and donor sperm or becoming pregnant with multiples. These patients may find themselves depleted of finances, emotional energy, and other resources as they embark towards their long-awaited dream of parenthood. Further issues to explore include self-esteem, marital communication and satisfaction, social support, relationships with family and friends, and overall quality of life. The good news is that infertility has the potential to teach individuals and couples life-long skills and resiliency to deal with future adversity. Long-term studies have indicated overall good psychological adjustment in both couples who achieved parenthood with medical assistance as well as those who remained childless [90].

Conclusion

As a final note, practicing as a fertility counselor presents numerous challenges and competent practice cannot take place in isolation. When a fertility counselor establishes a practice, there are many things to consider from preparing consents, releases, reports and so on, and not least of which is "what constitutes competency" to practice. Chapter 26 on legal issues provides a hands-on approach to clinical management. As one's practice grows, fertility counselors are continually presented with ethical dilemmas and struggles in their work, and Chapter 27 offers a valuable platform to address these complex issues. Membership and participation in the Mental Health Professional Group (MHPG) of the ASRM, the Psychology and Counselling Special

Interest Group of ESHRE, the British Infertility Counselling Association (BICA), Australia/New Zealand Infertility Counselling Association (ANZICA), BKiD (Germany) or other professional organizations representing the field of fertility counseling is essential. This specialization is a dynamic and continually expanding field in tandem with the technology, and fertility counselors must stay up-to-date.

References

1. Boivin J, Gameiro S. The evolution of psychology and counseling in infertility. *Fertil Steril* 2015;**104** (2):251–259.

2. Norre J, Wischmann T. The position of the fertility counselor in a fertility team: a critical appraisal. *Hum Fertil* 2011;**14**(3):154–159. Epub July 7, 2011.

3. Gameiro S, Boivin J, Domar A. Optimal in vitro fertilization in 2020 should reduce treatment burden and enhance care delivery for patients and staff. *Fertil Stertil* 2013;**100**(2):302–309.

4. Covington SN. Infertility counseling in practice: a collaborative reproductive healthcare model. In: Covington SN, Burns LH, Eds. *Infertility Counseling: A Comprehensive Handbook for Clinicians,* 2nd edn. Cambridge: Cambridge University Press, 2006: 493–507.

5. Van Empel IWH, Aarts JWM, Cohlen BJ, et al. Measuring patient-centredness, the neglected outcome in fertility care: a random multicentre validation study. *Hum Reprod* 2010;**10**:2516–2526.

6. Boivin J, Domar AD, Shapiro DB, Wischmann TH, Fauser BC, Verhaak C. Tackling burden in ART: an integrated approach for medical staff. *Hum Reprod* 2012;**27** (4):941–950.

7. Evers JL. Female subfertility. *Lancet* 2002;**360**:151–159.

8. Zegers FZ, Adamson GD, Dyer S, et al . The International Glossary on Infertility and Fertility Care: Led by ICMART in Partnership with ASRM, ESHRE, IFFS, March of Dimes, AFS, GIERAF, ASPIRE, MEFS, REDLARA, FIGO. *Fertil Steril* 2017;**108**(3):393–406.

9. te Velde ER, Eijkemans R, Habbema HD. Variation in couple fecundity and time to pregnancy, an essential concept in human reproduction. *Lancet* 2000;**355**:1928–1929.

10. Snick HKA, Snick TS, Evers JLH, Collins JA. The spontaneous pregnancy prognosis in untreated subfertile couples. The Walcheren primary care study. *Hum Reprod* 1997;**12**:1582–1588.

11. Leridon H. A new estimate of permanent sterility by age: sterility defined as the inability to conceive. *Popul Stud* 2008;**62**:15–24.

12. Boivin J, Bunting L, Collins JA, Nygren KG. International estimates of infertility prevalence and treatment-seeking: potential need and demand for infertility medical care. *Hum Reprod* 2007;**22**(6):1506–1512.

13. Gurunath S, Pandian Z, Anderson RA, et al. Defining infertility – a systematic review of prevalence studies. *Hum Reprod Update* 2011;**17**(5):575–588.

14. Wallace WH, Kelsey TW. Ovarian reserve and reproductive age may be determined from measurement of ovarian volume by transvaginal sonography. *Hum Reprod* 2004;**19**:1612–1617.

15. Hendershot GE, Mosher WD, Pratt WF. Infertility and age: an unresolved issue. *Fam Plan and Perspect* 1982;**14** (5):287–289.

16. Zinaman MJ, Clegg ED, Brown CC, O'Connor J, Selevan SG. Estimates of human fertility and pregnancy loss. *Fertil Steril* 1996;**65**:503–509.

17. te Velde ER, Pearson PL. The variability of reproductive aging. *Hum Reprod Update* 2002;**8**:141–154.

18. Nybo Andersen A-M, Kjaer Urhoj S. Is advanced paternal age a health risk for the offspring? *Fertil Steril* 2017;**107** (2):312–318.

19. Practice Committee of the American Society for Reproductive Medicine. Obesity and reproduction: a committee opinion. Birmingham, Alabama. *Fertil Steril* 2021;**116**:1266–1285.

20. Oscan Dağ Z, Dilbaz B. Impact of obesity on infertility in women. *J Turk Ger Gynecol Assoc* 2015;**16** (2):111–117.

21. Practice Committee of the American Society for Reproductive Medicine in collaboration with the Society for Reproductive Endocrinology and Infertility. Optimizing natural fertility: a committee opinion. *Fertil Steril* 2013;**100**:631–637.

22. Mahony M, Mottla GL, Richter KS, Ball GD, Ansari S, Hayward B. Infertility patient clinical journey outcome depends on initial treatment, starting with ovulation induction vs in vitro fertilization (IVF): results from a large real-world database. ASRM Abstracts P-734, e-396. *Fertil Steril* (Suppl. September) 2019; **112**(3): e396–e397.

23. World Health Organization. Endometriosis Fact Sheet. Available from: www.who.int/news-room/fact-sheets/deta il/endometriosis [last accessed June 15, 2022].

24. Schlegel PN, Sigman M, Collura B, et al. Diagnosis and treatment of infertility in men: AUA/ASRM guideline part II. *Fertil Steril* 2020;**115**(1):62–69.

25. Practice Committee of the American Society for Reproductive Medicine. American Society for Reproductive Medicine, Birmingham, Alabama. Fertility evaluation of infertile women: a committee opinion. *Fertil Steril* 2021;**116**:1255–1265.

26. Schlegel PN, Sigman M, Collura B, et al. Diagnosis and treatment of infertility in men: AUA/ASRM guideline part I. *Fertil Steril* 2020;**115**(1):54–61.

27. Practice Committee of the American Society for Reproductive Medicine, Birmingham, Alabama. Testing and interpreting measures of ovarian reserve: a committee opinion. *Fertil Steril* 2020;**114**:1151–1157.

28. World Health Organization. WHO Laboratory Manual for the Examination and Processing of Human Semen, 6th edn. Published July 27, 2021. Available from: www.who .int/publications/i/item/9789240030787 [last accessed June 15, 2022].

29. Schlegel PN, Sigman M, Collura B, et al. Diagnosis and treatment of infertility in men. AUA/ ASRM Guideline. American Urological Association. October 2020.

30. Oei SG, Helmerhorst FM, Bloemenkamp KWM, Hollants FAM, Meerpoel DM, Keirse MJNC. Effectiveness of the postcoital test. *BMJ* 1998;**317**:502–505.

31. Practice Committees of the American Society for Reproductive Medicine and the Society for Assisted Reproductive Technology. The use of preimplantation genetic testing for aneuploidy (PGT-A): a committee opinion. *Fertil Steril* 2018;**109**:429–436.

32. World Health Organization (WHO) and World Bank. WHO Report on Disability. Available from: www.who .int/teams/noncommunicable-diseases/sensory-functions- disability-and-rehabilitation/world-report-on-disability [last accessed June 15, 2022].

33. Covington SN, Ed. *Fertility Counseling: Clinical Guide and Case Studies*, 1st edn. Cambridge: Cambridge University Press, 2015.

34. Griel AL, Slausen-Belvins K, McQuillan J. The experience of infertility: a review of recent literature. *Social Health Illn* 2010;**32**(1):140–162.

35. Kenrick DT, Griskevicius V, Neuberg SL, Schaller M. Renovating the Pyramid of Needs: contemporary extensions built upon ancient foundations. *Perspect Psychol Sci* 2010;**5**(3):292–314.

36. Petok WD. The psychology of gender-specific infertility diagnosis. In: Covington SN, Burns LH. *Infertility Counseling: A Comprehensive Handbook for Clinicians*, 2nd edn. Cambridge: Cambridge University Press, 2006: 37–60.

37. Jordan C, Revenson TA. Gender differences in coping with infertility: a meta-analysis. *J Behav Med* 1999;**22**:341–358.

38. Pasch LA, Holley SR, Bleil ME, et al. Addressing the needs of fertility treatment patients and their partners: are they informed of and do they receive mental health services? *Fertil Steril* 2016;**106**(1):209–215.

39. Boivin J, Takefman J, Braverman A. Development and preliminary validation of the fertility quality of life (FertiQoL) tool. *Fertil Steril* 2011;**96**:409–415.

40. Verhaak CM, Lintsen AME, Evers AWM, Braat DDM. Who is at risk of emotional problems and how to know? Screening of women going for IVF treatment. *Hum Reprod* 2010;**25**:1234.

41. Newton CR. The Fertility Problem Inventory: measuring perceived infertility-related stress. *Fertil Steril* 1999;**72**:54–62.

42. Hakim LZ, Newton CR, MacLean-Brine D, Feyles V. Evaluation of preparatory psychosocial counselling for medically assisted reproduction. *Hum Reprod* 2012;**27** (7):2058–2066.

43. Boivin J. A review of psychosocial interventions in infertility. *Soc Sci Med* 2003;**57**:2325–2341.

44. Covington SN. Group approaches to infertility counseling. In: Covington SN, Burns LH, Eds. *Infertility Counseling: A Comprehensive Handbook for Clinicians*, 2nd edn. Cambridge: Cambridge University Press, 2006: 156–168.

45. Aarts JWM, van den Haark P, Nelen WLDM, Tuil WS, Faber JJ, Kremer JAM. Patient-focused Internet interventions in reproductive medicine: a scoping review. *Hum Reprod Update* 2012;**18**(2):211–227.

46. Roudsari RL, Allan HT, Smith PA. Looking at infertility through the lens of religion and spirituality: a review of the literature. *Hum Fertil* 2007;**10**(30):141–149.

47. American Society for Reproductive Medicine. Guidance for Providers Caring for Women and Men of Reproductive Age with Possible Zika Virus Exposure (Modified from CDC, FDA and WHO Published Guidance). Updated July 2019.

48. American Society for Reproductive Medicine. COVID-19 Updates and Resources. www.asrm.org/news-and- publications/covid-19/ [last accessed June 15, 2022].

49. Scarpa B, Dunson DB, Colombo B. Cervical mucus secretions on the day of intercourse: an accurate marker of highly fertile days. *Eur J Obstet Gynaecol Reprod Biol* 2006;**125**:72–78.

50. The Practice Committee of the American Society for Reproductive Medicine. Use of clomiphene citrate in infertile women: a committee opinion. *Fertil Steril* 2013;**100**:341–348.

51. Teede HJ, Misso ML, Costello MF, et al., on behalf of the International PCOS Network Recommendations from the international evidence-based guideline for the assessment and management of polycystic ovary syndrome. *Fertil Steril* 2018;**110**(3):364–379.

52. Practice Committee of the American Society for Reproductive Medicine, Birmingham, Alabama. Role of metformin for ovulation induction in infertile patients with polycystic ovary syndrome (PCOS): a guideline. *Fertil Steril* 2017;**108**:426–441.

53. Practice Committee of the American Society for Reproductive Medicine, Birmingham, Alabama. Fertility drugs and cancer: a guideline. *Fertil Steril* 2016;**106**:1617–1626.

54. The Practice Committee of the American Society for Reproductive Medicine, Birmingham, Alabama. Current evaluation of amenorrhea. *Fertil Steril* 2008;**90**:S219–S225.

55. Practice Committees of the American Society for Reproductive Medicine and Society for Reproductive Endocrinology and Infertility. Use of exogenous gonadotropins for ovulation induction in anovulatory women: a committee opinion. *Fertil Steril* 2020;**113**:66–70.

56. Mulders AG, Laven JS, Eijkemans MJ, Hughes EG, Fauser BC. Patient predictors for outcome of gonadotrophin ovulation induction in women with normogonadotrophic anovulatory infertility: a meta-analysis. *Hum Reprod Update* 2003;**9**:429–449.

57. Reindollar RH, Regan MM, Neumann PJ, et al. A randomized clinical trial to evaluate optimal treatment for unexplained infertility: the fast track and standard treatment (FASTT) trial. *Fertil Steril* 2010;**94**:888–899.

58. Wang R, Danhof NA, Tjon-Kon-Fat RI, Eijkemans MJ, Bossuyt PM, Mochtar MH, van der Veen F, Bhattacharya S, Mol BWJ, van Wely M. Interventions for unexplained infertility: a systematic review and network meta-analysis. *Cochrane Database Syst Rev*. 2019 Sep 5;**9**(9):CD012692. doi: 10.1002/14651858.CD012692.pub2. PMID: 31486548; PMCID: PMC6727181.

59. Goldman MB, Reindollar, Neumann PJ, et al. A randomized clinical trial to determine optimal infertility treatment in older couples: the Forty and Over Treatment Trial (FORT-T). *Fertil Steril* 2014;**101**:1574–81.e2.

60. Practice Committee of the American Society for Reproductive Medicine, Birmingham, Alabama. Removal of myomas in asymptomatic patients to improve fertility and/or reduce miscarriage rate: a guideline. *Fertil Steril* 2017;**108**:416–425.

61. The Practice Committee of the American Society for Reproductive Medicine, Birmingham, Alabama. Role of tubal surgery in the era of assisted reproductive technology: a committee opinion. *Fertil Steril* 2021;**115**:1143–1150.

62. The Practice Committee of the American Society for Reproductive Medicine. Endometriosis and infertility: a committee opinion. *Fertil Steril* 2012;**98**:591–598.

63. Adamson GD, Pasta DJ. Endometriosis fertility index: the new, validated endometriosis staging system. *Fertil Steril* 2010;**94**(5):1609–1615.

64. Vesali S, Razavi M, Rezaeinejad M, Maleki-Hajiagha A, Maroufizadeh S, Sepidarkishf M. Endometriosis Fertility Index for predicting nonassisted reproductive technology pregnancy after endometriosis surgery: a systematic review and meta-analysis. *BJOG* 2020;**127**(7):800–809.

65. The Practice Committee of the American Society for Reproductive Medicine. Report on varicocele and infertility. *Fertil Steril* 2008;**90**:S247–S249.

66. Practice Committee of the American Society for Reproductive Medicine in collaboration with the Society for Male Reproduction and Urology. Evaluation of the azoospermic male: a committee opinion. *Fertil Steril* 2018;**109**:777–782.

67. Steures P, van der Steeg JW, Hompes PG, et al. Effectiveness of intrauterine insemination in subfertile couples with an isolated cervical factor: a randomized clinical trial. *Fertil Steril* 2007;**88**:1692–1696.

68. Practice Committee of the American Society for Reproductive Medicine, Birmingham, Alabama. Evidence-based treatments for couples with unexplained infertility: a guideline. *Fertil Steril* 2020;**113**:305–322.

69. The Practice Committee of the American Society for Reproductive Medicine. Evaluation and treatment of recurrent pregnancy loss: a committee opinion. *Fertil Steril* 2012;**98**:1103–1111.

70. Genest G, Almasri W, Banjar S, et al. Immunotherapy for recurrent pregnancy loss: a reappraisal. *F&S Reviews* 2021 (online). https://doi.org/10.1016/j.xfnr.2021.11.002

71. Wald K, Hariton E, Morris JR, et al. Changing stimulation protocol on repeat conventional ovarian stimulation cycles does not lead to improved laboratory outcomes. *Fertil Steril* 2021;**116**:757–765.

72. Practice Committee of the American Society for Reproductive Medicine, Birmingham, Alabama. Comparison of pregnancy rates for poor responders using IVF with mild ovarian stimulation versus conventional IVF: a guideline. *Fertil Steril* 2018;**109**:993–999.

73. Kamath MS, Mascarenhas M, Franik S, Liu E, Sunkara SK. Clinical adjuncts in in vitro fertilization: a growing list. *Fertil Steril* 2019;**112**:978–986.

74. Farquhar C. Add-ons for assisted reproductive technology: can we be honest here? *Fertil Steril* 2019;**112**:971–972.

75. Practice Committee of the American Society for Reproductive Medicine, Birmingham, Alabama. Prevention and treatment of moderate and severe ovarian hyperstimulation syndrome: a guideline. *Fertil Steril* 2016;**106**:1634–1647.

76. Zhang Y, Guo X, Guo L, Chang H-M, Shu J, Leung PCK. Outcomes comparison of IVF/ICSI among different trigger methods for final oocyte maturation: a systematic review and meta-analysis. *FASEB Journal* 2021;**35**(7):e21696. https://doi.org/10.1096/fj.202100406r

77. Practice Committee of the American Society for Reproductive Medicine and Practice Committee of the Society for Assisted Reproductive Technology. Blastocyst culture and transfer in clinically assisted reproduction: a committee opinion. *Fertil Steril* 2018;**110**:1246–1252.

78. Practice Committee of the American Society for Reproductive Medicine and the Practice Committee for the Society for Assisted Reproductive Technologies, Birmingham, Alabama. Guidance on the limits to the number of embryos to transfer: a committee opinion. *Fertil Steril* 2021;**116**:651–654.

79. Practice Committee of the American Society for Reproductive Medicine and Practice Committee of the Society for Assisted Reproductive Technology, Birmingham, Alabama. Role of assisted hatching in in vitro fertilization: a guideline. *Fertil Steril* 2014;**102**:348–351.

80. Bonanno GA, Westphal M, Mancini AD. Resilience to loss and potential trauma. *Annu Rev Clin Psychol* 2001;**7**:511–535.

81. Herrmann D, Scherg H, Verres R, von Hagens C, Strowitzke T, Wischmann T. Resilience in infertile couples as a protective factor against infertility-specific distress and impaired quality of life. *J Assist Reprod Genet* 2011;**28**:1111–1117.

82. Kong L, Fang M, Ma T, et al. Positive affect mediates the relationships between resilience, social support and posttraumatic growth of women with infertility. *Psychol Health Med* 2018;**23**:707–716.

83. Ockhuijsen H, van den Hoogen A, Eijkemans M, Macklon N, Boivin J. The impact of a self-administered coping intervention on emotional well-being in women awaiting the outcome of IVF treatment: a randomized controlled trial. *Hum Reprod* 2014;**29**(7):1459–1470.

84. Practice Committee of the American Society for Reproductive Medicine and the Practice Committee for the Society for Assisted Reproductive Technology, Birmingham, Alabama. Guidance regarding gamete and embryo donation. *Fertil Steril* 2021;**115**:1395–1410.

85. Practice Committee of the American Society for Reproductive Medicine and Practice Committee of the Society for Assisted Reproductive Technology, Birmingham, Alabama. Recommendations for practices utilizing gestational carriers: a committee opinion. *Fertil Steril* 2017;**107**:e3–e10.

86. Practice Committee of the American Society for Reproductive Medicine, Birmingham, Alabama. Interpretation of clinical trial results: a committee opinion. *Fertil Steril* 2020;**113**:295–304.

87. Covington SN, Burns LH. Pregnancy after infertility. In: Covington SN, Burns LH, Eds. *Infertility Counseling: A Comprehensive Handbook for Clinicians*, 2nd edn. Cambridge: Cambridge University Press, 2006: 440–458.

88. Daniluk JC. Reconstructing their lives: a longitudinal, qualitative analysis of the transition to biological childlessness for infertile couples. *J Counsel Develop.* 2001;**79**:439–449.

89. Takefman JE. Ending treatment. In: Covington SN, Burns LH, Eds. *Infertility Counseling: A Comprehensive Handbook for Clinicians*, 2nd edn. Cambridge: Cambridge University Press, 2006: 429–439.

90. Wischmann T, Korge K, Scherg H, Strowitzki T, Verres R. A 10-year follow-up study of psychosocial factors affecting couples after infertility treatment. *Hum Reprod* 2012;**27** (11):3226–3232.

Chapter 2

Reproductive Psychology and Fertility Counseling

Susan Klock

The English language lacks the words to mourn an absence …. But for an absence for someone who was never there at all, we are wordless to capture that particular emptiness. For those who deeply want children and are denied them, those missing babies hover like silent ephemeral shadows over their lives. Who can describe the feel of a tiny hand that is never held?
Laura Bush, Spoken from the Heart

This was not how it was supposed to be. This was not what you dreamed it would be. And you don't know how it will end. It's okay if you don't know how to wrap your mind around your emotions. Be gentle with yourself for not totally having control of how you feel from moment to moment.
Steve Wiens, Huffington Post, May 28, 2013

The dream of having a baby is deeply embedded in most cultures, religious traditions and throughout time. As much as Western culture has evolved to include numerous roles for women, having a child continues to be an important life goal for the majority of women of childbearing age. The majority of women and couples who desire to become pregnant will conceive naturally, have a successful pregnancy and experience the transition to parenthood. But for a minority of individuals, the desire to become pregnant will be met with frustration, failure and unexpected challenges. Additionally, for single women and men, gay, lesbian, bisexual and transgender individuals, the quest for a family is increasingly available via the reproductive technologies, but having a child is a labyrinth of individuals (donors and gestational carriers), medical staff, money and emotions navigated over time. The experience of infertility prompts unique psychological reactions and adjustment. Mental health professionals (MHPs) are frequently called upon to provide psychological assessment and counseling to individuals and couples who are experiencing infertility and its psychosocial sequelae.

The purpose of this chapter is to provide an overview of the psychology of infertility as an aspect of reproductive psychology, and the field that has emerged of fertility counseling. Reproductive psychology refers to the psychological, behavioral and societal aspects of reproductive potential, fertility control and infertility, pregnancy and birth, and parenting. Each of these areas is a focus of clinical and scientific inquiry. An area of reproductive psychology that has significantly developed in the past 30 years is the psychology of infertility. The psychology of infertility focuses on the intrapersonal and interpersonal emotional, cognitive and behavioral factors related to the experience of infertility. After the provision of some background information, a review of two leading theoretical frameworks for understanding the psychology of infertility will be presented then, an introduction to the history and practice of fertility counseling will be provided. The aim of this chapter is to provide a broad review of the psychology of infertility, and to provide context for the specific counseling topics presented in this volume.

Background

Reproduction is a biological imperative for humans to perpetuate their continued existence but in the twenty-first century, in developed cultures, the wish for a child carries other meanings. In earlier times, (and still existing today in developing countries) children were needed for economic survival, providing accessible and free labor for a largely agrarian culture. As such, children were valued for their economic contributions to the family and the wider social context for their contributions to the labor force. After the Industrial Revolution and the implementation of child labor laws, children were displaced from the work force. The economic value of children diminished but the social and emotional value of children grew as the child's role shifted to one of providing affection, connection, stimulation and companionship for the parents. As Griel [1] noted, children became valuable as emotional investments, providing emotional warmth and affection, particularly to their mothers.

In modern cultures, having a child represents the desire to pursue happiness and the belief that having a child is a key component to personal happiness. Hoffman and Hoffman [2] discussed the motivation for parenting and described nine categories of motivation for parenting. These value categories describe the needs that a child fulfils in a parent, including adult status and social identity, expansion of the self, moral values, group ties and affection, stimulation and fun, achievement and creativity, power and influence, social comparison, and economic utility. Parenthood represents an important developmental milestone in most adults' lives, indicating that they have reached a point of stability and maturity and an arrival into adulthood.

Despite the strong motivation to have a child, some individuals will face a diagnosis of infertility. It is estimated that one in eight women are unable to become pregnant after a year of trying. According to Speroff, it is estimated that approximately 50% of infertility problems are attributed to the female partner, 35% to the male and 15% unexplained or rare [3].

There are numerous factors that affect the overall infertility rate, including the trend in the US and Western cultures to delay childbearing due to increased work, educational or financial goals [4]. The development and wide-spread availability of assisted reproductive technologies, including ovulation induction, in vitro fertilization (IVF), gamete donation and gestational surrogacy, have all contributed to the effective treatment of infertility, with nearly half of infertile couples seeking medical treatment for their infertility [5]. As the medical technology has developed and become more widespread, the psychological aspects of infertility have become an important field of study. The psychological adjustment to infertility and its treatment are the focus of the next sections of this chapter.

Reproductive Psychology and Infertility

For decades, clinicians believed that infertility, particularly "unexplained" infertility, was caused by psychic distress. This psychosomatic conceptualization was largely based in psychoanalytic thinking and focused on psychogenic conflict as a cause of infertility. Possible conflicts, such as conflict about the maternal role or feminine identity, were frequently cited as causes of female infertility. In the 1980s, MHPs began to question the assumption that psychological distress caused infertility, but instead posited that infertility caused psychological distress. This change of causal direction provided a new paradigm for conceptualizing the psychological aspects of infertility. Two theoretical perspectives have guided much of the clinical and research activity since this time: grief and loss theory and the stress and coping model.

Grief and Loss

Bowlby [6] described the four stages of grief after an "affectional bond" had been broken and proposed that grief was a normal adaptive response after a loss. The four stages of grief are described as: (1) shock and numbness; (2) yearning and searching; (3) despair and disorganization and; (4) reorganization and recovery. Shock and numbness is the phase during which the loss is not perceived as real and feels impossible to accept. There is physical distress during this phase, which can result in somatic symptoms. Yearning and searching is the stage during which one becomes aware that the loss has been experienced and the future that had been imagined or counted on is realized as no longer a possibility. Attempts at trying to fill the void that the loss has left are common, and preoccupation with the loss can persist. The third stage of grief is despair and disorganization. During this stage, the individual realizes that the loss has occurred and that life will not go back to the way it was or the way it was imagined. It is during this stage that despair and hopelessness may set in. Finally, reorganization and recovery occur as one develops new routines, plans and goals. The loss recedes and adjustment to the changed life develops. Bowlby 's classic model is useful in understanding the grieving that infertile individuals and couples undergo as they face the diagnosis of infertility.

A further exploration of grief and loss theory in the context of infertility was provided by Menning [7]. Menning applied Kubler-Ross's five stages of death and dying (shock, denial, anger, bargaining and acceptance) to describe the typical thoughts and feelings associated with the infertility experience. Although the grief and loss models are focused around the death of a loved one, in the infertility context the loss is of the imagined or dreamed of child.

Expanding on the grief and loss model, an important paper on the psychological aspects of infertility was by Patricia Mahlstedt [8]. In this manuscript, based on extensive clinical observation, Mahlstedt described a series of losses experienced by infertile individuals and couples, among them: the loss of self-esteem, relationships, health, and financial security. The adaptation to these losses can be conceptualized through the stages of grief theory provided above. Mahlstedt's paper provides important descriptive information for any clinician working with infertile individuals.

According to Mahlstedt, the infertile person experiences a loss of self-esteem by failing to achieve a desired goal of having a baby despite a concerted effort. The loss of the dreamed-for child can directly diminish the person's sense of self-efficacy, generativity and prompt existential anxiety. The inability to meet the goal of having a child challenges and erodes the person's self-esteem. The problem may worsen significantly if the individual has been highly successful in other areas of life and has not developed the coping skills to deal with failure and loss.

The second loss is the real or feared loss of important relationships. This includes not only the intimate partner relationship but also relationships with family, friends, co-workers and others. Significantly, the infertile partner may worry that their partner might leave them. They may also experience difficulties in discussing their thoughts and feelings about infertility and its treatment, blame one another for the infertility and have difficulty adjusting to the changes in sexual activity due to the infertility and its treatment. The changes in an infertile couple's sexual interactions have been written about extensively (see Wischmann for a review, [9]) but constitute a significant loss for the couple. In addition to the perceived losses in the intimate relationship, the individual(s) may also experience changes or losses in their relationships with family. Women may withdraw from relationships with siblings or friends who are pregnant or who have recently given birth. Infertile individuals may avoid social gatherings during which pregnancy and childrearing are discussed, and family gathering during the holidays is notoriously difficult for the infertile couple, in that the focus on family and children is very pronounced, thus highlighting the infertile person's loss. Withdrawal from others and loss of relationships diminishes social support and can compound feelings of isolation and depression.

The third loss discussed by Mahlstedt is the loss of health. The infertile couple initially undergoes numerous tests and procedures to assess their reproductive system. These tests are time consuming and often require numerous, specifically timed visits to the medical clinic. During the course of the infertility diagnostic evaluation and treatment, women and men can take on the patient role and begin perceiving themselves as ill or at times, serious medical problems, such as cancer, may be identified and they become ill. Moreover, for women taking fertility medications, the side effects of the medications can produce significant symptoms that undermine a woman's feeling of health. IVF can feel like the complete medicalization of reproduction.

A fourth loss can be the loss of financial security. At the time of writing, 19 states in the US mandate coverage for some type of infertility treatment, although the extent of the coverage is variable [10]. In the EU and UK, national coverage is provided but wait times are often lengthy. IVF can cost between $10,000 and $15,000 and often several cycles are needed. Couples may assume significant debt in order to finance their infertility treatment.

Related to the loss of self-esteem and the loss of relationships is the perceived stigma of infertility [11]. Stigma, the idea of a negative sense of social difference that is so outside the social norm that it devalues the individual, is experienced by the individual and in the context of the family, social group or larger society. The infertile individual may feel different, inferior, defective or worthless. Despite the advancement of women's rights in many areas, the predominance of childbearing as a primary value of women in culture is still the norm. Additionally, the experience of infertility for men is equally stigmatizing in masculine-dominated cultures. The stigma of infertility is evident in Western cultures but is even more pronounced in developing countries and nonsecular cultures. The experience of infertility in this context can prompt stigmatization of the individual by their family and society in addition to by the individual him or herself. This can lead to social isolation, which can compound feelings of loss, isolation and grief.

Stress and Coping

Another model that has provided a framework for conceptualizing the psychological aspects of infertility has been the stress and coping model. In the 1980s, as it became clear that psychological stress did not cause infertility but instead, infertility caused psychological distress, the stress and coping model became useful for understanding the emotional response and for providing a theoretical framework to study the psychological aspects of infertility. The stress and coping model refers to the theories put forward by Lazarus and Folkman and others (see Stanton for a review, [12]) to describe an individual's reaction to a stressful life event such as infertility.

A stressful event or experience is defined as one in which the person appraises the event or experience as challenging or exceeding one's abilities or endangering one's well-being. Using this model, the infertility experience is the stressful event and the individual's characteristics (appraisal, personality style, coping) influence their response or adjustment. The appraisal of infertility can mediate the severity of a person's response. Appraisal consists of primary and secondary appraisal. Primary appraisal refers to how important the person perceives the event. Secondary appraisal consists of the person's evaluation of their ability to affect or change the event. In the infertility context, a primary appraisal has a large magnitude of importance for a person who has tailored their life choices around parenting. It this case, the perceived threat to the person's sense of self caused by the infertility would be high because parenthood is of high importance to them. The secondary appraisal relates to the individual's perception of their ability to change the event. For the infertile woman, she may ask herself, "Can I see my doctor?"; "Can I undergo IVF?" Further, responses to stress can be both adaptive and maladaptive. In general, those events that are appraised as more threatening or important to an individual and those that are perceived as unchangeable, are more likely to impair adjustment [12].

Personality characteristics can also affect a person's adjustment or response to infertility. Traits such as locus of control, trait anxiety, optimism and resilience have all been studied in reference to infertility adjustment [13].

In addition to appraisal and personality factors, adjustment to infertility is also mediated by coping strategies and behaviors. There are four types of coping [14]. *Problem-focused coping* can be activity-related and includes activity engagement, restraint from activity and active planning. *Emotion-focused coping* includes psychological denial, avoidance, distancing, disengagement via alcohol or drugs, or mental disengagement. *Social coping* includes seeking instrumental support and seeking emotional support. *Meaning-focused coping* can include cognitive restructuring such as positive reinterpretation, humor and acceptance. As Folkman and Moskowitz point out, there are no inherently good or bad coping strategies; instead, the effectiveness of the coping is context-dependent [14].

Using the stress and coping model, the infertile person becomes aware of their infertility and appraises how challenging or threatening it is to them. For a woman for whom motherhood is a very important life goal, her appraisal of infertility is very challenging or threatening.

She may ask herself, "Who will I be if I am not a parent?" or "What will I do with my life if I can't have a child?" If her answers to those questions are unsatisfactory, then she may begin to formulate ways to cope. Problem-focused or active coping may include seeking information from her doctor, talking to friends, modifying her health behaviors (quit smoking, lose or gain weight), all in an attempt to alter her infertility situation. Seeking medical intervention in the form of infertility treatment can be viewed as a type of active coping. Emotion-focused coping could include avoidance, such as the person who avoids going to the shopping mall, religious services or other places where pregnant women are likely to be seen. Alternatively, an example of social-coping is an individual going to an infertility support group or an adoption education meeting, thereby creating connections with others to help cope with infertility. Meaning-based coping represents deeper cognitive reframing, attaching meaning to the infertility experience. A common example of this is a comment such as, "Going through infertility has made my marriage a lot stronger" or "Through infertility I have realized how much I value relationships with my extended family and friends."

Since the 1990s there have been hundreds of studies that have used this conceptual framework to improve our understanding of the psychology of infertility. These studies have investigated coping style and personality variables as they relate to psychological distress in the forms of anxiety, both state and trait, and depression, and treatment outcome as they relate to assisted reproductive technologies (ART) (see Boivin et al. for a review [15]). In general, studies have concluded that in the infertility situation, active coping is more adaptive than emotion-focused coping. Optimism and internal locus of control are more adaptive than pessimism and internal locus of control.

An additional framework to consider with the adjustment and coping to infertility is offered by Tedeschi and Calhoun in their concept of posttraumatic growth (PTG) [16]. In this framework, the authors posit that there can be positive psychological changed experienced as a result of the struggle with a highly challenging life circumstance. The experience of infertility is traumatic, but instead of a maladaptive reaction, positive changes could follow the experience of the trauma. PTG is mediated by several factors including resilience, managing distressing emotions and obtaining social support. This conceptual framework has been used in recent years by researchers investigating the psychological adjustment to infertility. Schmidt et al. [17] found that two-thirds of their sample of men and women undergoing fertility treatment reported PTG related to strengthening the couple's relationship. Kong et al. [18] found that perceived social support, resilience and positive affect were all related to PTG in a sample of women undergoing infertility treatment. The concept of PTG may provide an additional perspective in the stress and coping framework through which to view the adaptation to infertility and its treatment.

Fertility Counseling

History

With the advent of IVF in 1979 and the broad application of ART in developed countries in the 1980s and 1990s, the field of fertility counseling developed. For the past 30-plus years, psychologists, social workers, psychiatrists, marriage and family therapists and other mental health professionals, have been providing fertility counseling. Fertility counseling offers individuals an opportunity to explore their thoughts, feelings, beliefs and relationships to better understand the meaning and consequences of their choices; counseling may also offer support to them as they undergo treatment and may help them to process their feelings about the outcome of any treatment. The need for specialized fertility counseling has been identified since the widespread use of ART began in the late 1980s. Some countries mandate the provision of fertility counseling in relationship to specific types of ART (New Zealand, South Australia,) and some countries require fertility counseling to be available (UK, New South Wales and Western Australia), whereas in the majority of other countries there are professional society recommendations for fertility counseling but no legislative or other mandates for its provision (see Blyth for a review, [19]).

Fertility counselors can come from many different backgrounds. Psychologists, social workers, marital and family therapists and psychiatrists are common professions for fertility counselors. Currently the UK is the only country that has a training and credentialing program for infertility counselors. Professional societies in the US, the EU and Canada describe their recommendations for training and experience. The qualification guidelines from the Mental Health Professional Group (MHPG) and the American Society for Reproductive Medicine (ASRM) are provided in Table 2.1 [20]. This guidance document provides a summary of the types of services a fertility counselor should be able to provide as well as recommended qualifications and training. The five

Table 2.1 Qualification guidelines for fertility counselors (Adapted from the Practice Committee and the MHPG of the ASRM [20])

A qualified fertility counselor should be able to provide or refer patients appropriately to, the following services:

- Diagnosis and treatment of mental disorders
- Grief counseling
- Supportive counseling
- Crisis intervention
- Education/information counseling
- Decision-making counseling
- Third-party evaluation and implications counseling
- Psychometric test administration and interpretation
- Sexual counseling
- Support group counseling
- Psychotherapy
- Couple and family therapy
- Referral/resource counseling
- Staff education and consultation

The guidelines suggest minimum qualifications and training of mental health professionals providing fertility counseling and psychological services. The mental health professional should have:

1. Graduate degree in a mental health profession
2. Psychological testing proficiency associated with third-party reproduction
3. License to practice
4. Knowledge of the medical, legal and psychological aspects of infertility
5. Post-license supervised clinical experience
6. Continuing education

components of qualification and training include a graduate degree in a mental health discipline, proficiency in psychological testing associated with third-party reproduction, a license to practice, knowledge of the medical, legal and psychological aspects of infertility, supervised clinical experience in fertility counseling and participation in continuing education.

The Human Fertilisation and Embryology Authority Code of Practice [21] enumerated four aspects of infertility counseling: (1) information gathering and analysis; (2) implications and decision-making counseling; (3) supportive counseling and; (4) therapeutic counseling. In addition, the Australian and New Zealand Infertility Counselors Association have described five types of infertility counseling [22]. These five types have been described by Blyth (see Table 2.2 and [19]) and include implications counseling, support counseling, therapeutic counseling, decision-making counseling and crisis counseling. In addition to considering these types of counseling with the infertile individual or couple, this counseling is also appropriate and relevant to third-party

Table 2.2 Types of fertility counseling
(Adapted from Blyth [19])

1. **Implications counseling**: the exploration of personal and family implications of infertility and infertility treatments and gamete donation, requiring the skills of a trained psychosocial counselor. Undertaken prior to beginning treatment to allow sufficient time for reflection before making any irrevocable decision. Implications counseling may also be necessary after treatment.

2. **Support counseling**: the provision of emotional and psychological support throughout the process of diagnosis, investigation, and treatment and gamete donation, to assist patients to deal appropriately with the experience and/or consequences of their treatment.

3. **Therapeutic counseling**: focused on mediating the more pervasive, upsetting and stressful consequences of both impaired fertility and fertility treatment. Much like traditional psychotherapy, focusing on a specific problem or issue to be worked through.

4. **Decision-making counseling**: counseling available to patients at significant points in their decision-making around management of fertility treatment.

5. **Crisis counseling**: for patients experiencing a crisis or adverse outcome while undertaking fertility treatment.

reproduction participants, such as egg or sperm donors, gestational carriers and their partners. The provision of counseling to infertility patients can also be conceptualized and offered based on the type of treatment the individual or couple is receiving; for example, in a clinic it may be determined that all patients undergoing IVF, gamete donation or gestational surrogacy have counseling. Providing counseling based on the type of treatment being offered minimizes concerns of discrimination to particular subgroups of patients.

The most recent version of the European Society for Human Reproduction and Embryology (ESHRE) Psychology and Counseling Special Interest Group counseling guidelines offer best practice advice on how psychosocial care can be incorporated and implemented in infertility and medically assisted reproduction [23]. The aim of the guidelines is to provide evidence-based best practice advice to all fertility clinic staff on how to incorporate psychosocial care into routine infertility care.

The Canadian Fertility and Andrology Society Counseling Special Interest Group has also developed counseling guidelines [24]. The guidelines were written to meet the mandate of developing standards of practice for Canadian fertility counselors. The purpose is to define the provision of care to support individuals and couples experiencing infertility and to help them examine the emotional, psychosocial,

relational and ethical aspects of treatment options and to assist in informed decision-making. Additionally, the goals of counseling include helping individuals set realistic goals and prepare for and cope with treatment and its outcome. The Canadian guidelines also describe the multiple roles of the fertility counselor, which include psychosocial support and education, crisis counseling, psychotherapy, serving as a liaison between the patient and her treatment team, providing referrals, addressing ethical issues, development of counseling protocols and interventions, documentation of services, training of others in the field and research and writing.

All of the guidelines describe the two basic types of services provided by fertility counselors: assessment and counseling. Assessment includes a clinical interview and often the administration of measures of depression, anxiety, coping, quality of life, personality, and other relevant measures to provide initial assessment of individuals or couples presenting for fertility treatment. The information gathered from the clinical interview and any ancillary measures can provide useful information regarding the psychological functioning of the individual and guide further interventions, if needed. Assessment also may uncover the diagnosis of a psychological disorder requiring treatment; this may be a contraindication for, or a reason to delay, fertility treatment. Although the overall prevalence of a mental illness is low, women who have experienced infertility have been shown in population-based studies to be at an increased risk for dysthymia and anxiety disorders [25]. Assessment also includes the psychological assessment of third-party reproduction participants such as gamete donors, gestational carriers and intended parents.

In addition to assessment, the fertility counselor can provide various forms of counseling. The format, timing and type of counseling is highly individualized and dependent on the needs of the client, the availability of the counselor and the situation. Each patient has their own reproductive history and their own reproductive story that changes over time and based on the type of treatment and other experiences they have had [26]. Hearing the patient's full reproductive story provides important background information for the counseling relationship.

Peterson et al. provide a useful schemata for conceptualizing the stepwise process to determine the provision of psychological counseling [27]. They describe a stepwise progression, with the initial phase including information gathering and analysis and decision-making. If further intervention is needed, then additional implications counseling and decision-making counseling may be indicated as well as support counseling and short-term crisis counseling as the individual or couple moves through their medical treatment. Last, psychotherapy with crisis counseling and/or therapeutic counseling may be needed on a longer-term basis for some individuals. Peterson et al. also usefully point out the risk factors for high distress among infertile individuals that may require psychotherapy (Table 2.3).

There are pros and cons of whether the fertility counselor should be part of the treatment team or whether an outside consultant should have been considered. The advantages to having the mental health professional as part of the infertility treatment team are ease of access, decrease of stigmatization and facilitated communication with the medical staff. Disadvantages include perceived bias toward medical interventions and concern regarding communication boundaries with medical staff.

The impact of psychological counseling on the well-being and adjustment of infertile individuals has also been studied. A review of the studies of the effectiveness of psychosocial interventions in infertility was published by Boivin [28]. In this review, Boivin reported that of the 380 studies reviewed, only 25 assessed the impact of the intervention on a psychological outcome measure. Of these 25 studies, it was found that psychosocial interventions were effective in reducing negative affect but did not change interpersonal functioning. In addition, psychological interventions have not consistently been shown to change pregnancy rates in controlled studies. The need for large, theory-based, controlled trials for fertility counseling interventions is needed and presents a goal for the next stage in the development of the field of fertility counseling.

Fertility counseling is a dynamic and ever-changing field. Significant advancement has occurred since its inception almost 40 years ago, but change is inevitable as medical technology advances and individuals seek out advanced fertility care. Gameiro et al. described their view of optimal provision of care for IVF patients, which included recommendations specifically for the MHP [29]. These authors recommend routine pre-treatment psychological screening to identify at-risk or vulnerable individuals and offer them referral to psychological care early in the treatment process. Additionally, they recommend providing clear, easy to obtain information on how to access psychosocial help and urge the provision of general psychosocial support in daily care in the IVF treatment process. Counseling can also be used to promote healthy lifestyle choices among fertility patients to improve their health and decrease negative health behaviors that may affect fertility. There are many possible innovations and changes ahead for fertility counselors as we continue to improve and expand our efforts in assisting infertile individuals and couples achieve their goal of building a family. Whether in the context of assessment or the provision of therapy, providing empathy, knowledge and acceptance will continue to be the foundation of the care MHPs provide.

References

1. Griel AL. *Not Yet Pregnant: Infertile Couples in Contemporary America*. New Brunswick, NJ: Rutgers University Press, 1991.

2. Hoffman LW, Hoffman M. The value of children to parents: In: Fawcett JT, Ed. *Psychological Perspectives on Population*. New York, NY: Basic Books, 1973: 19–73.

3. Fritz M, Speroff L, Eds. *Clinical Gynecology, Endocrinology and Infertility*, 8th edn. Philadelphia, PA: Lippincott, Williams & Wilkins, 2011: 1157.

4. Van Balen F. Late parenthood among subfertile and fertile couples: motivations and educational goals. *Patient Educ Couns* 2005;59:276–282.

5. Boivin J. International estimates of infertility prevalence and treatment seeking potential need and demand for infertility medical care. *Hum Reprod* 2007;22:1506–1512.

6. Bowlby J. The making and breaking of affectional bonds. *BJP* 1977;130:201–210.

7. Menning B. The emotional needs of infertile couples. *Fertil Steril* 1980;34:313–319.

8. Mahlstedt P. The psychological component of infertility. *Fertil Steril* 1985;43:335–342.

Table 2.3 Risk factors for high distress among infertile individuals (Adapted from Peterson et al. [27])

Personal factors	Situational	Treatment related
Pre-existing psychopathology	Poor marital relationship	Medication side-effects
Primary infertility	Poor social network	Miscarriage
Female	Frequent reminders	Prior treatment failure
Avoidance coping of infertility		

9. Wischmann T. Sexual disorders in infertile couples: an update. *Curr Opin Obstet Gynecol* 2013; **25**:220–222.

10. RESOLVE. Insurance coverage in your state. Available from: www.resolve.org [last accessed June 15, 2022]].

11. Miall CE. Perceptions of informal sanctioning and the stigma of involuntary childlessness. *Deviant Behav* 1985;**6**:383–403.

12. StantonA. Cognitive *appraisal,* coping processes and adjustment to infertility. In: Stanton A and Dunkel-Schetter C, Eds. *Infertility: Perspectives from Stress and Coping Research.* New York, NY: Plenum Press, 1992: 87–108.

13. Verhaak C, Smeenk J, Evers A, Kremer J, Kraaimaat F, Braat D. Women's emotional adjustment to IVF: a systematic review of 25 years of research. *Hum Reprod Update* 2007;**13**:27–36.

14. Folkman S, Moskowitz J. Coping: pitfalls and promises. *Annu Rev Psychol* 2004;**55**:745–774.

15. Boivin J, Griffiths E, Venetis CA. Emotional distress in infertile women and failure of assisted reproductive technologies: meta-analysis of prospective psychosocial studies. *BMJ* 2011;**23**(342):223.

16. Tedeschi R, Calhoun L. Posttraumatic growth: conceptual foundations and empirical evidence. *Psychological Inquiry* 2004;**15**:1–18.

17. Schmidt L, Holstein C, Chistensen U, Boivin J. Does infertility cause marital benefit? An epidemiological study of 2250 women and men in fertility treatment. *Patient Educ Counsel* 2005;**59**:244–251.

18. Kong L, Fang M, Ma T, et al. Positive affect mediates the relationships between resilience, social support and posttraumatic growth of women with infertility. *Psychol Health Med* 2018;**23**:707–716.

19. Blyth E. Guidelines for infertility counseling in different countries: is there an emerging trend? *Hum Reprod* 2012;**27**:2046–2057.

20. Practice Committee and the Mental Health Professional Group, American Society for Reproductive Medicine. Guidance on Qualifications for Fertility Counselors, 2021. www.fertstert.org [last accessed June 15, 2022].

21. Human Fertilization and Embryo Authority. Code of Practice. London: HFEA, 1991.

22. Australian and New Zealand Infertility Counselor's Association Guidelines for Professional Standards of Practice in Infertility Counseling. 2003.

23. Psychology and Counseling Special Interest Group. Guidelines on psychosocial care by healthcare professionals in infertility and medically assisted reproduction. Available from: www.eshre.eu/Specialty-Groups/Special-Interest-Groups/Psychology-Counselling/ [last accessed June 15, 2022].

24. Counseling Special Interest Group, Canadian Fertility and Andrology Society. Assisted Human Reproduction Counseling Practice Guidelines. December 2009. Available from: https://cfas.ca/counsellors-sig.html [last accessed June 15, 2022].

25. Baldur-Felskov B, Kjaer S, Albieri V, et al. Psychiatric disorders in women with fertility problems: results from a large Danish register-based cohort study. *Hum Reprod* 2013;**28**:683–690.

26. Jaffee J. Reproductive trauma: psychotherapy for pregnancy loss and infertility clients from a reproductive story perspective. *Psychotherapy* 2017;**54**:380–385.

27. Peterson B, Boivin J, Norre J, Smith C, Thorn P, Wischmann T. An introduction to infertility counseling: a guide for mental health and medical professionals. *J Assist Reprod Genet* 2012;**29**:243–248.

28. Boivin J. A review of psychosocial interventions in infertility. *Soc Sci Med* 2003;**57**:2325–2341.

29. Gameiro S, Boivin J, Domar A. Optimal in vitro fertilization in 2020 should reduce treatment burden and enhance care delivery for patients and staff. *Fertil Steril* 2013;**100**:302–309.

Chapter

3

Fertility Counseling for Individuals

Linda Applegarth

Introduction

The practice of individual counseling or psychotherapy is both a science and an art. True understanding of this art and science can only come with real-time exposure to therapist–patient interactions, regardless of the amount of empirical knowledge someone may have about a specific psychotherapeutic theory or technique. Psychotherapy and counseling techniques are rational and systematic procedures designed to improve the patient's mental health [1]. Ideally, counseling techniques are applied within a theoretical framework or approach. In this chapter, the terms "counseling" and "psychotherapy" will be utilized interchangeably.

In general, individual counseling or psychotherapy includes interactive processes between a person and a qualified mental health professional (psychiatrist, psychologist, clinical social worker, marriage and family therapist, licensed counselor or mental health practitioner). Its purpose is the exploration of thoughts, feelings and behavior with the goal of problem solving or achieving higher levels of functioning. Psychotherapy aims to increase the individual's sense of personal well-being. Psychotherapists employ a range of techniques based on experiential relationship building, dialogue, communication and behavioral change, all of which are intended to improve the mental and emotional health of a client or patient, or to improve relationships. Although society typically has been somewhat skeptical of what is considered a "soft science," it is encouraging to note that in a 2014 study in Germany [2] about attitudes toward psychotherapy, it was found that a significant majority of the population (ranging in age from 14 to 92 years) indicated a positive belief and approach regarding counseling. A later study [3] also found that attitudes towards seeking help from mental health professionals has greatly improved over the last 25 years, and that psychotherapy is consistently preferred over psychotropic medication.

Broadly speaking, psychotherapy may also be performed by practitioners with different qualifications. It may be legally regulated, voluntarily regulated, or unregulated, depending on the country, state, or district jurisdiction. Requirements of these professions vary, and often require graduate school and supervised clinical experience.

In the United States (US), for example, "psychotherapist" is a general term used to describe an individual who has been professionally trained in an advanced degree (i.e., psychiatry, psychology, social work, nursing or counseling) and licensed by a state professional board to treat mental, emotional and behavioral disorders by psychological means [1]. Criteria for such licensure vary from state to state. In general, the practice of "psychotherapy" or "psychological counseling" may sometimes be vague and ill-defined. For those who have met their district, state or country's requirements as a "psychiatrist," "psychologist," "social worker," "psychiatric nurse," "professional counselor" or "marriage and family therapist," there is usually a requirement of additional education and clinical training on psychotherapeutic theory and technique.

Within the framework of a broad number of therapeutic approaches to individual counseling, fertility counseling also takes an important place – one that requires not only training and experience, but also a knowledge of the many (and ever-developing) medical components of fertility treatment. Individual counseling is, in fact, the cornerstone of fertility counseling, and a solid knowledge and skill-base of psychotherapeutic approaches and clinical techniques are critical to treating the infertile population effectively.

Individual fertility counseling is defined as psychotherapeutic interaction or treatment contracted between a trained mental health professional and a client or patient who is struggling emotionally to achieve parenthood. This struggle usually includes issues that are psychological in nature and can vary in terms of their causes, influences, triggers and potential resolutions. Accurate assessment of these and other variables depends on the practitioner's experience, capability and understanding of the psychological and medical components of infertility and its treatment. Psychotherapy strategies and techniques can also change or evolve as the practitioner acquires greater knowledge and more insight into the patient's issues and conflicts. As Van den Broeck and colleagues point out, "infertility counseling has become a specialist form of counseling requiring professional expertise and qualification" [4, p. 422].

This chapter will present three key approaches to individual fertility counseling and each will be explained. These theoretical approaches include: (1) psychodynamic psychotherapy; (2) cognitive–behavioral therapy (CBT), including a discussion of dialectical behavior therapy (DBT) and trauma-focused therapy; and (3) supportive counseling. They will be described as they pertain specifically to fertility counseling and are intended to help to elucidate the theories and techniques within the context of assisting fertility patients to understand, manage and/or mitigate the emotional and psychological consequences of their condition.

Psychodynamic Psychotherapy

The theoretical foundations of psychodynamic psychotherapy can most appropriately be understood within an historical context. First and foremost, psychodynamic therapy has grown out of early psychoanalytic theory. But, as McWilliams has pointed out, psychoanalysis has never been a static theory, and is also ever-evolving [5]. Nonetheless, there are several key influential concepts in psychoanalysis that have significantly impacted psychodynamic psychotherapy: (1) early Freudian theory and practice; (2) ego psychology; (3) object relations theory and interpersonal psychoanalysis and (4) the self-psychology movement.

Briefly, the early work of Freud was an effort to understand and to reduce psychopathology for those diagnosed with severe "neuroses." The patients who initially "captured Freud's attention suffered from what we would now term posttraumatic, borderline, and somatoform disorders" [5, p. 72]. Although he originally used hypnosis to relieve psychiatric symptoms, Freud later began to value free association as a treatment methodology. It was within this context that the "talking cure" was born. From his patients' free associations, Freud inferred that many of their "neuroses" were the result of the expression of two contradictory internal attitudes, one or both of

which were unconscious. For example, wishes for sexual gratification existing in tandem with moral rejection of such wishes. He thus adopted the concept of "dynamism" from physicists and began referring to the dynamic unconscious; thus, the source of the term "psychodynamic" [5].

Interestingly, Freud's form of psychoanalysis did not point to qualitative differences between healthy and sick, or normal and abnormal. Rather, psychoanalysis views psychological problems on a continuum, as a matter of degree, and as different aspects and expressions of universal human struggles. Although contemporary analytic therapies have diverged considerably from their Freudian base, the core ingredients in Freud's early work remain present in one form or another in almost all current psychodynamic therapies: an appreciation of dynamic unconscious processes, the assumption of a direction or tilt to all mental life, a developmental viewpoint, a sense of the ubiquity of conflict and defense and an attention to the transference process [6].

Ego psychology is a psychoanalytic approach that developed in North America in the 1930s. It was based on Freud's notion that the mind is a competing arena of demands from the id (primitive impulse), ego (sense of "I") and super ego (conscience and personal values/ideals). The ego is seen as mediating between id, super-ego and reality – using both conscious coping skills and unconscious defenses such as repression, denial, displacement and projection. Psychological and emotional health is thus equated with ego strength, the ability to cope realistically, flexibly and adaptively with life's challenges [7]. In treatment, ego psychological therapists work to make clients aware of their defenses so that they can consciously choose more adequate ways to cope. In so doing, the analyst also works to foster a strong working alliance so that the client experiences the therapist as a warm and caring collaborator [8]. In traditional ego psychology, in addition to a strong psychotherapeutic alliance, interpretation was considered to be the therapist's primary therapeutic activity, and insight was assumed to be the main agent of change. There is also now a greater attempt to address the needs of different populations, cultural contexts and other pressures on practice.

In the United Kingdom (UK) in the 1950s, several analysts such as Fairbairn, Winnicott and Klein began to focus on internalized relationships and their affective themes. This body of work was called object relations theory, and in the US a similar movement led by Harry Stack Sullivan and colleagues called itself interpersonal psychoanalysis. As a result of this movement, the Freudian focus on drive, conflict and defense was considered less relevant to a client's problems than were primary relationship issues [9]. Most notably, the focus is often on one's sense of self more than, for example, on Freudian issues of gratification and frustration. Similarly, issues of basic security, closeness and an internal sense of effectiveness and control are more critical than issues of drive satisfaction. Psychotherapists who adhere to object relations theory recognize what earlier relationships the client has internalized or "introjected." McWilliams [5] notes that from an object relations viewpoint, one group of patients whom psychotherapists found easier to understand included those who are often diagnosed as borderline personality disorder. Specifically, clients with a borderline diagnosis often feel controlled and engulfed in relationships; hence, those who adhere to the object relations theory understand the significance of primary relationships and attachments in the client's life and are able to maintain empathy with them, as well as boundaries, and to be a stabilizing presence.

The self-psychology movement of the 1970s appears to have evolved from broad cultural changes, particularly in the West: rapid technological change, splintered extended families and communities, and increased mobility. As a result, psychoanalysts began seeing more clients who suffered from feelings of emptiness, low self-esteem and confusion about their identity and direction in life. These clients seemed to have a broken or stunted sense of self and tended to crave validation from outside. Ironically, Freud had considered these patients as untreatable [5]. In self-psychology, the dynamic of shame was seen to play a significant role in the patient's inner experience. Hans Kohut was instrumental in the self-psychology movement because his attention to empathy, nonjudgmental acceptance and authenticity, along with a focus on the client's early childhood shame experiences, played out in the therapeutic relationship [10]. Of interest, the notion of shame as described in self-psychology may be a particularly useful one in relation to psychotherapeutic work with fertility patients. Shame is often a central emotional construct in infertility, and the therapist can assist the patient in addressing what is experienced as a broken or diminished sense of self-worth.

Over time, psychoanalysts have become increasingly aware of self-esteem issues and have seen the applicability to all clients of the self-psychology orientation. Kohut and colleagues, then and now, see empathy as an important treatment technique, and have urged clinicians to choose interventions based on whether or not they will be experienced as "empathically attuned" [5].

In sum, many approaches to psychodynamic psychotherapy have evolved in response to different clinical and societal challenges. Most contemporary psychoanalytic therapists now draw from all or most of the approaches described previously in response to the distinct psychological needs of each patient. Psychodynamic therapy can be effective as both a long-term or a short, time-limited modality. It should be noted, however, that perhaps the greatest difference between this psychotherapeutic approach and others has to do with the attention to transference and countertransference. Psychodynamic psychotherapy focuses on the "here and now" – both in the session and in the patient's life. The patient may project painful feelings and negative attributions (as well as loving ones) from past key relationships onto the counselor. At the same time, the therapist must also be alert to their own feelings about the patient. The countertransference may relate either to the therapist's personal issues (such as unresolved infertility), or to the patient's issues and behaviors that engender strong feelings in the therapist. These can inform treatment issues and strategies. Countertransference, regardless of one's theoretical treatment orientation, is significant to the treatment process, especially if the counselor has had personal experience with infertility. (Additional discussions of transference and countertransference are provided throughout this text and are directly addressed in Chapters 20 and 24.)

Cognitive–Behavioral Therapy

Cognitive–behavioral therapy (CBT) is an active, here and-now focused psychotherapeutic approach. The goal is to help clients understand the ways in which their thinking and behavior contribute to their distress, to help them develop strategies to overcome problematic cognitive and behavioral patterns, to solve their current life difficulties and ultimately to apply learned strategies to manage life's challenges after therapy has ended [10]. For the purposes of this chapter, the terms "cognitive therapy" and "cognitive–behavioral therapy" will be used interchangeably.

Aaron Beck, considered by many to be the father of cognitive therapy, initially developed this therapeutic approach to treat depression. It has since become a treatment for a wide range of psychiatric disorders, including personality disorders, anxiety, substance abuse, eating disorders and suicidal behavior. In addition, there are "many more psychiatric disorders, psychological problems, and medical conditions with psychological components" [11, p. 130] for which cognitive therapy has been demonstrated to be efficacious by empirical research. The emotional and psychological components of infertility would certainly be included in this list. A study by Faramarzi and colleagues found that CBT improved the social concerns, sexual concerns, marital concerns, rejection of a child-free lifestyle and need for parenthood more than the use of psychotropic medication. They indicate that CBT is a reliable alternative to antidepressant medication and suggest that it is superior to psychotropic medication (i.e., fluoxetine) in resolving and reducing infertility stress [12].

Cognitive–Behavioral Theory and Principles

Craske notes that the theories and principles of CBT are derived from several different sources that have become interwoven with one another over time [13]. Thus, the CBT practitioner will draw from both learning theories and cognitive appraisal theory to conceptualize a problem and develop a treatment plan. Underlying the basic goal of CBT is the idea that problem cognitions, behaviors and emotions have been acquired in some part through learning and experience, and are likely therefore to be modified by new experiences and learning – notwithstanding other contributing factors such as genetics and temperament. CBT aims to teach new ways of responding and to build new learning experiences that together promote more adaptive ways of cognitive, affective, and behavioral responding. Specifically, cognitive therapy, within the broader context of CBT, has the greatest breadth and depth of empirical research that supports its efficacy and effectiveness [14,15].

Most important, however, is the development of a solid understanding of the client's clinical presentation that takes precedence over the use of any specific techniques. Unlike other approaches to counseling, the client is actively engaged in the process of experimentation and ongoing evaluation of the effectiveness of any interventions. Evaluation of the intervention strategies not only permits revision where applicable, but also assessment of the overall progress of treatment. A key to CBT treatment is the active involvement of the client, as well as client–therapist collaboration in formulating and implementing a treatment plan.

Cognitive–Behavioral Therapy Strategies and Process

The process by which psychotherapists work collaboratively with clients is generally known as cognitive restructuring. Clients and therapists thus work to identify, to evaluate and, if necessary, to modify cognitions that are experienced in situations in which the client also experienced emotional distress [16]. The aim of this process is to assist clients to: (1) recognize the ways in which their cognitions affect their mood, and (2) modify inaccurate or unhelpful cognitions that are exacerbating emotional distress. Cognitive restructuring with patients is done during psychotherapy sessions to coach clients in acquiring and practicing these skills. The therapist also encourages clients to apply these skills systematically in their daily lives outside of the sessions.

In CBT, *self-monitoring* is a tool for evaluating the working relationships between thoughts, behaviors and emotions, including antecedents and consequences in real time. Self-monitoring is especially valuable for recording subjective experience (e.g., "all of my friends ask when I am going to announce that I am pregnant") along with levels of subjective distress [13]. This strategy begins with the notion that emphasizes the importance of observing one's own reactions by using objective terms rather than emotionally loaded terminology. Work sheets and diaries are common forms of recording, and feedback from the counselor about the self-monitoring positively influences compliance as well as emphasizing progress or identifying relationships between behavior, thoughts and emotions that can be further targeted in treatment. There is seldom a contraindication to self-monitoring, but the technique may need to be modified to suit an individual patient's needs or personality [17].

Another primary technique in CBT is *relaxation*. This can include a broad array of strategies such as autogenic training, progressive muscle relaxation, breathing retraining, as well as meditation and yoga. Muscle relaxation is generally anxiety-reducing, and has been used for a number of disorders such as headaches, sleep disturbance, asthma, hyperactivity and so on, as well as various forms of anxiety, including specific concerns that center on various aspects of the fertility treatment process.

A third CBT technique involves behavioral *rehearsal of social skills and assertiveness*. This treatment technique initially involves an evaluation of the client's skills in several social and assertive situations. The rationale for this useful technique emphasizes how learning more effective social and assertive skills will help patients to achieve greater personal control and respect for self and others. For example, many patients present to the fertility counselor acknowledging fears of asking specific questions to the medical team about treatment protocols or decisions; or are often at a loss as to how to manage questions from family or friends about fertility status. Their anxiety, self-consciousness and emotional sensitivity leave them feeling helpless, overwhelmed, or angry – or all of the above. In such cases, the fertility counselor may assist the patient in developing specific behaviors for the purposes of role-playing and behavioral rehearsal. Notably, there are circumstances in which behavioral rehearsal of social skills and assertiveness must be limited. Assertiveness training, for example, should be undertaken in a culturally responsive manner. Many CBT strategies are based on North American/European norms of autonomy and independence. For example, in other cultures such as Asia, the Middle East, South America and Africa, assertiveness may conflict with values of the importance of family and collectivism [18]. Culturally sensitive assertiveness, instead, can include prefacing assertive communication with more traditional forms of deference and respect or by using other CBT strategies.

A fourth, and important, CBT skill that has been utilized for a wide array of difficulties including anxiety, depression, couples' conflict and stress management, is *problem-solving* [13]. As with other strategies described above, cognitive–behavioral therapists use a guided discovery approach to problem-solving, and create an environment for clients to acquire skills that will help them to solve specific problems in their lives. The focus is for clients to draw their own conclusions on the basis of problem-solving, and gain confidence so that they can address other problems in their lives that arise when they are no longer in treatment [11].

In essence, problem-solving is a skill-building intervention. The work of D'Zurilla and Nezu [19] has become the framework for many CBT therapists' problem-solving approaches. The process includes approximately four distinct steps to problem-solving: (1) the CBT therapist works with the client to identify the problem using objective language, to separate facts from assumptions and to set realistic goals; (2) alternatives are developed by generating as many solutions as possible, and a list of action plans are set forth for the enactment of each solution; (3) a cost–benefit analysis is conducted of each solution to determine which are most likely to be implemented; and (4) the action plan that is associated with the most effective solution is implemented, and the success of the implementation is evaluated so that modifications can be made if necessary.

Table 3.1 provides an overview of the previously described CBT strategies or techniques that can be

Table 3.1 Cognitive–behavioral strategies for individual fertility counseling

Self-monitoring The patient records events or images (such as failed IVF treatment or the sight of pregnant woman) that create emotional distress. The patient then records resulting negative thoughts and feelings, along with cognitive distortion utilized, and alternative, more balanced ways of thinking and responding.

Relaxation and stress management: The patient learns an array of physiologic strategies for managing anxiety and stress. Often utilized before or during medical treatments or receiving bad or difficult news. Includes muscle relaxation, breathing exercises, meditation or yoga. This provides the patient with a greater sense of self-mastery.

Behavioral rehearsal and assertiveness: This technique emphasizes learning more effective social and assertive skills for achieving a greater sense of personal efficacy and respect for self. It enables infertility patients to ask questions and discuss treatment options more effectively with medical staff, and/or manage inappropriate or probing questions or comments from family, friends, work colleagues and so on.

Problem-solving: A skill-building intervention that allows the patient to identify the problem so as to separate fact from assumption, develop useful, alternative descriptions or solutions to the problem, and implement a more effective plan of action to deal with the problem. This treatment strategy can be very helpful for infertility patients who must consider alternative medical treatments or who must confront alternative family building options other than biologic or genetic parenthood.

Trauma-focused CBT (TF-CBT): A treatment that directly addresses the impact of traumatic events – specifically as they pertain to reproductive trauma. There are three main types of TF-CBT that have been proven in research studies to be effective for PTSD. The therapy can also address depression and anxiety that accompanies PTSD.

applied to the specific needs of infertility patients. These patients can ultimately apply these skills not only to concerns, conflicts and difficulties that arise during their infertility experience, but also to other difficult or stressful challenges in their lives.

Wenzel notes that a final important aspect of CBT is the "extensive empirical basis for its efficacy and effectiveness" [11, p. 173]. Clients not only acquire strategies for managing the cognitive and behavioral aspects of their current distress, but also develop a solid understanding of the components of their life problems. Many infertile patients seeking individual psychotherapy request CBT. Most who enter counseling, in fact, do not wish to explore deep-seated issues or resolve past conflicts, nor remain in therapy long term. Rather, they are asking for tools with which to manage the anxiety, fear and depression that stem from infertility diagnoses and treatment outcomes within a short-term parameter.

Dialectical Behavioral Therapy and Trauma-focused Therapy

There are also fertility patients who can benefit from other specific forms of CBT. These include *dialectical behavioral therapy* (DBT) and *trauma-focused therapy*. DBT has a greater focus on emotional and social components and was originally developed by Marsha Linehan, PhD to treat patients with extreme or unstable emotions and harmful behaviors. Often, these individuals are diagnosed with borderline personality disorder (BPD). It is an evidence-based treatment that helps people deal with emotional dysregulation. As this treatment method has evolved, there is also recent research that shows DBT may help with many other mental health concerns, including self-harm. The infertility experience, depending on the patient's personality structure, can lead to severe emotional responses as well as suicidality in rare cases. DBT attempts to integrate four essential elements in a comprehensive way by addressing the biological, environmental, spiritual, and behavioral elements of a person's struggle [20]. There is an effort to balance the need for the individual to change while also being fully accepted for who one is in the moment. DBT teaches the patient that their experiences are real, and also teaches self-acceptance, regardless of the challenges or difficult experiences.

The relationship between the therapist and the patient is very important, and it is important that the therapist maintain ongoing supervision/consultation with other mental health professionals. Of note, Galen and Aguirre [20] point to "ten ways to live an antidepressant life" as part of DBT treatment that are helpful to all fertility patients (and everyone!). These include: (1) exercise; (2) meditation; (3) eating a less-refined, less processed, and less calorie-rich diet; (4) being careful regarding alcohol and drug use; (5) getting adequate sleep; (6) maintaining social interaction and connection; (7) adding recreation and relaxation into one's routine; (8) accessing green space and a healthy environment; (9) taking care of pets or other animals; and lastly, (10) making time for faith and prayer (spirituality). See Chapter 8 for more information on the use of spirituality in fertility counseling.

For some individuals, the infertility experience is clinically traumatic. There are patients who, as a result, will experience significant anxiety, depression, shame, fear, helplessness or other intense emotion in response to certain fertility-related experiences or "triggers," and/or as the result of pregnancy loss. The individual's usual coping abilities will be ineffective, and the condition continues for a pro-longed time. Emotional dysregulation is also symptomatic of the trauma associated with fertility challenges. As a result, these persons can benefit from trauma-focused psychotherapy – an umbrella term that includes trauma-focused cognitive–behavioral therapy (TF-CBT) and eye movement desensitization reprocessing (EMDR). Both have been reported effective in adults [21], and each requires specific techniques for successful outcomes. The goal of treatment is to lower distress, help put the traumatic experience into perspective, and help with the return to normal functioning. TF-CBT generally involves three therapy approaches that address the impact of the traumatic event on the individual [22]. These include: (1) cognitive processing therapy (CPT), focusing on unrealistic or unhelpful thoughts and beliefs; (2) common elements treatment approach (CETA), targeting specific symptoms; and (3) prolonged exposure (PE), reducing intense negative emotions that are caused by memories or being reminded of the trauma. These forms of trauma-focused therapy work primarily because the patient is participatory, and actively trying to change in-between therapy sessions by utilizing key strategies that assist with symptom reduction. (Please note that Chapter 20 in this text provides an in-depth discussion of the issues of reproductive trauma and PTSD along with treatment implications.)

Supportive Counseling

Individual supportive psychotherapy is defined as a treatment modality designed to ameliorate or reduce symptoms, to maintain or improve the client's self-esteem, and to maximize one's adaptive capacities. It is used primarily to reinforce a patient's ability to cope with stressors through a number of key activities, such as the counselor attentively listening and encouraging expression of feelings and thoughts, in an effort to help the individual gain a greater understanding of their situation and alternatives. Some consider supportive psychotherapy to be the most widely used psychotherapy and treatment modality provided to the majority of patients seen in mental health centers and psychiatric clinics [23]. Supportive psychotherapy bases much of its approach on psychoanalytic, cognitive–behavioral and learning theories [24]. It is also humanistic and client-centered. Those who primarily practice supportive psychotherapy must, according to Winston and Goldstein, be able to integrate successfully various other therapeutic approaches to best meet the needs of the patient. Many fertility counselors will do supportive psychotherapy, in part because it tends to focus less on unconscious drives and conflicts, and in part because it is often consistent with the desires and needs of those seeking treatment. It is a common form of therapy that may be provided over the short or long term, depending on the individual and the specific set of circumstances.

Winston [23] points out, however, that decreasing levels of ego function and increasing levels of psychopathology are also indications for a more supportive stance. Although this is generally not the case with infertility patients, who seldom present with significant psychopathology, this type of intervention and the techniques utilized still rely on patient assessment. If supportive psychotherapeutic interventions are indicated, the techniques include "alliance building, skills building, reducing and preventing anxiety, and awareness expanding" [23, p. 7]. As in psychodynamic psychotherapy, the importance of the therapeutic relationship is also stressed in supportive psychotherapy. However, supportive psychotherapy tends to focus more on the real relationship between patient and therapist, and less on the transference as is traditionally done in psychodynamic approaches. The real relationship exists in the here and now of the therapeutic alliance and includes a genuine liking for each other without the distortions that are a critical part of the transference. Thus, the real relationship will include the patient's hopes and aspirations for help, care, understanding and love, as well as daily interactions that occur between individuals on a social level.

The specific interventions or techniques utilized in supportive psychotherapy will again depend on the assessment of the client. For example, alliance-building on the part of the therapist may include expressions of interest, empathy and conversational style. Esteem-building can involve reassurance, normalizing and encouragement. Skills-building includes teaching, advice and guidance through anticipation. Importantly, normalizing, reframing and rationalizing techniques can reduce anxiety. Interventions such as clarification, confrontation and interpretation can also be helpful in expanding the patient's awareness of his or her problem or situation. Winston [23] stresses, however, that interpretation is used sparingly in supportive psychotherapy; and, when it is used, it is in a more general or indirect way. A treatment strategy in supportive therapy is to strengthen defenses, as opposed to that of psychodynamic psychotherapy, which as noted previously attempts to challenge defenses so that more in-depth conflicts, feelings and wishes become more available for exploration.

Winston and Goldstein [24] also point out that cognitive–behavioral techniques are a critical component of supportive psychotherapy and can be utilized for specific problems such as panic, depression, obsessive–compulsive symptoms and dysfunctional thinking. The authors state that the therapeutic process in supportive psychotherapy involves identifying and challenging automatic thoughts and testing them empirically. Patients are taught to monitor their automatic thoughts, validate these thoughts and develop alternative ways of thinking. Reframing is an additional technique often utilized to correct cognitive distortions.

Similarly, therapeutic interventions used in supportive psychotherapy are seen as a form of teaching – a way of imparting knowledge. Within the context of a supportive psychotherapeutic approach, patients may be encouraged to seek out additional resources, and develop strategies for using those resources to achieve objectives.

Resources may be libraries, the Internet, articles, books, videos and so forth [24]. In the process, the patient can also be involved in evaluating their own learning, and ultimately promoting the skill of critical reflection, that is, the process in which the patient questions and then replaces or reframes an assumption. Alternative perspectives are developed from previously taken-for-granted ideas or forms of reasoning. Like CBT, the goal of this technique is to enable the patient to devise alternative ways of thinking, relating to others and problem-solving.

Supportive psychotherapy has many practical and effective applications in fertility counseling. Most infertility patients presenting for assistance from a fertility counselor are anxious and depressed – fearful that they cannot tolerate treatment or that they will never become parents. Often, the fertility counselor is asked to take on multiple roles within the psychotherapeutic interaction – roles that include not only traditional forms of psychotherapy, but also that of providing education and information about common responses to treatment options, perspectives on parenting alternatives, as well as information on how best to access additional support resources.

In sum, through supportive psychotherapy, counselors assist patients in learning how to move forward and make decisions or changes that may be necessary to adapt, either to an acute change, such as a pregnancy loss or a failed infertility treatment cycle, or to a chronic situation, such as depression resulting from lengthy and ongoing infertility and treatment. In this form of therapy, a trusting relationship between the patient and therapist is integral to the patient's healing process, particularly if the patient needs to come to terms with his or her life circumstances and related losses. Chapter 19 on resiliency offers more information on the importance of the therapeutic relationship in healing.

Conclusion

In this chapter there has been an attempt to review some central foundations, values and techniques of three fertility counseling approaches: psychodynamic psychotherapy, cognitive–behavioral therapy and supportive psychotherapy. I have not gone into specific detail about many of the techniques given the limitations of this chapter. However, the goal has been to provide basic information as to how each of these individual treatment approaches can apply most effectively to patients experiencing infertility and its treatment, as well the aftermath (see Table 3.2).

Each of these approaches also has bodies of research that support it and provide data on "evidenced-based" effectiveness. At the same time, although it is important for the mental health community to appreciate the value of qualitative and process research as well as accumulated clinical experience, it may often be easier empirically to study more discrete elements of practice than the more subtle aspects of therapeutic process and relationship. It has been this author's longstanding conclusion that the personal qualities and experience of the individual counselor are key to a successful psychotherapy outcome. In fact, Wampold and Imel [25], in their latest book, *The*

Great Psychotherapy Debate, have effectively delineated pathways within a contextual model that make psychotherapy effective. They report that:

1. The initial therapeutic relationship is critical and must be created before treatment can be effective.
2. The personal relationship between therapist and patient ("the real relationship") must be genuine, empathic and caring. The personality of the therapist is a significant factor.
3. The creation of expectations through explanation of the problem and the treatment involved establishes a restoration of morale in the patient.
4. The theoretical bases of the techniques used, and the strictness of adherence to those techniques, are *not* factors. Rather, the therapist's ability to elicit healthy patient actions which, in turn, can lead to psychological improvement, is important.
5. The counselor's realistic optimism and strength of belief in the efficacy of the technique is also an important factor.

Despite the availability of valuable resources to a person experiencing the emotional distress of infertility – friends, family, religious and spiritual guides, personal reading, healthy eating and exercise, to name a few – psychotherapeutic intervention can still be most effective at healing this profound psychological and emotional injury. Critical to the psychotherapeutic treatment is the therapist's knowledge and understanding of the available resources in reproductive technology, medical treatments and options that patients must confront and make decisions about on a regular basis.

There are many therapeutic treatment approaches that the practitioner may utilize during individual fertility counseling. This unique population, although generally psychologically healthy, often lacks sufficient coping strategies for managing the many complex, unpredictable and potentially devastating aspects of fertility treatment and outcomes. Depression and anxiety are the two most frequent emotional sequelae of the infertility experience. However, these psychological states may stem from very different sources, depending on the personality factors and coping styles of any particular client. The type of psychological intervention will therefore vary not only because of various personality types, but also because of the severity of the distress. Specific requests from the patient as to what approach and treatment length is most suitable for them will also determine the counseling approach and may mean that the individual will need to

Table 3.2 Individual fertility counseling: three approaches to psychotherapy

Psychodynamic psychotherapy: Patient is appropriate for and wishes to explore longstanding emotional conflicts and concerns, significant relationships, and issues of self-esteem within the context of understanding and managing infertility. Treatment can be long- or short-term.

Cognitive–Behavioral Therapy: Patient requests skills-building assistance and techniques for managing anxiety, depression, anger and other negative feelings associated with the infertility experience. Treatment is generally focused and time limited. A specific subset of individuals may benefit from *dialectical behavioral therapy* or *trauma-focused therapy*, depending on the special emotional or psychological issues/needs of the patient.

Supportive psychotherapy: Patient requests emotional support through understanding and empathy. Patient may ask to be seen on an "as-needed" basis. The individual may be emotionally vulnerable or resistant to self-exploration. Psychoeducational information and resources may be provided along with CBT strategies for managing the infertility experience. Treatment is generally short-term.

be referred to a suitable psychotherapist, not only with expertise in fertility counseling but also specialized training in the required treatment modality.

Many infertility patients, however, have had little or no prior experience with psychotherapy or counseling, and are unsure of how the fertility counselor will be able to assist them. As Peterson and his colleagues have suggested, psychological care for infertility patients can include implications and decision-making counseling, support counseling and short-term crisis counseling [26]. This author has found clinically that most are responsive to a supportive counseling approach, in that this approach tends to be time-limited, provides strategies for managing anxiety and depression (including crisis intervention), depends on a strong therapeutic alliance and can include an important psycho-educational component as well. Commonly, a supportive counseling approach can sometimes move into a more psychodynamic treatment approach, or likewise into a more definitive cognitive–behavioral approach, depending on the personality characteristics and stated needs of the patient.

In recent years, in response to the COVID-19 pandemic, the call for psychological treatment via telehealth has dramatically increased. It should be noted that levels of anxiety and depression have led to a greater need for professional mental health assistance, not only for fertility patients, but also for the general population. As a result, the author stresses that the therapeutic approaches for individuals described here can not only be delivered via telehealth in meaningful and effective ways, but teleconferencing also allows mental health clinicians the ability to reach a broader base of those suffering from fertility challenges. Of note, Chapter 25 in this text addresses the importance of the appropriate and effective use of telepsychology in fertility counseling.

This chapter is intended to provide a solid overview of three individual fertility counseling approaches, and it hopefully also provides a useful glimpse into what is believed to be the breadth, depth and richness of fertility counseling as it is practiced today.

References

1. Greenberg LS, McWilliams N, Wenzel A. *Exploring Three Approaches to Psychotherapy*. Washington, DC: American Psychological Association, 2014.

2. Petrowski K, Hessel A, Korner A, Weidner K, Brahler E, Hinz A. Attitudes toward psychotherapy in the general population. *Psychother Psychosom Med Psychol* 2014;**64** (2):82–85.

3. Angemeyer MC, Van Der Auwera S, Carta MG. Public attitudes towards psychiatry and psychiatric treatment of the 21st century: a systematic review and meta-analysis of population surveys. *World Psychiatry* 2017;**16**(1):50–61.

4. Van den Broeck U, Emery M, Wischmann T, Thorn P. Counselling in infertility: individual, couple and group interventions. *Patient Educ Counsel* 2010;**81**:422–428.

5. McWilliams N. Psychodynamic therapy. In Greenberg LS, McWilliams N, Wenzel A, Eds. *Exploring Three Approaches to Psychotherapy*. Washington, DC: The American Psychological Association, 2014:71–127.

6. Pincus D. Who is Freud and what does the new century behold? *Psychoanalytic Psych* 2006;**23**:367–372.

7. Hartmann H. *Ego Psychology and the Problem of Adaptation*. (D. Rapaport, Trans.) New York, NY: International Universities Press, 1958.

8. Greenson R. *The Technique and Practice of Psychoanalysis* (Vol. **1**). New York, NY: International Universities Press, 1967.

9. Guntrip H. *Psychoanalytic Theory, Therapy, and the Self: A Basic Guide to the Human Personality*. New York, NY: Basic Books, 1971.

10. Kohut H. *The Restoration of the Self*. New York, NY: International Universities Press, 1978.

11. Wenzel A. Cognitive therapy. In: Greenberg LS, McWilliams N, Wenzel A, Eds. *Exploring Three Approaches to Psychotherapy*. Washington, DC: The American Psychological Association, 2014: 129–182.

12. Faramazi M, Pasha H, Esmailzadeh S, Kheirkhah F, Heidary S, Afshar Z. The effect of the cognitive behavioral therapy and pharmacotherapy on infertility stress: a randomized controlled trial. *Int J Fertil Steril* 2013;**7** (3):199–206.

13. Craske MG. Cognitive-behavioral therapy. In: Vandenbos GR, Meidenbauer E, Frank-McNeil J, Eds. *Psychotherapy Theories and Techniques: A Reader*. Washington, DC: The American Psychological Association, 2014.

14. Dobson KS. *Cognitive Therapy*. Washington, DC: The American Psychological Association, 2012.

15. Epp AM, Dobson KS. The evidence base for cognitive-behavioral therapy. In: Dobson KS, Ed. *Handbook of Cognitive-Behavioral Therapies*, 3rd edn. New York, NY: The Guilford Press, 2010: 3915.

16. Fairburn GC. *Cognitive Behavior Therapy and Eating Disorders*. New York, NY: The Guilford Press, 2008.

17. Heide JM, Mara BP. Self-monitoring as a treatment vehicle. In: O'Donohue W, Fisher JE, Hayes SC, Eds. *Cognitive Behavior Therapy: Applying Empirically Supported Techniques in Your Practice*. New York, NY: Wiley & Sons, 2003: 361–367.

18. Hays PA, Iwamasa GY. *Culturally Responsive Cognitive-Behavioral Therapy: Assessment, Practice, and Supervision.* Washington, DC: The American Psychological Association, 2006.

19. D'Zurilla TJ, Nezu AM. *Problem-Solving Therapy: A Social Competence Approach to Clinical Intervention*, 2nd edn. New York, NY: Springer Publishing Company, 1999.

20. Galen G, Aguirre B. *DBT for Dummies.* New Jersey, NJ: John Wiley & Sons, Inc., 2021.

21. Mavranezouli I, Megnin-Viggars O, Daly C, et al. Psychological treatments for post-traumatic stress disorder in adults: a network meta-analysis. *Psychol Med* 2020;**50** (4):542–555.

22. *Trauma-Focused Cognitive Behavioral Therapy for Adults.* Publication of the University of Washington, Harborview Medical Center, Center for Sexual Assault and Traumatic Stress, 2017.

23. Winston A. The nuts and bolts of supportive psychotherapy. *Psychiatric News* 2012;**47**(12):6b–7.

24. Winston A, Goldstein M. Theory of supportive psychotherapy. In Gabbard GO, Ed. *Textbook of Psychotherapeutic Treatments.* Arlington, VA: American Psychiatric Publishing Inc., 2009: 393–416.

25. Wampold B, Imel EZ. *The Great Psychotherapy Debate: The Evidence for What Makes Psychotherapy Work*, 2nd edn. New York, NY: Routledge, 2015.

26. Peterson B, Boivin J, Norre J, Smith C, Thorn P, Wischmann T. An introduction to infertility counseling: a guide to mental health and medical professionals. *J Assist Reprod Genet* 2012;**29**(3):243–248.

Fertility Counseling for Couples

Brennan Peterson and Kristy Koser

Over the past several decades, the field of fertility counseling for couples has undergone a remarkable evolution. Advances in clinical training and empirically supported research have provided fertility counselors with improved tools and knowledge to effectively guide couples through this challenging experience. Couples experience psychological distress, confusion about the future, and a loss of control over their lives. In addition, they question their assumptions about masculinity and femininity, their identities, and the value they place on parenthood. While some couples grow closer because of the infertility experience [1], it can also erode the strength and stability of even the most satisfied relationships. However, even though the infertility journey can be full of adversity and struggle, it can also lead to unexpected discoveries of resilience, purpose and meaning.

Because biological parenthood is a central life goal for many couples, infertility can be conceptualized as a nonnormative lifecycle transition that represents a significant developmental interruption in a couple's expected life course [2]. This unexpected turn of events in a couple's life can often be destabilizing and emotionally unsettling. Fortunately, fertility counselors are familiar with the emotional terrain and are thus in a unique position to help couples navigate this journey.

This chapter will guide fertility counselors in the assessment and treatment of couples experiencing infertility. Fertility counselors will learn strategies to help couples strengthen their relationships, reduce psychological and infertility-related distress, and regain a sense of purpose and meaning in their lives. The chapter will review empirically supported research about the impact of infertility on couple relationships and provide an overview of best practices and clinical treatment interventions. Fertility counselors will learn techniques to help couples improve communication, coping, and joint decision-making that promote relational well-being. The chapter will also highlight the impact of infertility on a couple's sexual

relationship, examine the connection between age and fertility, and help couples share infertility-related treatment information with others that effectively balances the need for privacy with the benefits of seeking and receiving social support. Finally, the chapter will discuss ways to help couples grieve the many losses they experience, while also helping them transform their adversity into meaning and resilience.

Fertility Counseling for Couples

The field of fertility counseling encompasses a wide variety of services, including therapeutic counseling aimed at helping couples cope with the psychosocial challenges of infertility, as well as implications counseling that assists couples in decision-making and considerations of third-party reproduction [3]. The form of counseling provided, whether it be therapeutic counseling or implications counseling, will be determined by the needs of the couple, the timing of treatment and the couple's level of distress.

Counseling services may be most beneficial at the beginning or end of treatments, when couples are considering varying options or coping with significant loss. Less distressed couples may require brief counseling approaches that emphasize education, while supportive counseling can be used when couples are moderately distressed. Longer-term therapeutic counseling can be used when psychological stressors and symptoms are more severe or after failed fertility treatments or pregnancy loss. Couples who are considering third-party reproduction (donor insemination, egg donation, embryo donation or gestational surrogacy) as well as issues unique to lesbian, gay, bisexual, transgender, and queer (LGBTQ) couples, are explored in-depth in several other chapters of this volume.

Dyadic Conceptualization and the Effectiveness of Couple Counseling

Because infertility is a shared stressor, it is important to conceptualize the couple as the unit of analysis in

The addenda referred to in this chapter are available for download at www.cambridge.org/covington-clinical-guide

research, as well as the unit of treatment in clinical settings [4]. Recent systemic conceptualizations of the couple's journey highlight the need for conjoint assessment and provide fertility-focused recommendations for treating low-distress, moderately distressed, and highly distressed couples [5]. Other conceptualizations call for increased emphasis on using couple therapy models grounded in theoretical approaches such as emotion-focused couple therapy (EFT) and attachment theory [6].

The effectiveness of couple counseling for infertility has long been supported by clinical consensus. However, a lack of outcome research for conjoint treatment highlights a need for more studies in this area. In 2021, the first systematic review was published examining the effectiveness of therapy with couples and infertility. The findings provide fertility counselors with confidence that systemic interventions for couples lowers infertility stress, reduces depression, decreases anxiety, and improves marital and sexual satisfaction [7]. Emotion-focused therapy (EFT), cognitive–behavior therapy (CBT), and behavior couple therapy (BCT) produced superior results when compared with other models. In addition, couples with lengthier infertility histories benefited more from fertility counseling, and couples receiving six or more counseling sessions reported increased effectiveness compared to couples having fewer treatment sessions.

Cultural and Contextual Considerations

A couple's response to infertility is highly contextualized by dominant cultural, societal, and religious norms regarding childbearing, parenthood, and family. In pronatalist societies and religious communities where childbearing is highly encouraged, couples can feel marginalized as they are excluded from normative parenting and social experiences. Well-intentioned but unhelpful friends and family can offer unsolicited advice and make insensitive comments about a couple's plans for children.

The significance of broader cultural influences cannot be overstated. In African countries where childbearing is highly valued, infertility is highly stigmatized and carries intense pressure from family. A study of 12 married Nigerian women, 10 of which were in polygamous marriages, found that infertility was related to depression, isolation, social stigma, social pressure and marital problems [8]. Most of the women reported being treated poorly by their mother-in-law and husband's relatives, with many encouraging the man to divorce the woman or marry another spouse.

Broader cultural beliefs about childbearing also impact men's experience with infertility. A 2018 qualitative study of men in Ghana found that men's reactions to infertility were contextualized by traditional beliefs that women were responsible for infertility and that a man's masculinity was linked with his ability to father a child [9]. These cultural forces led men to report feeling intense guilt that their wives bared a heavier burden because of infertility, particularly when it was a male-factor diagnosis.

In traditional Chinese culture, having a biological child who can continue the family bloodline creates a powerful context for the infertility experience. Chinese women often feel intense pressure and familial obligations to have a child [10]. They also report being excluded from social situations, leading to feelings of marginalization. Chinese men report feelings of shame if they are unable to have a biological child.

Fortunately, new definitions of femininity and masculinity provide more favorable cultural contexts for those experiencing infertility. For example, research with men in the Middle East and Mexico, two regions with long-standing cultural traditions of male dominance and patriarchy, found that these traditions have led to widespread stereotyping of men's roles and reactions to stress. However, less constricting narratives of masculinity are providing men in these cultures with new ways to break old scripts that offer greater flexibility to historically rigid male behavior [11]. See Chapters 15 and 19 for further discussion.

For religious couples, beliefs and communities that once provided nurturance and support can become a source of stress and strain. Religious couples may question their faith and feel anger at the unfairness of infertility – especially if they believe that having a child is a religious expectation. Couples may also experience loneliness and marginalization as others in their faith community become parents (see also Chapter 8).

Assessment

Fertility counselors should use assessment interviews and measures to gain a more complete understanding of the broader forces and systemic nature of the couple's response to infertility which can help determine the type of counseling needed. The most vital assessment method is an in-person conjoint psychosocial interview that obtains the perspectives and experiences of both members of the couple. Table 4.1 provides an overview of the main areas of assessment to cover during an

Table 4.1 Conjoint psychosocial fertility assessment

Relationship history
- Length of relationship
- Length of time trying to start a family
- Children from current or past relationships
  - If yes, conceived naturally or from fertility treatment

Fertility history and diagnosis
- Type of diagnosis
- Length of diagnosis

Treatment history
- Fertility treatments attempted
  - Medications/surgeries
  - IUI cycles (if yes, how many)
  - IVF treatments (if yes, how many)
- Medical stress (managing medications, doctor visits, 2-week waiting period)
- Treatment results
  - Failed treatment, miscarriage, stillbirth, live birth
- Consideration of third-party reproduction
  - Egg donation, sperm donation, surrogacy

Cultural/religious context
- Cultural or religious factors that add stress or strain
- Cultural or religious factors that provide support

Impact of infertility and treatment on:
- Communication (talked about too little, too much, agreement)
- Coping (impact of partner coping strategies)
- Decision-making about past and future treatments
- Partnership (has relationship been strengthened or weakened by infertility)
- Sexual relationship

Family history
- Family reaction to infertility
- Family network providing support or stress
- Impact of siblings having children
- Impact of family gatherings

Social support/social networks
- Friendship reactions to infertility – support or stress
- Friends having children? Impact of social gatherings
- Impact of sharing infertility-related information

Employment/financial factors
- Employer stressor or support – employer flexibility to accommodate fertility treatments
- Concerns about work disruption and loss of income

Goals and type of counseling needed
- Couple goals for treatment
- Implications/decision-making counseling
- Therapeutic counseling

interview. Fertility counselors should assess the couple's fertility history, including length of diagnosis, type of infertility, and attempted treatments and outcomes – as couples with longer infertility histories likely experience heightened emotional distress. The impact of infertility and treatment should be assessed by examining the couple's communication and coping patterns, treatment decision-making and how infertility influences the sexual relationship. The impact of contextual factors such as cultural/ethnic background, religious or spiritual factors, social class and financial position, as well as current levels of family and social support, should also be assessed. An often overlooked and critical area of assessment is the couple's relationship history prior to infertility, as the quality of their past relationship can be predictive of the couple's ability to manage the stress of infertility.

Fertility counselors can also use standardized assessment measures to determine the couple's levels of psychological distress. Assessing for infertility stress, depression, anxiety, relationship satisfaction and quality of life using standardized measures is important as couples consider treatment options. Knowing a couple's distress level is essential, as higher rates of psychological distress are related to increased risk of patient drop-out. In addition, men and women who experience severe depressive symptoms prior to undergoing fertility treatments are at risk of experiencing higher fertility stress levels.

Treatment

Historically, the main role of fertility counselors in reproductive clinics was to provide general support for patients in crisis and/or carry out psychological screening before treatment. Currently, fertility counselors are also called upon to provide counseling to decrease fertility and psychological distress, provide guidance in patient decision-making and improve relationship satisfaction. Fertility counselors use evidence-based, integrative approaches to provide comprehensive patient care using psychosocial interventions that effectively reduce depression, anxiety, and infertility stress [12].

Fertility counselors working with couples can integrate existing couples therapy models with fertility-focused interventions. Fertility counselors can help couples develop stress management techniques, provide educational support, challenge unhelpful thinking styles, promote relational support, facilitate emotional expression, and help couples create coherent, meaningful narratives to decrease infertility stress and increase relational satisfaction [5,7]. Emotion-focused approaches can strengthen a couple's connection through emotional awareness and expression, transforming problematic partner interactions into emotionally secure patterns of connection [6] (see also *Case Studies*, Chapter 4). Experiential behavior therapies that integrate mindfulness-based strategies can help couples confront previously avoided thoughts and feelings that result in decreased psychological distress and increased relational satisfaction [13].

Fertility counselors using empirically supported models of therapy can integrate fertility-specific treatment recommendations including:

- Helping couples improve communication
- Altering problematic dyadic coping patterns
- Facilitating joint decision-making
- Reducing sexual distress
- Helping couples create boundaries for sharing infertility-related information
- Increasing fertility awareness
- Assisting couples in grieving losses and creating new meaning.

Communication

Couples undergoing fertility treatment typically report high relationship satisfaction, most notably at the beginning of treatment. This can be due to selection bias – as more satisfied couples pursue treatment and participate in research studies. It can also be because infertility stress is more strongly related to emotional distress, and couples view infertility as a shared problem to be overcome. Regardless, prolonged infertility stress can take a toll on even the most satisfied relationships, as the rigors of treatment, emotional and physical exhaustion, and repetitive discussions about treatments and future decisions can deplete a couple's relational well-being.

Fertility counselors should routinely address a couple's communication style during the counseling process. Research has found that more empathic sharing was a key to improved communication and responsiveness towards one's partner in couples experiencing infertility [14]. Mutual decision-making and joint problem-solving are also key communication skills. To create positive cycles of communication that bond couples together, empathically attuned discussions – defined as communication that clearly sees and understands the needs of the other – are vital. On the other hand, misattuned infertility-related discussions over a significant period of time can create circular patterns of negative cycles of communication that push couples apart.

Fertility counselors can help couples create positive cycles of connection through in-session enactments, role-plays and at-home practice. Fertility counselors can promote empathically attuned communication patterns by helping both partners increase awareness of their own needs and emotions, and teaching couples to effectively communicate these needs to their partner when engaging in difficult infertility-related discussions. Since couple communication is always systemic, couples must manage and take responsibility for their contribution to the cycle, to create opportunities for new patterns of interaction to emerge. If one partner can communicate and express what they are needing from the other at the outset of fertility discussions, partners can increase the probability of mutual understanding and positive cycles that result in connection and support. Figure 4.1 provides an example of a couple doing their best to support each other, but are also inadvertently experiencing misattuned communication that results in a negative cycle.

In this example, Partner A is experiencing sadness and anger because of treatment failure and is seeking emotional support and validation from their partner, while Partner B is trying to help Partner A cope with the stress by looking to future treatments. However, because Partner B is misattuned to Partner A's needs, and because Partner A has not clarified these needs during the discussion, a negative communication cycle is likely to result.

Figure 4.2 provides an example of a couple who creates a positive interaction cycle where both partners feel connected, understood, and supported. In this example, Partner A brings awareness of their relational needs to an infertility discussion and couples this awareness with an expression of need, while Partner B uses attuned communication to meet the expressed need. An example of this type of interaction cycle using an EFT approach can be found in Koser's case study in Chapter 4 of the accompanying *Case Studies* volume.

For couples who need more concrete tools to manage communication differences, fertility counselors can use "The Twenty Minute Rule" [15] – an intervention aimed at helping couples set boundaries around fertility-related conversations. Before beginning a fertility-related discussion, couples agree on a time limit (many couples find 20 minutes works best) and start a timer when the conversation begins. When the timer is done, the couple stops the discussion.

This intervention has many potential benefits [15]. First, it provides partners who need to discuss fertility-related challenges the opportunity to do so, while also providing a time-limited structure for partners who feel overwhelmed by the frequency of these discussions. Second, because of the time-limit, the clarity of communication may improve for partners who share, while

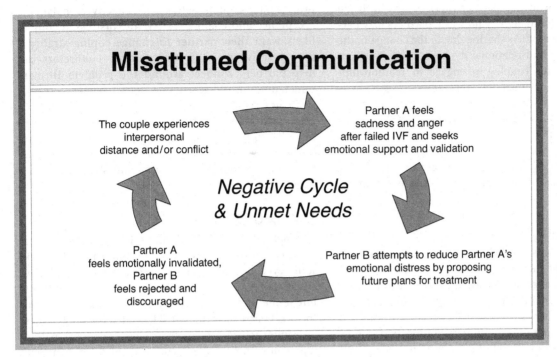

Figure 4.1 Misattuned communication.

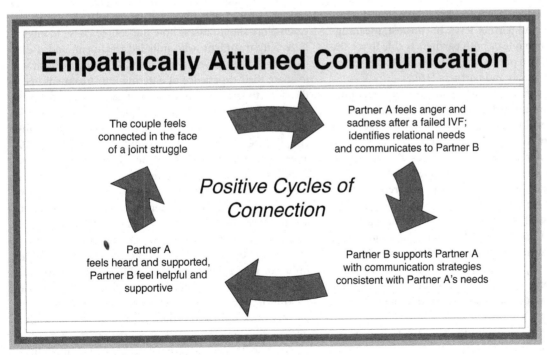

Figure 4.2 Empathically attuned communication.

previously overwhelmed partners may be able to listen more intently. Third, more withdrawn partners may paradoxically increase their sharing due to the change in the communication and relational dynamic. And fourth, it frees up time for couples to engage in relationship-enhancing activities they may have otherwise put aside. Although many couples find success implementing this strategy, fertility counselors should be mindful that this intervention is not recommended for use on days when more lengthy infertility-related conversations are needed – such as when receiving difficult treatment results or when needing to make future treatment decisions.

Dyadic Coping

Fertility counselors can help couples examine the relational impact of their preferred coping strategies. Over the past two decades, studies using the couple as the unit of analysis have found that one partner's coping strategies influence the other partner's fertility-related stress [16]. Thus, coping is not only an individual process (i.e., how one partner copes with infertility affects how they feel) but also a relational process (i.e., one partner's coping affects how their partner feels). For example, active avoidance coping strategies, in which one partner changes their behavior to avoid reminders and stressors related to infertility, are related to increased psychological distress at the individual and partner level. In contrast, meaning-based coping, when one or both partners is able to see the fertility problem in a positive light, is related to decreased distress for individuals and partners [16].

Fertility counselors can help couples identify coping strategies that are individually adaptive, but relationally problematic. Fertility counselors can encourage both partners to share their preferred coping strategies, while giving the partner a chance to discuss the relational implications of these coping strategies. For example, one partner emotionally distancing may reduce their individual distress; however, it may also increase their partner's distress if they feel alone in the struggle (the corresponding *Case Studies*, Chapter 4 describes this dynamic). By framing coping as a dyadic process, fertility counselors can help couples produce more positive systemic interactions, leading to new coping patterns that can create increased understanding, relational safety, and increased support.

Fertility counselors should be aware that while some coping patterns may be amenable to change, others may not. Thus, a key to working with problematic coping patterns is effectively balancing acceptance and change [17]. While distressed couples likely want their partner to change coping strategies they perceive as ineffective, fertility counselors can help partners connect around the problem through understanding and acceptance of each partner's coping strategies. This intervention can help couples remain connected despite partner differences and is supported by research that found that couples who reported having mutual respect and support for a partner's coping patterns experienced less blame and stronger marital benefit [14].

Joint Decision-making

Throughout a couple's fertility journey, couples are required to make a considerable number of decisions, some even beginning before they enter a reproductive clinic. These decisions are often complex and demand intentional thought and united agreement to determine the best course of treatment. The added pressure of these decisions can be taxing on the couple's relationship, leading to miscommunication, confusion or resentment. This is particularly true for couples who have low relationship satisfaction and lack an emotional connection prior to treatment [6].

Fertility counselors can help couples learn how to engage in productive treatment-related decisions. Counselors should assess how the couple chose to engage in fertility treatment, who initiated treatment, and if they considered alternatives to treatment. Allowing each partner to share their experience of entering into treatment opens the door to further conversation if one partner felt obligated, rushed or unheard in the initial decision-making.

Joint treatment decision-making is also vital because couples are faced with a multitude of ethical and life-altering treatment decisions, including embryo disposition, the number of eggs to fertilize, genetic testing, and their ability to financially and emotionally continue or progress through the treatment process. These decisions are often required of couples early in the reproductive treatment process, possibly when couples are already overwhelmed with a new medical diagnosis or the sudden influx of new information regarding their reproductive health. Couples may become stuck in their decision-making or may disagree about how to proceed. Some partners may have a considerable amount of fear heading into another treatment cycle or pursuing another course of treatment that involves more invasive modalities. Fertility counselors can help facilitate emotional sharing and coach partners on how to be supportive in making decisions that feel fair and minimize risk to the couple relationship.

Fertility counselors can also help couples with decision-making when they are considering stopping treatment, regardless if they have had a child or not. Couples at this stage may be considering the advantages and disadvantages of additional attempts. They may also need assistance in decision-making regarding the disposition of frozen embryos. Couples who have been unsuccessful in treatment must confront the possibility that they may never have a biological child. In instances where couples experience regret about previous treatment decisions (i.e., we should have started treatment sooner; we should have stopped sooner), fertility counselors help cultivate compassionate responses, both to oneself and one's partner.

Decreasing Sexual Stress

The stress of infertility can impact a couple's sexual relationship. Both partners can experience decreased sexual desire, lower sexual satisfaction, lower sexual desirability, and feelings of marginalization when the sole purpose of sex is for conception. A 2020 study of 94 Croatian couples found that women and men who reported higher levels of infertility-stress, also reported lower levels of sexual satisfaction. In addition, lower sexual satisfaction was related to lower sexual self-esteem and challenges with scheduling infertility-related sex for both women and men [18].

Sexual difficulties related to infertility are much more likely to be a consequence rather than a cause of an infertility diagnosis. As with coping strategies, sexual stress in one partner can impact sexual stress in the other, supporting an emerging view that sexual stress is systemic instead of solely an individual problem [18]. Ironically for couples, increased sexual strain in the relationship can lead to reduced frequency of sexual relations, which lowers the chance of achieving a pregnancy.

If one or both members of the couple are experiencing heightened levels of sexual stress, fertility counselors should make this a focus of treatment. Fertility counselors can normalize sexual stress through education and help couples differentiate between 'procreational' and 'recreational' sex (e.g., sex for the sole purpose of pregnancy, compared to sex for pleasure, intimacy and connection). Couples whose sexual relationship is strained may also benefit from taking a break from sex during treatment, when sex is not necessary for conception.

Unfortunately, for many couples, there does not seem to be an optimal time to focus on improving a strained sexual relationship once the infertility journey has begun. During fertility treatments, couples are commonly too focused on achieving a pregnancy and have little interest in recreational sex because it is too closely linked with painful reminders of infertility. For couples who achieve pregnancy, they are often nervous that sex may cause pregnancy complications or miscarriage. For couples who give birth to a child, the demands and challenges of parenting take priority over renewing the sexual relationship. It is common for the stress on the sexual relationship to continue long after treatments end. Therefore, fertility counselors should help couples reclaim the intimacy and closeness they once achieved through sex prior to the infertility diagnosis. See Chapter 6 for more information on sex therapy in fertility counseling.

Sharing Infertility-related Information with Family and Friends

A frequent component of couple counseling involves discussing to what degree and with whom the couple shares information about their infertility-related struggles. While some couples may agree on how best to do this, others may disagree, which can lead to relational strain. Fertility counselors can help couples openly discuss these issues, promote acceptance of differences in partner disclosure patterns, and help couples find mutually agreeable strategies to disclose their infertility-related struggles to family and friends.

Helping couples balance their privacy needs with their needs for sharing their infertility journey is an important counseling goal. When a couple is first diagnosed with infertility, they may find they are more open to sharing treatment details with family and friends because they are optimistic about their chances of success. However, if treatments fail, the couple may take a more closed position regarding sharing, to avoid repeatedly sharing painful treatment details with those in their social network. On the other hand, a couple may initially decide to take a more closed position on sharing information with others in the hopes of rapid success. Later, they may recognize a need for extra support from friends and family if treatments continue unsuccessfully. This is particularly true with couples who experience added emotional pressure on their relationship because they are managing painful infertility-related emotions in isolation.

Regardless of the disclosure strategies couples choose, couples will benefit most by remaining flexible as they balance disclosure with clearly articulating the support they hope to receive from those closest to them. Fertility counselors should also be aware that disclosure becomes a more complicated issue when third-party reproduction is involved, and this is discussed in more depth in Chapters 9 and 11 of this volume.

Fertility Awareness and Age-related Infertility

There is significant evidence that fertility awareness in men and women worldwide is low [19]. Combined with delayed childbearing, couples who lack fertility awareness are at greater risk for infertility due to age-related fertility decline. Fertility counselors should be aware that because of decreased egg quality and quantity, female fertility begins to decline between 28–32 years of age and markedly declines at approximately age 37. In addition, male infertility increases with age, but not at the same rate as women. Advanced maternal age at first birth is also associated with increased rates of miscarriage, stillbirth, and health risks for the mother and child, while advanced paternal age is associated with decreased fertility and increased incidence of miscarriage, birth defects, schizophrenia and autism in children [20].

It is important for fertility counselors to help couples understand the limitations of fertility treatments for those in their late thirties and early forties (or older) [21]. Fertility counselors should educate couples that even the most advanced medical treatments often cannot overcome age-related decline in fertility. Helping couples make informed decisions based on their age and treatment success rates is an important clinical responsibility for the fertility counselor. Couples dealing with age-related fertility decline may face unique challenges, including guilt, self-blame and marital conflict revolving around how postponement decisions were made or sadness that they did not find their partner earlier in life. Older couples who have high achieving, goal-oriented personalities may find infertility particularly challenging because it is a long-term, low-control stressor. For couples who equate hard work with success, infertility is a struggle because it cannot be solved with more effort, and they are likely to feel anger, frustration, guilt and helplessness during the treatment process.

Fertility counselors can assist couples in this situation by assessing the process and context of prior decision-making. Both partners need to feel heard and understood by the other partner, particularly regarding their motivations for delaying childbearing. If one partner encouraged a delay while the other strongly felt they should begin sooner, the couple might find themselves experiencing increased tension or conflict in the relationship until this issue is discussed and resolved.

Secondary infertility (when a couple can have one biological child but cannot have a second) may also be an issue in older couples. Because secondary infertility can be just as disruptive as primary infertility, fertility counselors can ask couples about their motivations to have a second child, how they view the role and importance of a sibling in their child's life, and what their lives might look like if their future family size consists of only one child.

Secondary infertility may also occur with remarried couples in their newly formed marital system [22]. For these couples, secondary infertility often results from one's spouse's decision to have a vasectomy or a tubal ligation after having children in a prior relationship. Remarried couples often begin trying to have a child within the first two years of the union, while the stabilization of the blended family unit can take several more years. Thus, the overlap of this timing can take a toll on the couple's relationship, stressing a family system that is not yet cohesive and is vulnerable to disruption. In addition to helping these couples with the stresses of infertility, fertility counselors should also be aware of the challenges that arise in a newly formed blended family. Even if the couple has been together several years, fertility counselors must help both partners explore the implications of prior reproductive decisions, and the status of their current family unit as they relate to the stress of infertility.

Processing Losses, Posttraumatic Growth and Meaning Creation

To experience infertility is to experience loss. Lifelong expectations of parenthood, relationships with family and friends, financial savings intended for other life goals and meaningful connections to cultural and religious groups are just a few of the losses couples experience. Losses can become most pronounced if couples experience failed treatment, miscarriage or stillbirth.

Fertility counselors can help couples grieve through the sharing of stories that allow couples to connect with the losses they have experienced. Experiential exercises such as expressive writing techniques can help couples process painful emotions of sadness and grief that are necessary for the healing process [23].

Therapeutic rituals can also help couples grieve invisible losses, which are not often recognized by traditional social ceremonies. Therapeutic rituals are co-created with couples and use elements of existing cultural traditions such as funerals, weddings, and other ceremonies to express affect and create new meaning. A fertility counselor, for example, may help a couple create a ritual acknowledging the anniversary of a failed IVF attempt, miscarriage or stillbirth to provide a context for mourning and letting go, allowing new meaning to emerge.

Perhaps the most significant outcome of processing loss is an increased ability to accept one's emotional reactions and challenging life circumstances. This process can be conceptualized as posttraumatic growth (PTG) – a process where new perspectives, beliefs and strength stem from adverse life circumstances [24]. While changing long-held beliefs and expectations is a psychologically painful experience for most people, couples who are successful in doing so are in a stronger position to make new meaning of the infertility experience and move towards acceptance. This process is the foundation for creating resilience and can lead couples to discover a new sense of purpose in their life, even if treatments are unsuccessful.

Another potential benefit for couples emerging from the shared experience of infertility is the opportunity to address ruptures in the relationship that occurred during the fertility treatment process. Fertility counselors can help couples repair broken relational bonds by working to establish safe and secure connection even amid grief and fear, creating a firm foundation for safety throughout pregnancy and parenthood. For couples who end treatment without a child, these bonds can be essential in helping couples faced with future family building decisions such as adoption or childfree living.

Finally, although infertility is a stressful life experience, studies have found it can strengthen a couple's relationship, a phenomenon known as marital benefit [14]. In a five-year longitudinal study of 239 Danish couples who ended fertility treatment without having a child, one-third reported marital benefit [1], highlighting the possible positive effect of infertility on marital relationships. Qualitative studies have also found marital benefit in couples experiencing infertility through themes of being engaged in a shared hardship, feeling close to one another, developing satisfying communication and support, and having faith in their ability to face adversity [14].

Conclusion

Fertility counselors play a vital role in helping couples navigate the infertility journey. Helping couples understand the impact of cultural and social factors is critical in a couple's adjustment, as is helping couples improve communication patterns, coping strategies, joint decision-making and their sexual relationship. Interventions based on empirically supported couple therapies can help couples reduce distress, improve satisfaction and grieve the many losses they experience. Although the couple's infertility journey can be a long and arduous struggle, it can also lead to unanticipated discoveries and resilience born of adversity. Couples who find acceptance through the infertility journey can also discover a renewed sense of purpose and meaning in life, regardless of whether or not they have a child.

References

1. Peterson BD, Pirritano M, Block JM, Schmidt L. Marital benefit and coping strategies in men and women undergoing unsuccessful fertility treatments over a 5-year period. *Fertil Steril* 2011;**95**(5):37606313.

2. Peterson B, Place JMS. The experience of infertility: an unexpected barrier in the transition to parenthood. In: *Pathways and Barriers to Parenthood: Existential Concerns Regarding Fertility, Pregnancy, and Early Parenthood.* New York, NY: Springer International Publishing, 2019, pp. 19–37.

3. Peterson B, Boivin J, Norré J, Smith C, Thorn P, Wischmann T. An introduction to infertility counseling: a guide for mental health and medical professionals. *J Assist Reprod Genet* 2012;**29**(3):243–248.

4. Peterson BD, Pirritano M, Christensen U, Boivin J, Block J, Schmidt L. The longitudinal impact of partner coping in couples following 5 years of unsuccessful fertility treatments. *Hum Reprod* 2009;**24**(7):1656–1664.

5. Shreffler K, Gallus K, Peterson B, Greil A. Couples and infertility. In: Wampler KS, Blow AJ, Eds. *The Handbook of Systemic Family Therapy.* New York, NY: John Wiley & Sons Ltd, 2020, pp. 385–406.

6. Koser K. Fertility counseling with couples: a theoretical approach. *Family J* 2020;**28**(1):25–32.

7. Thompson J. The effectiveness of couple therapy on psychological and relational variables and pregnancy rates in couples with infertility: a systematic review. *Aust N Z J Fam Ther* 2021;**42**(2):1–25.

8. Naab F, Lawali Y, Donkor ES. "My mother in-law forced my husband to divorce me": experiences of women with infertility in Zamfara State of Nigeria. *PLoS One* 2019;**14**(12):e0225149.

9. Naab F, Kwashie AA. 'I don't experience any insults, but my wife does': the concerns of men with infertility in Ghana. *S Afr J Obstet Gynaecol* 2018;**24**(2):45–48.

10. Ying LY, Wu LH, Loke AY. The experience of Chinese couples undergoing in vitro fertilization treatment: perception of the treatment process and partner support. *PLoS One* 2015;**10**(10):e0139691.

11. Inhorn MC, Wentzell EA. Embodying emergent masculinities: men engaging with reproductive and sexual health technologies in the Middle East and Mexico. *American Ethnologist* 2011;**38**(4):801–815.

12. Boivin J, Gameiro S. Evolution of psychology and counseling in infertility. *Fertil Steril* 2015;**104**(2):251–259.

13. Peterson BD, Eifert GH. Using acceptance and commitment therapy to treat infertility stress. *Cogn Behav Pract* 2011;**18**(4):577–587.

14. Sauvé MS, Péloquin K, Brassard A. Moving forward together, stronger, and closer: an interpretative phenomenological analysis of marital benefits in infertile couples. *J Health Psychol* 2020;**25**(10–11):1532–1542.

15. Volmer L, Rösner S, Toth B, Strowitzki T, Wischmann T. Infertile partners' coping strategies are interrelated – implications for targeted psychological counseling. *Geburtshilfe und Frauenheilkunde* 2017;**77**(1):52–58.

16. Bombardieri M. Coping with the Stress of Infertility. Fact Sheet 15 (online). Available from: www.resolve.org

17. Vazirnia F, Karimi J, Goodarzi K, Sadeghi M. Effects of integrative behavioral couple therapy on infertility self-efficacy, dyadic adjustment, and sexual satisfaction in infertile couples. *J Client-Centered Nurs Care* 2021;**7**(1):43–54. Available from: http://jccnc.iums.ac.ir/article-1-295-en.html

18. Nakić Radoš S, Soljačić Vraneš H, Tomić J, Kuna K. Infertility-related stress and sexual satisfaction: a dyadic approach. *J Psychosom Obstet Gynecol* 2020;**23**:1–8.

19. Pedro J, Brandão T, Schmidt L, Costa ME, Martins M v. What do people know about fertility? A systematic review on fertility awareness and its associated factors. *Ups J Med Sci* 2018;**123**(2):71–81.

20. Hultman CM, Sandin S, Levine SZ, Lichtenstein P, Reichenberg A. Advancing paternal age and risk of autism: new evidence from a population-based study and a meta-analysis of epidemiological studies. *Mol Psychiatry* 2011;**16**(12):1203–1212.

21. Schmidt L, Sobotka T, Bentzen JG, Andersen AN. Demographic and medical consequences of the postponement of parenthood. *Hum Reprod Update* 2012;**18**(1):29–43.

22. Hafkin N, Covington S. The remarried family and infertility. In: Burns LH, Covington SN, Eds. *Infertility Counseling: A Comprehensive Handbook for Clinicians.* New York, NY: Parthenon Publishing, 2000, pp. 297–312.

23. Frederiksen Y, O'Toole MS, Mehlsen MY, et al. The effect of expressive writing intervention for infertile couples: a randomized controlled trial. *Hum Reprod* 2017;**32**(2):391–402.

24. Duraskova G, Peterson B. Posttraumatic growth in women with a long-standing experience of involuntary childlessness in the Czech Republic. *J Humanist Psychol* 2022 (online). https://doi.org/10.1177/00221678211068291

Fertility Counseling with Groups

Landon Zaki and Rachel Rabinor

Introduction

Therapy conducted in a group context can be a healing and transformational experience. For those grappling with fertility struggles and loss, this can be especially true. Individuals and couples facing infertility are often grief-stricken and in mourning for the child that they do not yet have. Single parents by choice, LGBTQ+ couples, and others undergoing third-party reproduction also face many unique challenges, with few places to turn for answers and emotional support. Groups offer a remarkably soothing and effective medicine for fertility-related distress, while providing a safe venue for information sharing as well as a powerful antidote to the stigma and isolation of childlessness.

This chapter provides an overview of fertility counseling with groups and offers a primer for counselors interested in forming a group for those experiencing infertility and other fertility-related struggles. We review the benefits of group counseling for fertility issues, relevant research literature, the role of the fertility group counselor, practical and clinical considerations in providing fertility counseling with groups, and common themes and challenges that emerge in the fertility group context. The goal of this chapter is to provide fertility counselors with the background necessary to build a successful fertility group in their specific work setting.

Background

The ability to reproduce and the desire for children is valued by cultures around the world. In the West, families and friends commonly "shower" expectant parents with celebration when a child is on the way. In many Eastern cultures, new mothers and fathers are nurtured with special foods and comforts in the first month after a baby is born. In each case, new parents advance into the next phase of adult development, bolstered by the

The addenda referred to in this chapter are available for download at www.cambridge.org/covington-clinical-guide

support of loved ones and validated by society's respect for their new social status. In contrast, the inability to have a child has long been socially stigmatized, with childless individuals being alienated from loved ones and their communities [1]. Imagine then the profound heartache and isolation of those blocked from achieving their dreams of parenthood because of infertility or other reproductive challenges. Where do they go for support? What communities provide recognition for their experience and comfort for their pain?

Increasingly, group counseling has provided a haven for emotionally distressed and socially isolated individuals. As a method of treatment, group approaches originated in the early 1900s when American physician, Joseph Hersey Pratt, taught classes to groups of medical patients on how to manage their physical illnesses [2]. Through this process, he observed that patients' psychological symptoms also improved, a serendipitous discovery that led him and others to conclude that group connection and mutual support are beneficial in the treatment of psychosomatic illnesses. In Europe, Freud and his protégés also experimented with group approaches to psychic problems. Group modalities eventually became an established method of psychosocial treatment when, during World War II, the mental health needs of soldiers far exceeded the supply of help available. The remainder of the twentieth century saw the proliferation of groups for various types of medical and psychological problems, including cancer, HIV, alcoholism, depression and anxiety.

The application of group treatment for fertility problems eventually came to fruition. One of the first mentions of group therapy for infertility came in 1959 when Abarbanel and Bach proposed adding short-term group psychotherapy as an adjunct to the medical treatment of infertile couples [3]. A decade later, this proposal was put into practice by Barbara Eck Menning, a visionary counselor who invited infertile women into her Boston kitchen to share their experiences and provide one another with support [4]. From these humble origins, Menning founded *Resolve: The National Infertility Association*, and became a staunch advocate for the inclusion of psychosocial support in the treatment of fertility patients. Menning's work, although centered around peer support, helped pave the way for the development of professionally led support groups for fertility patients.

Today, professionally led fertility counseling groups are offered in diverse settings including fertility clinics, hospitals and independent mental health practices. These groups focus on a variety of reproductive topics, including primary and secondary infertility, choice parenting, third-party reproduction, adoption, LGBTQ+ families, recurrent pregnancy loss, and many more. They may be time-limited, with a closed membership, or ongoing, accepting members on a rolling basis. Increasingly, fertility counseling groups are held virtually, allowing counselors to expand the reach of their services and connect members from disparate and underserved areas. The overall goal of fertility counseling groups is to decrease distress and isolation, increase active coping, facilitate the exchange of information, and nurture supportive connections among individuals and couples facing the same, or similar, fertility struggles.

Fertility counseling groups broadly fall into one of three categories: support, psychoeducational, and cognitive–behavioral [2]. Support groups have traditionally been the most common group modality used with fertility patients. Support groups focus on emotional expression and discussion of thoughts and feelings around specific fertility topics, which members themselves typically initiate. They tend to be less directive and open-ended, and may be time-limited or ongoing. Support groups may be peer-led, as through organizations like *Resolve*, or professionally led through clinics and independent mental health practices. In general, leaders of support groups, particularly peer-led ones, may use greater self-disclosure during the group process.

Psychoeducational groups are time-limited, professionally led groups focused on imparting information, education, preparation and resources around a specific fertility topic. An example of such a group might include a seminar designed to educate intended parents using donor gametes about the medical, psychological and legal aspects of this path to parenthood. Such groups may be co-led and include other relevant professionals, such as a reproductive endocrinologist or an attorney specializing in third-party reproduction.

Cognitive–behavioral groups for fertility are also professionally led. These groups impart knowledge and provide skills training, are more structured, directed, and goal-oriented, and typically have a closed membership and set number of meetings. Facilitators of such groups must possess specific training and clinical experience using cognitive–behavioral techniques to alleviate distress in a group setting. Examples of such groups include the "Mind-Body Program for Infertility" and the "Eastern Body-Mind-Spirit Group," which will be discussed in greater detail later in this chapter [5,6].

As an approach to treatment, fertility groups offer the counselor, client and clinic many distinctive benefits. For fertility counselors, groups provide a time-efficient and practical way to help a broader and more diverse spectrum of clients, with a potentially greater financial return for their time investment. For clients, fertility groups offer an excellent way to obtain affordable psychosocial support, a non-trivial advantage given the significant financial costs of fertility treatments. Finally, groups benefit reproductive medical clinics because they provide a cost-effective way to engage patients and reduce the emotional burden of infertility which often causes early drop-out from treatment [7]. Beyond these practical benefits, however, the fundamental superpower of fertility counseling groups is their ability to normalize difference, relieve shame, and empower those stigmatized by childlessness. Building on sociologist Erving Goffman's concept of stigma as a devalued social attribute [8], we provide one theoretical perspective on the unique effectiveness and suitability of groups for treating the fertility patient.

Theoretical Perspective

Infertility as Social Stigma

Infertility as social stigma is as ancient as time. From the early biblical period, infertility has been stigmatized with barren women shunned from society and labeled as "defective," "inferior," and "other." Infertility and childlessness continue to remain stigmatized conditions in modern times, with parenthood encouraged, rewarded and considered the norm in pronatalist societies around the world. In his classic work on stigma, Goffman defines stigma as "an attribute that is deeply discrediting" and one that produces a "spoiled identity" for the possessor. The word "stigma" has linguistic and cultural origins in ancient Greece, where it meant a "tattoo mark" used to brand "deviant" people considered by society to be "morally tainted" in some way. Importantly, Goffman distinguished between two types of stigmas: visible and invisible. Visible stigmas are devalued traits that are obvious to others (such as being disabled in an able-bodied society), whereas invisible stigmas are not readily apparent to others. Both are associated with negative psychological and relational consequences for the individual; however, possessing an invisible stigma – such as infertility or other reproductive disadvantage – is unique in that individuals can choose to conceal their stigma from others [8].

Indeed, it is not uncommon for fertility clients to have told no one about their reproductive struggles. To avoid social stigma and judgment, fertility clients may engage various "information management strategies," including fully or selectively concealing their stigma, providing medical disclaimers, or otherwise practicing forms of "deception." These stigma concealment practices, while understandable, can unfortunately lead to a host of negative consequences for the individual [9]. Those who conceal a stigma keep a secret, and keeping secrets is costly for the psyche as they are shame-based. Cognitively, stigma concealment is associated with preoccupation with the stigmatized attribute, thought intrusions and vigilance around stigma discovery. Emotionally, individuals who avoid talking about their stigmatized attribute experience elevated levels of anxiety, depression, guilt and shame. Behaviorally, concealment of a stigmatized attribute is associated with social avoidance, isolation and impaired relationship functioning. Ultimately, the negative consequences of stigma concealment contribute to a diminished sense of self-efficacy and a damaged view of the self – all unfortunate psychological impacts that fertility counselors regularly treat in their practices.

Groups Destigmatize Infertility

We believe that group approaches to fertility problems offer an ideal antidote to the negative consequences of possessing (and concealing) an invisible stigma, such as infertility or other reproductive challenges. Group interventions take advantage of the fact that humans are a social species who value and seek comfort and support from other humans during times of stress and loss. Groups provide an immediate and powerful sense of belonging that serves to reduce isolation, stigma and shame. In the fertility group setting, individuals and couples facing infertility and other reproductive challenges may safely disclose their stigmatized attribute to a group of supportive and inclusive others. In doing so,

they can obtain relief from the cognitive preoccupation, emotional distress and behavioral isolation that characterizes the experience of stigma concealment. Indeed, research on perceived stigma, disclosure and distress in infertility patients supports this idea. Studies from around the globe have found that higher levels of perceived infertility-related stigma are associated with lower fertility status disclosure, poorer social support, and higher levels of emotional distress in both men and women with infertility [10, 11, 12, 13]. Importantly, the social context in which an individual or couple discloses their fertility struggle matters. Disclosure to nonsupportive others can exacerbate distress and increase isolation, whereas disclosure to empathetic and supportive others can reduce stigma and shame and increase well-being. This point may be particularly salient for certain cultural or familial contexts where the revelation of fertility struggles could cause more harm than help. Fertility counseling groups fill a desperately needed void of empathetic and compassionate support for many individuals and couples stigmatized by fertility challenges.

Fertility Group Models

As previously described, fertility counseling groups may be categorized as supportive, psychoeducational or cognitive–behavioral in approach. While evidence suggests both supportive and cognitive–behavioral groups are effective in reducing fertility-related distress, group interventions that emphasize education and skills training (e.g., relaxation training) were found to be significantly more effective in producing positive changes across broader outcomes, when compared to supportive group interventions focused more on emotional expression [14]. This section therefore highlights relevant cognitive–behavioral and psychoeducational group approaches to fertility counseling that have been evaluated and described in the literature.

Mind–Body Program for Infertility (US)

One of the first group cognitive–behavioral interventions to demonstrate efficacy in treating fertility-related distress was "The Mind–Body Program for Infertility" created by psychologist Alice Domar in the US [5]. This ten-week program for infertile women was adapted from "The Mind–Body Basic Program" at Harvard, a behavioral medicine group intervention designed to treat individuals with stress-related medical symptoms, primarily by eliciting the relaxation response through various techniques. The Mind–Body Program for Infertility built on this intervention by supplementing additional stress management techniques, cognitive restructuring, exercise/yoga, nutrition education, unstructured group support time and partner participation. Mind–Body group sessions are held weekly, with eight of the ten group sessions lasting 2 hours in length. The group also includes one half-day session focused on nutrition and exercise, and one whole-day session geared towards exercise, yoga, and couples' cognitive–behavioral exercises (see Table 5.1 for a list of session topics). Studies comparing the Mind–Body cognitive–behavioral fertility group to traditional fertility counseling support groups in women with infertility have found that the Mind–Body group produced the greatest improvement in stress management skills, depressive symptoms and self-esteem at a 6-month follow-up [15]. Some evidence suggests that completion of the Mind–Body Program may also improve pregnancy rates; however, such data are inconclusive and confounded by fertility treatment factors [16]. For a more detailed review of the Mind–Body Program for Infertility, see [5,15,16].

Eastern Body–Mind–Spirit Group (China)

The Eastern Body–Mind–Spirit group is another structured, psychoeducational group intervention, which has demonstrated efficacy in treating state anxiety in women undergoing in-vitro fertilization (IVF) [6]. Developed at the University of Hong Kong, this four-session group program represents a holistic Eastern approach to treatment, specifically geared towards the needs of Chinese patients. The Eastern Body–Mind–Spirit group uses Traditional Chinese Medicine and Chinese philosophies of life to honor the belief that mind, body and spirit must be balanced for optimal health and harmony during stressful times. Like the Mind–Body Program for Infertility, the Eastern Body–Mind–Spirit Group is grounded in stress-reduction training, but incorporates Eastern therapeutic practices including tai-chi, meditation and discussion of Chinese philosophical writings (see Table 5.1). In a randomized controlled study comparing the Eastern Body–Mind–Spirit Group with a no-treatment control group for women undergoing their

Table 5.1 Summary of session topics for general infertility groups

Week	Mind–Body Program for Infertility [5]	Eastern Body–Mind–Spirit Program [6]	Fertility Group Intervention [17]
1	Introduction to the physiology of stress, relaxation response and relationship between stress and reproduction	Mini-lectures on Traditional Chinese Medicine and mind–body harmony	Emotions – acceptance and tolerance
2	Diaphragmatic breathing and mini-relaxation-response exercises	Stress-reduction training, coupled with Tai-chi, meditation and breathing techniques	The wish for a child – where is the previous life?
3	Cognitive restructuring and affirmations	Discovering positive meaning from negative experiences through activities such as singing, journal writing, and drawing	Coping with stress due to the reactions of others – communication with outsiders
4	Developing self-empathy and compassion	Ancient Chinese philosophical writings on suffering and the meaning of life	Enjoy life and feel good
5	Half-day session – nutritional lunch, exercise and nutrition		Attitude towards medical treatment
6	Mindfulness		Self-esteem strengthening
7	The emotions		Meaning of the wish for a child
8	Anger and forgiveness		Disappointment and hope
9	Whole day session (Sunday) – yoga, exercise, couples' cognitive–behavioral exercises		Waiting period
10	Review and follow-up information		We are the champions!

first IVF cycle, Chan and colleagues [6] found that Eastern Body–Mind–Spirit Group participants had significantly lower state anxiety on the first day of ovarian stimulation and on the day of embryo transfer, as compared to those who received no psychosocial treatment at all. For more information on the content and structure of the Eastern Body–Mind–Spirit Group, see [6].

Fertility Group Intervention (Switzerland)

The Fertility Group Intervention is an evidence-based approach to group fertility counseling designed for couples with primary or secondary infertility undergoing assisted reproductive technologies (ART) [17]. Developed in Switzerland for fertility patients at the Fertility Centre of the University Hospital of Bern, the Fertility Group Intervention is a ten-session program aimed at improving the mental health and quality of life of patients undergoing infertility treatment. Sessions are organized around specific fertility-related topics, such as stress management, communication with others and coping with difficult emotions (see Table 5.1). Like the previously outlined group approaches, the Fertility Group Intervention teaches relaxation training in a structured group setting that incorporates both educational and supportive therapeutic elements. Preliminary data suggest the Fertility Group Intervention benefits the mental health of infertility patients and is feasible for fertility counselors to implement. Future research on this group intervention is needed to uncover specific mental health and relationship benefits, including benefits that may differ by sex. For a more detailed description of this intervention, including how to implement it in your fertility clinic setting, see [17].

Donor Insemination Seminar (Germany)

Developed in Germany, the Donor Insemination (DI) Seminar is a groupwork approach designed to empower couples undergoing donor insemination to build their family [18]. The goals of each seminar are two-fold: (1) to prepare couples with comprehensive information on the medical, psychological and legal aspects of donor insemination, and (2) to actively challenge the stigma associated with donor-assisted reproduction. Seminars are team taught by a fertility counselor, reproductive endocrinologist and legal professional, and are held over both days of the weekend. Day one of the seminar is devoted to education and group discussion, with day two focused entirely on whole group and separate, sex-based group discussions. Seminars also include learning

from couples about their experiences of parenting and talking to their donor-conceived children about their conception. Research on participants completing the Donor Insemination Seminars suggest that it provides vital information and support, diminishes feelings of isolation and shame, and increases confidence in talking to one's child and others about donor conception. For a more detailed review of this intervention, see [18] and [19].

The above fertility counseling group approaches demonstrate that structured, psychoeducational and skills training groups for infertility are effective in reducing anxiety, depression, stigma and shame, while improving overall coping, stress management, self-esteem and confidence. However, these studies, as well as others, have focused almost exclusively on the psychological experience of women diagnosed with infertility. While this dovetails with robust evidence that women suffer greater psychological distress (symptoms of anxiety and depression) and poorer coping with infertility and reproductive challenges, as compared to men, future research is needed to investigate the acceptability of fertility group counseling approaches for men. See Chapter 15 on the male experience with infertility for further discussion. Moreover, research on racially and ethnically representative samples of individuals and couples suffering reproductive challenges is sorely needed. Chapter 18 on racial and cultural diversity issues in fertility counseling provides a more in-depth review of these issues.

Starting a Fertility Counseling Group

Starting a fertility counseling group can be a rewarding but daunting task that requires patience, creativity and persistence. Each phase of the group cycle presents important logistical and clinical issues for the counselor to consider. Below we highlight some of the most common issues, themes and challenges counselors may confront when building and facilitating a fertility counseling group.

Group Preparation

The success of any new professionally led fertility counseling group can be traced in part to the amount and quality of group preparation. The old adage "If you build it, they will come" applies, but perhaps with the caveat that "building it can take some time." This includes the time needed to obtain a graduate degree in mental health and sufficient supervised clinical experience facilitating groups. Counselors interested in forming a fertility support group must also possess specialized education and training in different aspects of reproductive mental health. Once these professional qualifications are met, fertility counselors can begin planning for the group they hope to run.

As an early step, it can be wise for the fertility counselor to devote some time to reflecting on the specific needs, feelings, questions, concerns and goals of their group population. For example, a group designed for women grieving infertility will look and feel different from a group geared towards LGBTQ+ couples seeking information on third-party family building. What are the primary needs of the population you hope to serve? How will a group setting meet these needs? What is the primary group goal – to impart information, teach coping skills, facilitate emotional expression? What will participants learn or feel upon completion of the group? Having thoughtful, clear answers to these basic questions helps ensure targeted treatment and informs practical decisions that must be made regarding group membership, structure, content, fees and recruitment, if applicable.

Another significant preparatory task involves the selection of members for the group. Who will be included, who will be excluded, and why? How homogeneous versus heterogeneous will group membership be? Answers to these questions have significant implications for the functioning and dynamic of the group. For example, a more homogeneous general infertility support group for women might include only women trying to conceive for less than two years and with the intention of using their own gametes. A more heterogeneous version of this group might include women with fertility journeys lasting (potentially much) longer than two years, those considering or pursuing third-party reproduction or women with a wide age range.

Neither version is better or worse than the other, but each presents unique benefits and potential challenges to consider. More homogeneous groups can benefit clients due to similarities in diagnosis, age, stage of treatment or psychological reactions to infertility, and as such, can be easier for the counselor to manage. However, high levels of group member similarity can also present a challenge, as group members may engage more readily in negative social comparison and over-identification. Fertility counselors can address and normalize the tendency for social comparison, while teaching members how to positively reframe what the loss or success of another group member means for them. Heterogeneous groups, on the other hand, benefit from the richness and diversity of group member experiences. Important interpersonal learning

and healing can happen when wisdom of more "seasoned" group members is passed to those newer in the fertility journey. However, such groups can present challenges for the counselor, who must integrate and hold varied experiences and psychological reactions to infertility while simultaneously monitoring group process and meeting group goals.

Additional membership concerns involve screening potential group members and deciding on the number of participants. If possible, scheduling a brief phone or video consultation with each interested group member is advisable. This initial screening serves several purposes: (1) to establish a therapeutic relationship and enhance motivation for group work; (2) to provide information, answer questions and allay any concerns about the group; and (3) to screen for psychopathology that may require a higher level of care or otherwise be counter-indicated for group participation (e.g., current suicidality, active substance abuse, severe depression or other personality pathology). Potential members not suitable for group work can then be referred for appropriate care.

Regarding number of group participants, the ideal number generally falls between 5–12 participants; however, this can vary based on the group population, type of group (e.g., supportive, psychoeducational, cognitive–behavioral), and any workspace limitations. For example, psychoeducational groups designed primarily to educate and prepare individuals for some aspect of ART may be larger and can effectively include up to 15–20 or more participants. In contrast, supportive or cognitive–behavioral groups are likely to be smaller, commonly including between 5–12 participants, to help facilitate emotional vulnerability and sharing or effective skills training and support.

Other significant logistical considerations pertain to group structure. Will the group operate as a closed or open group? Will it be time-limited or ongoing? What about session frequency, time of day, and duration? Is there particular benefit, or need, to hold the group virtually versus in-person? What fee, if any, will be charged for the group? Again, the needs and goals of the specific group population can guide answers to these questions.

Choosing a group name can also be an important and creative task that requires some careful thought and intention. Consider how certain names or words might feel for the members of the group. For example, "support group for infertile women" might deter those reluctant to accept the infertility label, whereas "fertility resilience group" might be a more attractive option. Consider names that focus on strengths or inspire specific feelings or skills that the group may impart.

A last structural consideration involves whether the group facilitator will encourage or discourage contact among group members outside of sessions. Given the stigma and isolation of infertility and other reproductive challenges, it is common for fertility counselors to encourage this outside contact to support the development of relationships that endure beyond group termination. Of course, counselors should obtain proper participant consent to share contact information and in what format (i.e., email, texts, phone number, etc.).

Finally, it is important to know that establishing a successful group with a steady stream of referrals can take some time. Depending on your work setting and the population being served, it may take up to several weeks or even months before enough participants have been assembled to form a group. Invest time in advertising your group to potential referral sources, including fertility clinics, therapists, acupuncturists and other community groups likely to overlap with the population you are seeking to recruit. Counselors may create written or electronic fliers to post in these venues and can seek out opportunities to share information about their services in community presentations, talks, as well as on social media. Remember: If you build it, they will come – eventually!

Role of the Group Facilitator

The fertility counselor must be prepared to wear multiple hats to facilitate a successful fertility counseling group. According to Yalom, the first basic task of the group therapist is to establish a cohesive group [20]. This involves both the physical reality of the group (outlined in the previous section) and its psychological safety. To create and maintain a psychologically safe space, the facilitator must be able to "recognize and deter any forces that threaten" this safety. Examples of such threats include continual lateness, monopolizing of the group, or in the case of a fertility counseling group – participant pregnancy. While adequate group preparation and screening can limit some threats, the fertility counselor must be flexible and prepared to manage these challenges with curiosity, genuine concern, empathy, respect and cultural attunement. As we describe further, there are times when group level needs will outweigh individual ones. Additionally, the fertility counselor can create group safety and cohesiveness by ensuring accurate understanding of confidentiality. Group participants should appreciate that confidentiality applies to all members of the group and that information shared within the group will be protected and not shared with outsiders (e.g., the reproductive medical clinic staff). Participants should sign a consent for group treatment which details confidentiality. Additionally, it can be helpful for participants to sign a document outlining expectations for group participation and behavior (e.g., "group agreements"), both of which help facilitate the formation of a cohesive group. See Addendum 5.1 and 5.2 for sample group consents and agreement forms.

Another significant task for the group facilitator involves building the group culture. As the group leader, the fertility counselor is responsible for establishing and shaping the norms of the group. This work begins with the initial client contact and extends into the group process where the counselor models therapeutic factors, including active listening, nonjudgment, validation, compassion, empathy, support and hope. According to Yalom, therapists shape group culture by embodying the dual roles of "technical expert" and "model-setting participant." The "technical expert" wears their traditional "counseling hat," and employs various techniques (e.g., explicit instruction, nonverbal and verbal reinforcement of altruistic behaviors) to achieve the goals of the group. Simultaneously, the "model-setting participant" embodies desirable group behavior such as spontaneous participation, appropriate self-disclosure and acknowledgment of missteps to demonstrate humanity and vulnerability.

The last significant role of the group facilitator involves the "activation and illumination of the here and now." This role describes attention to and intervention around the dynamics and nuances of interpersonal group relationships. While this role may assume greater prominence in true psychotherapy groups (as compared to educational or skills-training groups), fertility group counselors should be aware of common themes and challenges that may impact the dynamic and functioning of the fertility group. In the following, we outline several themes and challenges that typically arise in the fertility group context.

Group Themes and Challenges

Grief and Loss

Infertility and other reproductive challenges fundamentally involve loss. These losses include loss of health, esteem, body image, control, finances, relationships, intimacy and the imagined child, to name just a few. It is important to recognize that the normal, human psychological response to loss is grief, which may present in complex and overlapping forms. Feelings of shock, disbelief, anger, anxiety, sadness, shame, blame, guilt, depression and hopelessness are all common in fertility clients. The group counselor can validate, normalize, accept, and soothe this grief, as the group members provide solidarity, belonging and support. By working in the "here and now," the fertility group counselor must also monitor the impact of such intense emotions on the group process. Ideally, the group counselor strikes a balance between catharsis and helpful expression of negative emotion so that the safety, engagement and integrity of the group is maintained [2]. The group counselor can also focus on amplifying positive emotions through contemplative practices (e.g., mindfulness and compassion-focused meditations) and explicit techniques, which can create an encouraging and hopeful energy in the group. Such practices focused on amplifying strengths and psychological resilience can be especially helpful as a closing to a difficult group.

Stress and Coping

Reproductive challenges and their treatment are inherently stressful experiences that can test the coping capacities of even the strongest client. Indeed, fertility clients often seek professional support to learn new stress management techniques when their usual methods of coping fall short. Cognitive–behavioral techniques such as cognitive restructuring, relaxation training and mindfulness can be especially beneficial to fertility clients who often experience significant anxiety, worry or fear during the process of trying to conceive. In the group context, such intense emotions can easily become contagious, threatening group process and safety, if not addressed with concrete anxiety management strategies. The professional group counselor is ideally poised to teach fertility clients valuable evidence-based stress management techniques, with the group setting providing an ideal space to practice these new skills.

Pregnancy

Pregnancy can provoke strong reactions in fertility patients, triggering intense emotions (e.g., anger, devastation, envy, hopelessness) and urges to avoid. Therefore, when a member of a fertility support group becomes pregnant, it presents a complex challenge for the fertility counselor to address. How can the fertility counselor preserve the psychological safety and cohesiveness of the group, while balancing the need for the newly pregnant person to have support? While there are no "hard

and fast" rules, some considerations can guide the fertility counselor in managing this delicate situation. Yalom [20] highlights how strong client and therapist alignment around therapy expectations predict good therapy outcomes. It can therefore benefit the group counselor to develop some "policy" or approach to managing pregnancy that can be clearly communicated to group members early in the therapeutic relationship. This could occur during the initial phone contact with a potential group member and can be a welcome conversation that allays participant anxiety about the "elephant in the room" and enhances motivation for group work. Another approach might include having participants sign a "group agreements" document outlining how pregnancy will be managed in the group. These agreements can be revisited during the life cycle of the group to maintain group safety, engagement and cohesion. See Addendum 5.1 and 5.3 for a sample group agreements form. For a detailed review of how the fertility counselor can manage pregnancy in a group setting, see the *Case Studies* volume companion to this chapter.

Interpersonal Relationships

Reproductive challenges can impact every aspect of a client's life, starting with their relationships. Fertility clients often report dissatisfaction with the interpersonal support they receive from partners, friends, extended family, colleagues and even the medical treatment team. They may be surprised and hurt by the lack of sensitivity and understanding for the problems they are facing. The fertility support group can be a haven for these under-supported individuals, as fertility clients naturally "get it" and require no complicated explanation for their struggles. This emotionally attuned and accurate interpersonal support can be incredibly healing and freeing for many. Furthermore, the fertility group counselor can enhance this emotional support with education and interpersonal effectiveness training. Fertility counselors can provide education on the widely documented gender differences in how men and women experience and cope with reproductive challenges. Counselors can also teach skills to increase interpersonal effectiveness through role play and assertiveness training to help clients get their needs for emotional and practical support met.

Resilience and Hope

The journey to the goal of a healthy child can be an emotionally exhausting and arduous one for many. It is important to help clients learn how to draw on their strengths, build upon their natural resilience, and find hope for the uncertain future that lies ahead. The fertility group counselor can help clients uncover these innate abilities and orient them towards positive goals by structuring sessions to include explicit discussion of these topics. In addition, the group counselor can encourage realistic goal setting, altruism and the deepening of one's sense of self and relationships as ways to find purpose or meaning in adversity. In the end, the inherent wisdom of the group can provide irreplaceable hope for those struggling to find it in their fertility journey. For further discussion, see Chapter 19.

Summary

Group counseling as a psychosocial approach to fertility problems is an effective treatment method for reducing emotional distress, social stigma and isolation in fertility clients. By providing group treatment, professional fertility counselors magnify the impact of their work, save time and reach a broader and more diverse spectrum of clients. Fertility clients benefit from the affordability, solidarity and belonging that groups inherently provide. Most of all, fertility counseling groups provide a rarely found space for individuals and couples facing infertility and reproductive challenges to find true nurturing, comfort and support. The bottom line is groups work!

References

1. Miall CE. The stigma of involuntary childlessness. *Soc Probl* 1986;**33**:268–282.

2. Covington SN. Group approaches to infertility counseling. In: Covington SN, Burns LH, Eds. *Infertility Counseling: A Comprehensive Handbook for Clinicians*, 2nd edn. Cambridge: Cambridge University Press, 2006: 156–168.

3. Abarbanel AR, Bach G. Group psychotherapy for the infertile couple. *Int J Fertil* 1959;**4**:151–155.

4. Menning BE. The emotional needs of infertile couples. *Fertil Steril* 1980;**34**:313–319.

5. Domar AD, Seibel MM, Benson H. The Mind/Body Program for Infertility: a new behavioral treatment approach for women with infertility. *Fertil Steril* 1990;**53**:246–249.

6. Chan CHY, Ng EHY, Chan CLW, et al. Effectiveness of psychosocial group intervention for reducing anxiety in women undergoing in vitro fertilization: a randomized controlled study. *Fertil Steril* 2006;**85**:339–346.

7. Domar AD, Rooney K, Hacker MR, et al. Burden of care is the primary reason why insured women terminate in vitro fertilization treatment. *Fertil Steril* 2018;**109**:1121–1126.

8. Goffman E. *Stigma: Notes on the Management of Spoiled Identity*. Englewood Cliffs, NJ: Prentiss Hall, 1963.

9. Pachankis JE. The psychological implications of concealing a stigma: a cognitive-affective-behavioral model. *Psychol Bull* 2007;**133**:328–345.

10. Martins MV, Peterson BD, Costa P, et al. Interactive effects of social support and disclosure on fertility-related stress. *J Soc Pers Relat* 2012;**30**:371–388.

11. Slade P, O'Neill CO, Simpson AJ, et al. The relationship between perceived stigma, disclosure patterns, support and distress in new attendees at an infertility clinic. *Hum Reprod* 2007;**22**:2309–2317.

12. Donkor ES, Sandall J. The impact of perceived stigma and mediating social factors on infertility-related stress among women seeking infertility treatment in Southern Ghana. *Soc Sci Med* 2007;**65**:1683–1694.

13. Zhang F, Lv Y, Wang Y, et al. The social stigma of infertile women in Zhejiang Province, China: a questionnaire-based study. *BMC Women's Health* 2021;**21**:1–7.

14. Boivin J. A review of psychosocial interventions in infertility. *Soc Sci Med* 2003;**57**:2325–2341.

15. Domar AD, Clapp D, Slawsby E, et al. The impact of group psychological interventions on distress in infertile women. *Health Psychol* 2000;**19**:568–575.

16. Domar AD, Clapp D, Slawsby EA, et al. Impact of group psychological interventions on pregnancy rates in infertile women. *Fertil Steril* 2000;**73**:805–811.

17. Haemmerli K, Znoj H, Burri S, et al. Psychological interventions for infertile patients: a review of existing research and a new comprehensive approach. *Couns Psychother Res* 2008;**8**:246–252.

18. Thorn P, Daniels KR. A group-work approach in family building by donor insemination: empowering the marginalized. *Hum Fertil* 2003;**6**:46–50.

19. Daniels K, Thorn P, Westerbrooke R. Confidence in the use of donor insemination: an evaluation of the impact of participating in a group preparation programme. *Hum Fertil* 2007;**10**:13–20.

20. Yalom ID, Leszcz M. *The Theory and Practice of Group Psychotherapy*, 6th edn. New York, NY: Basic Books, 2020.

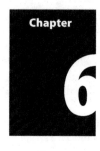

A Sexual Therapy Primer for Fertility Counselors

Erika Kelley and Sheryl Kingsberg

Definitions and Models of Sexual Response

Sexuality is an integral part of health and well-being and incorporates multiple dimensions, including gender roles and identities, sexual orientation, intimacy, sexual functioning, reproduction and pleasure. Sexual health not only encompasses the absence of dysfunction or disease, but also the ability to have safe and pleasurable sexual experiences [1] (WHO, 2006). This chapter provides an introduction to the identification of problems in sexual functioning in the context of fertility counseling and therapeutic approaches to treatment of sexual dysfunction.

Models of Sexual Response

Sexual functioning in all genders encompasses multiple domains including sexual desire (i.e., libido, sexual drive, or interest in and motivation to engage in sexual activity), cognitive arousal (i.e., feeling "turned on" or the mental excitement with sexual activity), genital or physiological arousal (i.e., genital engorgement and sensation associated with sexual stimuli/activity), and orgasm (i.e., transient peak of sexual pleasure sensation and release of sexual tension that typically coincides with involuntary muscle contractions, and ejaculation in men). Sexual satisfaction is also an important component of sexual health. Masters and Johnson developed a model of sexual response outlining a linear progression of physiologic stages consisting of excitement, plateau, orgasm and resolution [2]. This model implied the necessity of orgasm in sexual response. Later modifications highlighted the role of neurobiology and incorporated a psychological component, desire, to sexual response identifying desire, arousal and orgasm as the response stages [3].

Circular, non-linear models of sexual response later hypothesized that pleasurable and satisfying sexual experiences would lead to further sexual experiences. A model by Basson and colleagues indicated that many women may engage in sexual activity for reasons other than desire and highlighted the importance of other non-physiologic motivators for sexual activity (e.g., relationship satisfaction). Further, female sexual desire may include *spontaneous* desire that motivates engagement in, or initiation of, sexual activity, and/or *responsive* desire, which may occur following sexual arousal or in response to sexual stimuli and may be driven by motivations beyond desire for sexual activity (e.g., improved intimacy) [4].

Physiological factors also play a role and one's sexual response is determined by "excitatory" (e.g., dopamine, testosterone, norepinephrine) and "inhibitory" (e.g., serotonin, prolactin) neuromodulatory underpinnings [5]. An imbalance in the excitatory and inhibitory factors may disrupt sexual functioning, according to the "sexual tipping point" [6]. Thus, low excitatory factors and heightened inhibitory factors may contribute to distressing low levels of sexual desire.

As noted above, sexual functioning is best understood within a biopsychosocial framework determined by various etiological factors [7]. Biologic factors include neuroendocrine functioning, age, physical health, hormones and effects of medications or medical treatments. Psychological factors include presence/absence of mental health conditions (e.g., depression), body image concerns, beliefs related to sexuality and history of exposure to interpersonal violence (e.g., childhood sexual abuse). Sociocultural factors can include cultural norms, religious or societal beliefs about sexual activity and reproduction (e.g., gender role expectations, fertility related to masculinity/femininity and expectations to parent), family upbringing and relationship variables (e.g., presence of intimate partner violence, relationship communication). This framework highlights the importance of a multidisciplinary approach to assessment and treatment of sexual problems.

The addenda referred to in this chapter are available for download at www.cambridge.org/covington-clinical-guide

Sexual Dysfunction

Sexual dysfunction is characterized by a persistent impairment (i.e., at least 3 to 6 months in duration; occurring in at least 75% of sexual experiences in frequency) in a domain of sexual response (sexual desire, arousal or orgasm/ejaculation) or sexual pain that causes significant personal distress [7,8]. Sexual dysfunction is specified by *lifelong* (present across the lifespan) versus *acquired* (developed after a period of normal functioning) conditions, and *situational* (present in certain conditions, such as sexual activity with a specific partner) versus *generalized* (present across all sexual experiences/stimuli) conditions. A fertility counselor may encounter instances of acquired sexual dysfunction, such as a female patient with genitopelvic pain penetration dysfunction (GPPD) developing as an anxious response to trying to satisfy her partner's needs. Similarly, situational sexual dysfunction may present in the fertility counselor's setting, such as a male patient with "performance anxiety" who has difficulty achieving orgasm during timed intercourse for the goal of pregnancy, but is able to reliably achieve orgasm during non-ovulatory times or with masturbation. Severity or distress and impairment of the dysfunction is often classified as mild, moderate or severe. An individual may experience more than one sexual dysfunction concurrently.

There exists a variety of classification systems and nomenclatures for male and female sexual dysfunction (see Addendum 6.1 for references). Some of the most commonly used are described below.

Male Sexual Dysfunction

The APA *Diagnostic and Statistical Manual of Mental Disorders*, fifth edition outlines criteria for four different male sexual dysfunction diagnoses: delayed ejaculation; erectile disorder; male hypoactive sexual desire disorder; and premature (early) ejaculation (see Table 6.1) [8]. More recently, a more comprehensive list of male sexual dysfunctions and definitions with varying levels of evidence supporting them was developed by expert committee at the fourth International Consultation of Sexual Medicine. These conditions and definitions include male hypoactive sexual desire disorder; erectile dysfunction, premature ejaculation; primary delayed ejaculation, acquired delayed ejaculation, retrograde ejaculation,

Table 6.1 Male sexual dysfunction definitions/classifications according to the *Diagnostic and Statistical Manual for Mental Disorders*, fifth edition (DSM-5; APA, 2013)

Male sexual dysfunction	
	DSM-5 criteria
Delayed ejaculation	Either of the following symptoms must be experienced on almost all or all occasions (approximately 75–100%) of partnered sexual activity (in identified situational contexts or, if generalized, in all contexts), and without the individual desiring delay: 1. Marked delay in ejaculation. 2. Marked infrequency or absence of ejaculation.
Erectile disorder (ED)	At least one of the three following symptoms must be experienced on almost all or all (approximately 75–100%) occasions of sexual activity (in identified situational contexts or, if generalized, in all contexts): 1. Marked difficulty in obtaining an erection during sexual activity. 2. Marked difficulty in maintaining an erection until the completion of sexual activity. 3. Marked decrease in erectile rigidity.
Male hypoactive sexual desire disorder	Persistently or recurrently deficient (or absent) sexual/erotic thoughts or fantasies and desire for sexual activity. The judgment of deficiency is made by the clinician, taking into account factors that affect sexual functioning, such as age and general and sociocultural contexts of the individual's life.
Premature (early) ejaculation (PE)	A persistent or recurrent pattern of ejaculation occurring during partnered sexual activity within approximately 1 minute following vaginal penetration and before the individual wishes it.

* The symptoms must persist for at least 6 months in duration (and occur in 75–100% of occasions for premature ejaculation), cause clinically significant distress, and not be better explained by another disorder, medical condition, substance/medication, or significant stressor.

** Specifiers are used to indicate if the disorder is (1) lifelong vs. acquired; (2) generalized vs. situational; and (3) mild, moderate or severe in severity.

anorgasmia, hypohedonic orgasm, painful ejaculation or orgasm, and post-orgasmic illness syndrome [9].

Female Sexual Dysfunction

The DSM-5 describes three diagnoses of female sexual dysfunctions that incorporate changes from the previously published edition [8]. These include female sexual interest-arousal disorder (combining the previous female hypoactive sexual desire disorder and female sexual arousal disorder diagnoses); female orgasm disorder; and genito-pelvic pain/penetration disorder (GPPD; combining the previous vaginismus and dyspareunia diagnoses). However, research and clinical guidance indicate that there are limitations to this classification system. For example, the combination of difficulties in female sexual desire and arousal into one diagnostic category has limited research support, and this combined condition may disrupt treatment efficacy, since treatment is best approached by targeting the primary domain of disrupted sexual dysfunction. This chapter uses nomenclature outlined in the International Society for the Study of Women's Sexual Health (ISSWSH) process of care for the identification and treatment of female sexual dysfunction that addresses some of the limitations in the DSM-5 classification system (see Table 6.2) [10]. This nomenclature retains the separation of hypoactive sexual desire disorder (HSDD) and sexual arousal disorders, and includes female orgasm disorders and genito-pelvic pain/penetration dysfunction. Less common, though distressing, conditions under further research investigation are also listed (e.g., persistent genital arousal disorder).

Prevalence

Prevalence rates of sexual dysfunction vary across studies, in part due to methodological differences, variation in sample characteristics, limited inclusion of the assessment of distress or impairment, and differences in nomenclature/definition used to assess sexual dysfunction. The International Consultation on Sexual Medicine summarized that approximately 20% to 30% of adult men and 40% to 45% of adult women have at least one manifest sexual dysfunction [11].

Among men, prevalence estimates of erectile dysfunction are between 12% and 19% and estimates of premature ejaculation are between 8% and 31% in men of reproductive age [12]. Although premature ejaculation may be more prevalent, erectile dysfunction is often perceived by a male patient as a more distressing or severe condition. Estimates also indicate that approximately 15% of men report low sexual desire, 10% report sexual arousal disorders (including erectile dysfunction), 30% report ejaculation problems, and 5% report sexual pain disorders [13]. Erectile dysfunction increases significantly with age among men.

Research on rates of female sexual dysfunction is more limited compared with male sexual dysfunction. A US-based population survey indicated that the most common distressing sexual concern in women was low desire (reported in 10% of women), followed by low arousal (5.5%), and orgasm difficulties (4.7%), however, sexual pain was not assessed [14]. A systematic review of 54 studies indicated that the incidence of painful intercourse in women ranged between 8% and 22% [15].

Table 6.2 International Society for the Study of Women's Sexual Health and International Consultation on Sexual Medicine female sexual dysfunctions: nomenclature and definitions

Hypoactive sexual desire disorder
Manifests as any of the following for a minimum of 6 months:
- Lack of motivation for sexual activity as manifested by either:
  - Reduced or absent spontaneous desire (sexual thoughts or fantasies)
  - Reduced or absent responsive desire to erotic cues and stimulation or inability to maintain desire or interest through sexual activity
- Loss of desire to initiate or participate in sexual activity, including behavioral responses such as avoidance of situations that could lead to sexual activity, that is not secondary to sexual pain disorders
  and is combined with clinically significant personal distress that includes frustration, grief, incompetence, loss, sadness, sorrow or worry.

Female sexual arousal disorder
Female cognitive arousal disorder
- Characterized by the distressing difficulty or inability to attain or maintain adequate mental excitement associated with sexual activity as manifested by problems with feeling engaged or mentally turned on or sexually aroused, for a minimum of 6 months.
Female genital arousal disorder
- Characterized by the distressing difficulty or inability to attain or maintain adequate genital response, including vulvovaginal lubrication, engorgement of the genitalia, and sensitivity of the genitalia associated with sexual activity, for a minimum of 6 months.

Table 6.2 (cont.)

Disorders related to:
- o Vascular injury or dysfunction and/or
- o Neurologic injury or dysfunction

Persistent genital arousal disorder
- Characterized by the persistent or recurrent, unwanted or intrusive, distressing feelings of genital arousal or being on the verge of orgasm (genital dysesthesia), not associated with concomitant sexual interest, thoughts, or fantasies, for a minimum of 6 months.
May be associated with:
- o Limited resolution, no resolution, or aggravation of symptoms by sexual activity with or without aversive or compromised orgasm
- o Aggravation of genital symptoms by certain circumstances
- o Despair, emotional lability, catastrophization, or suicidality
- Inconsistent evidence of genital arousal during symptoms

Female orgasm disorders
- Characterized by the persistent or recurrent, distressing compromise of orgasm frequency, intensity, timing, or pleasure associated with sexual activity, for a minimum of 6 months:
- o *Frequency*: orgasm occurs with reduced frequency (diminished frequency of orgasm) or is absent (anorgasmia)
- o *Intensity*: orgasm occurs with reduced intensity (muted orgasm)
- o *Timing*: orgasm occurs either too late (delayed orgasm) or too early (spontaneous or premature orgasm) than desired by the woman
- o *Pleasure*: orgasm occurs with absent or reduced pleasure (anhedonic orgasm, pleasure dissociative orgasm disorder)

Female orgasmic illness syndrome
- Characterized by the peripheral or central aversive symptoms that occur before, during, or after orgasm not related, per se, to a compromise of orgasm quality

Genito-pelvic pain penetration dysfunction
Persistent or recurrent difficulties with ≥1 of the following:
- Vaginal penetration during intercourse
- Marked vulvovaginal or pelvic pain during genital contact
- Marked fear or anxiety about vulvovaginal or pelvic pain in anticipation of, during, or as a result of genital contact
- Marked hypertonicity or overactivity of pelvic floor muscles with or without genital contact

FSD = female sexual dysfunction; ICSM = International Consultation on Sexual Medicine; ISSWSH = International Society for the Study of Women's Sexual Health.

Reprinted from Parish SJ, Hahn SR, Goldstein SW, et al. The International Society for the Study of Women's Sexual Health. Process of care for the identification of sexual concerns and problems in women. *Mayo Clin Proc* 2019;94:842–856, with permission from Elsevier.

Relationship Between Infertility and Sexual Functioning

Research regarding the specific relation between sexual dysfunction and infertility is limited, but growing. Variability in methodology, low statistical power or lack of comparison group, focus on heterosexual couples, and variability in definitions used contribute to limitations. It appears likely that the relationship between infertility and sexual dysfunction is bidirectional for some individuals or couples.

Male Sexual Functioning

A recent global review indicated that the prevalence of sexual dysfunction among infertile men ranges from 6.7% to 75% [12]. The same review indicated that, though it is rare, in about 0.4% to 4.6% of infertile men, sexual dysfunction could be the cause of male infertility. Based on the existing limited research, it appears that rates of male sexual dysfunction are higher among infertile men than men in the general population and infertility (including male factor infertility) is associated with lower sexual satisfaction in men [12].

Female Sexual Functioning

A global meta-analysis of 16 nonrandomized controlled and quasi-experimental studies found incidence rates of sexual dysfunction in women with infertility ranged from 43.3% to 90% [16]. The majority of studies indicated worse sexual function in women with infertility compared to women without infertility.

Potential Mechanisms

There are multiple mechanisms that may contribute to the relationship between sexual dysfunction and infertility and should be considered by the fertility counselor. However, further research is needed to better identify mediating and moderating factors of this relationship.

Decreased general health status, medications used to treat general health conditions, presence of psychological disorders (e.g., depression and anxiety), and age are independently associated with impairments in both reproductive and sexual health [12]. Moreover, the experience of increased mental health symptoms, psychological distress, financial stress, reproductive loss, and relationship strain that may accompany infertility treatment (e.g., see Chapter 7) are likely contributing factors to disruptions in sexual function in individuals or couples diagnosed with infertility. Thus, the fertility counselor is well suited to address such psychosocial factors contributing to sexual dysfunction in the context of infertility. The experience of infertility may contribute to general feelings of inadequacy, guilt, low self-esteem, and distress, which in turn can negatively affect sexual functioning. Some data also suggest that women are more negatively impacted by infertility status than men in terms of sexual dysfunction.

The fertility counselor may see cases whereby the presenting concern is a sexual dysfunction appearing as infertility. For example, a couple who has not had vaginal intercourse due to sexual problems (e.g., vaginal pain that has developed as an anxious response to sex; performance anxiety) may present for assisted reproductive technology (ART). In some cases, sexual dysfunction may develop as a defense against feeling coerced or pressured to reproduce, when an individual may not really want to. In such cases, resolution of the sexual problem may mitigate the need for ART.

In addition, there is some research indicating that ART can contribute to development of sexual dysfunction, in part due to expectations regarding ART/outcomes contributing to stress and anxiety and the engagement in sexual activity for reproductive purposes (e.g., on-demand masturbation to provide semen samples; scheduled sexual intercourse timed around ovulation). For couples undergoing fertility treatment, the focus on sexual activity for the purpose of procreation rather than recreation and the intrusive nature of medical requirements can negatively affect sexual function. Couples undergoing fertility treatment may feel as though their medical care providers are symbolically present during sexual activity. Alternatively, research also indicates that treatment for correctible causes of infertility can lead to improvement in sexual function [12]. In summary, the relationship between infertility diagnosis and treatment and sexual functioning is complex, and a thorough assessment of sexual functioning in the context of infertility is crucial.

Assessment

It is important to recognize that the etiology of most sexual dysfunction is likely multifactorial and although a specific contributing factor may be easily identified, a thorough assessment is useful for maximizing treatment. Screening for sexual problems should occur for every patient or couple and can be performed by the fertility counselor. Research consistently demonstrates that patients prefer their healthcare professional to initiate conversations regarding sexual problems, particularly given the personal nature of the topic. The fertility counselor is often well-suited to screen for sexual problems given the highly intimate topics covered in fertility counseling. Inquiry about sexual concerns is often best done via a ubiquity statement, in this case related to infertility/ART. For example, "Many couples (or individuals) undergoing infertility treatment experience difficulties with sexual function, what sorts of sexual concerns do you have?" This also reflects an open-ended question, which commonly nets more information with little effort compared to closed yes/no questions [17]. Table 6.3 presents brief screening questions. These questions open the door for further assessment, highlight the importance of acknowledging sexual activity with partners of the same or different gender identities/sex, and highlight the role of sexual problems in contributing to avoidance or lack of sexual activity.

Sexual History Taking

A standard operating procedure for sexual history taking presents a unified approach with three basic principles [17]. First, a *patient-centered paradigm* emphasizes the importance of building therapeutic alliance and understanding the whole person when assessing sexual health, with attention to personal values, expectations and ideas. Second, there is a need for *evidence-based practice* for developing recommendations, including staying up-to-date with relevant research and clinical guidelines regarding management

Table 6.3 Brief sexual function screening questions

Single-item screen
Do you have questions or concerns about your sexual functioning?

Three-item screen
"Are you currently in a relationship?" or *"Are you sexually active?"*

If yes:	If no:
"Have your partners identified as cis men, cis women, transgender, or nonbinary?" *"What sexual concerns do you have?"*	*"Do you have sexual concerns that you would like to discuss or that have contributed to lack of sexual behavior?"*

Adapted from Kingsberg SA. Taking a sexual history. *Obstet Gynecol Clin North Am* 2006;33:535–547.

Table 6.4 Contributing factors to sexual dysfunction

Medical conditions	• Cardiovascular disease • Diabetes • Thyroid disease • Chronic pain • Urinary incontinence • Spinal cord injury • Multiple sclerosis • Neuromuscular disorders • Prolactinoma • Malignancy/treatment: mastectomy, gynecologic/colorectal surgery, pelvic radiation • Gynecologic disorders: pelvic organ prolapse, endometriosis, fibroids, vulvar dermatoses, vulvodynia/vestibulodynia • Psychiatric disorders
Medications	• Anticonvulsants: carbamazepine, phenytoin, primidone • Cardiovascular medications: amiodarone, b-blockers, calcium channel blockers, • Clonidine, digoxin, hydrochlorothiazide, statins, methyldopa • Hormonal agents: antiandrogens (flutamide, spironolactone), gonadotropin releasing • Hormone agonists, combined hormonal contraceptives, tamoxifen, • Aromatase inhibitors • Pain medication: nonsteroidal anti-inflammatory drugs, opioids • Psychotropic medications: antipsychotics, benzodiazepines, lithium, selective • serotonin reuptake inhibitors, serotonin and norepinephrine reuptake inhibitors, • tricyclic antidepressants

Reprinted from Parish SJ, Hahn SR, Goldstein SW, et al. The International Society for the Study of Women's Sexual Health. Process of care for the identification of sexual concerns and problems in women. *Mayo Clin Proc* 2019;94:842–856, with permission from Elsevier.

of sexual problems (e.g., see Addendum 6.1). Third, the use of a *unified management approach* emphasizes the importance of sexual health to individuals across the gender spectrum, particularly as sexual function in gender minorities has been under-assessed and under-treated.

The primary goal of sexual history taking should be to obtain as much information about the presenting sexual problem, with attention to development of patient–physician alliance. Providers should assess all domains of sexual function and sexual pain and satisfaction. Contributing biopsychosocial factors should be assessed thoroughly (see Table 6.4). A list of validated self-report measures that can be valuable for screening and informing assessment is included in addenda for this chapter (see Addendum 6.2). Follow-up questions will assess the degree of distress or frustration associated with the impaired domain of sexual response or pain. History of treatment for the sexual concern should be assessed, as well as the partner's (if relevant) response to the patient's sexual problem. Relatedly, the patient's interest in, perceptions of, and motivations for treatment should be assessed.

Sexual history taking should be adapted to the individual or couple as needed. This requires respect for cultural differences and the need for the fertility counselor to build and maintain their cultural competence. Examples include: improving communication between the fertility counselor and patients (e.g., reducing language barriers); self-assessment of the fertility counselor's own perspectives, biases and experiences in relation to sexuality; improving knowledge of cultural differences in sexuality (e.g., differences in gender norms across

cultures, expectations regarding sexual activity); and specific skills [17].

It is important for the healthcare professionals to assess whether the sexual problem is lifelong or acquired and generalized or situational. It is particularly helpful to identify onset with fertility patients when considering a sexual problem as resulting from, or perhaps impacting, infertility. Thus, gathering a timeline of the individual or couple's sexual problems, and asking about a range of sexual activities or experiences (e.g., engagement in masturbation as well as coupled sexual activity) can be useful in conceptualization.

Female Sexual Function

The ISSWSH process of care presents a model for the identification and management of female sexual dysfunction in particular [10] (see Addendum 6.3). Many recommendations for a core sexual history assessment are consistent with the standard operating procedure described above. More thorough female sexual assessment may require referral to a sexual medicine specialist, and should include assessment of medical factors that commonly affect sexual functioning (see Table 6.4). Clinical interview and use of self-report measures is typically sufficient for identification of the most common sexual problems, but assessment of sexual pain may require referral to a specialist (e.g., in gynecology, urology, sexual medicine or dermatology) for physical examination. Laboratory testing may be useful for identification of vaginal pathogens and sexually transmitted infections that may contribute to sexual pain, or clarification of medical etiologic factors.

Special Considerations for the Fertility Counselor

The fertility counselor is particularly well-suited to assess behavioral health and psychiatric problems that contribute to sexual dysfunction. Factors to assess include past and current exposure to sexual abuse or other interpersonal trauma; conflict or violence in relationships; body image concerns; and psychiatric conditions commonly comorbid with sexual dysfunction (depression, anxiety, substance use and posttraumatic stress disorders). Attention to intrapersonal and sociocultural variables should be made (e.g., impact of religion on beliefs and expectations relevant to sex or reproduction, family of origin approaches to sexuality, and partner's expectations or beliefs regarding sexuality). Coordinating with a prescribing psychiatric healthcare professional can assist with addressing psychiatric treatment-emergent sexual dysfunction, as some medications used to treat mental health conditions may disrupt sexual functioning (e.g., antidepressants are associated with low sexual desire) [10]. Medication management in this context may be complex and warrant specialty care, particularly given risks associated with medication in context of fertility treatment, pregnancy and breastfeeding.

Moreover, fertility counselors are often faced with the all-too-common sexual problems resulting from sex for procreation. There are many reasons why sex for procreation leads to sexual problems. First, sexual activity is now a means to an end (pregnancy) and becomes associated with failure (to conceive), frustration and on-demand/pressured/timed sexual activity. In addition to draining the enjoyment and delicious anticipation, "tonight's the night" may now trigger anxiety in couples, with erectile dysfunction in men, or lack of genital arousal in women as well as decreased desire for sexual activity. Additional information regarding assessment can be found in the addendum for this chapter (see Addendum 6.1 and Addendum 6.4).

Treatments

Treatment of sexual dysfunction typically necessitates a multidisciplinary approach. Establishment of a strong network of sexual medicine referral sources can help with coordination of care for patients experiencing concurrent infertility and sexual dysfunction, including specialists in gynecology, urology, andrology, dermatology and pelvic floor physical therapy. This chapter focuses on psychological interventions within sex therapy and a discussion of medical/pharmacologic treatments for sexual dysfunction is beyond its scope. Further information is available in documents referenced in the addenda for this chapter (see Addendum 6.1 and Addendum 6.4). Fertility counselors who are interested in further training and education in sexual dysfunction and sex therapy, or identifying a healthcare professional trained in this area, are encouraged to consult the following associations and resources: the International Society for the Study of Women's Sexual Health (ISSWSH), the Sexual Medicine Society of North America (SMSNA), the Society for Sex Therapy and Research (SSTAR), and the American Association of Sexuality Educators, Counselors, and Therapists (AASECT).

Male Sexual Dysfunction

Sexual counseling and education, which may be conducted by the fertility counselor, are recommended for management of male sexual dysfunction and are likely maximized by an interdisciplinary approach. For example, psychological intervention in combination with phosphodiesterase type 5 inhibitor (PDE5i, e.g., Viagra,) tends to yield better outcomes than either intervention alone for treatment of erectile dysfunction.

Female Sexual Dysfunction

The ISSWSH process of care provides an algorithm for the treatment of female sexual dysfunction [10]. Core level treatment that could be provided by the fertility counselor includes education regarding common contributing factors of sexual dysfunction, the potential benefit of use of foreplay, sexual toys and devices, and nonpenetrative sexual activity to improve arousal and orgasm; addressing communication concerns with a sexual partner; and introductory education regarding lubricants, moisturizing, and local hormone therapy options for addressing dyspareunia due to genitourinary syndrome of menopause (GSM) (which likely requires further referral to a specialist; see the section "Special Populations") [10]. More advanced treatment may require referral to a sexual medicine specialist(s). While further discussion of pharmacologic and medical interventions for sexual dysfunction are beyond the scope of this chapter, it should be noted that research on, and availability of, treatments for female sexual dysfunction is lacking relative to male sexual dysfunction. There are only two current US FDA-approved medications available for the treatment of female sexual dysfunction (specifically, acquired, generalized HSDD in premenopausal women): flibanserin and bremelanotide. Flibanserin is a multifunctional 5-HT2a-receptor antagonist and 5HT1a-recepter agonist taken daily, orally at bedtime. Bremelanotide is a cyclic 7-amino acid melanocortin-receptor agonist, and is self-administered on demand 45 minutes before intended sexual activity, by subcutaneous injection using an auto-inject device into the thigh or abdomen.

Summary of Sex Therapy Approaches

Depending on the sexual dysfunction and the relationship status of the patient, sex therapy may be conducted in individual, couples, or group format. It should be noted that most insurance companies do not reimburse for treatment of sexual dysfunction, which may serve as a barrier to patient access to adequate treatment. The approaches described here may be utilized or adapted for individuals across the gender spectrum. The fertility counselor's attention to cultural competence within any sex therapy approach is critical, and requires continued self-awareness of one's own attitudes, beliefs and values regarding sexuality and attention to those of the patient or couple. Fertility counselors interested in learning more about sex therapy approaches are encouraged to access resources listed in the Addendum for this chapter, including further readings, organizations (many of which

provide trainings) and online resources (see Addendum 6.4 and Addendum 6.5).

Brief Sexual Counseling

Several models for brief sexual counseling exist and may be modifiable to patients with comorbid sexual dysfunction and infertility and facilitated by trained fertility counselors. These models typically include validation of the patient's sexual concern, provision of education regarding sexual functioning and contributing factors, and education regarding specific interventions (e.g., use of lubricant for vaginal pain due to dryness) and referrals to specialists as appropriate. Examples of existing sexual counseling models are referenced in the chapter addenda (see Addendum 6.1).

One of the most effective brief interventions for cis gender, heterosexual infertility couples struggling with decreased desire or anxiety-related dysfunction due to timed intercourse for procreation is differentiating sex for procreation from lovemaking. Many infertility patients worry they have lost interest in sex or in their partner because procreative sex has taken away the enjoyment of sexual activity. Encouraging couples to make love (not a baby) during nonovulatory times and with non-intercourse activities helps them restore desire and refocuses them on pleasure, not "work." Identifying and separating rooms or areas in their home for "baby-making" versus "love-making" may also be helpful.

Cognitive–Behavioral Therapy

Cognitive–behavioral therapy (CBT) for sexual dysfunction focuses on the identification and restructuring of maladaptive cognitions and maladaptive behaviors that contribute to sexual dysfunction. Imbalanced or unreasonable expectations regarding sexual activity should be addressed (e.g., that a woman must be the passive recipient of sexual activity). Patients are instructed in cognitive restructuring and the fertility counselor can provide accurate information to correct misperceptions. Communication skill deficits can be addressed, with psychoeducation regarding assertive communication and use of role play (e.g., to specifically assert one's sexual preferences). Avoidance behaviors should be addressed, such as a partner avoiding initiating sexual activity due to fear of not pleasing their partner sexually. In couples with infertility, the fertility counselor may specifically target beliefs associated with fertility or fertility treatment that are affecting sexual function (e.g., that one's worth is determined only by their ability to reproduce). Issues of performance anxiety that may affect fertility (e.g., men who have difficulty producing sperm samples on-demand due to anxiety) can be addressed using CBT [16].

Mindfulness-based Cognitive–Behavioral Therapy

Mindfulness-based therapy (MBT), and mindfulness-based CBT (MCBT) for sexual dysfunction focuses on increasing one's nonjudgmental awareness and acceptance of the present moment during sexual activity and awareness of sensation/touch and sexual response [18]. Whereas MBT approaches typically focus on awareness and acceptance of cognitive processes, MCBT also incorporates components of cognitive restructuring of maladaptive thoughts. Modified versions of MBT and MCBT protocols have been developed for treatment of sexual dysfunction using group and individual formats. Small, uncontrolled studies and clinical trials have demonstrated improvement in sexual desire/arousal problems and sexual pain.

Sensate Focus Therapy

Sensate focus sex therapy was originally developed by Masters and Johnson and remains a commonly used sex therapy for the treatment of sexual dysfunction and the enhancement of relationship satisfaction and intimacy [2]. Elements of sensate focus are commonly integrated into other therapeutic approaches (e.g., MCBT). Sensate focus is based on three foundational, attitudinal skill sets. First, the use of touch mainly for the self (rather than one's partner) promotes a patient's awareness of the sensations experienced and allows for natural sexual response to occur. Second, touching is guided by interest through focusing on sensations rather than one's own or a partner's sexual pleasure or arousal. Sensations that patients are instructed to focus on include temperature (cool or warm), texture (smooth or rough), and pressure (firm/hard or light/soft). Third, patients are taught to identify and manage any experience other than sensation as a distraction. Sensate focus consists of engagement in a series of nondemand, progressive touching and exploration exercises that teaches mindful awareness of the sensations of touch to redirect from distractions. Mindful awareness of touch sensations provides an alternative to distractions and to judgments, expectations and evaluations that can disrupt natural sexual response.

For at-home progressive exercises, couples are instructed to have one partner initiate the touching exercise and engage in exploratory touching of their partner using the principles above; typically for around 5 to 15 minutes. They are instructed to avoid intentionally trying to be orgasmic through this process. These touching exercises progress over time, beginning with nonsexual/genital touch and ultimately to genital-to-genital contact with insertion/penetration. Sensate focus can be modified to address specific sexual dysfunctions and for individual or group formats. *Sensate Focus in Sex Therapy: An Illustrated Manual* presents one such manual to guide sensate focus sex therapy [19].

Directed Masturbation

Directed masturbation has demonstrated evidence in small randomized trials for treatment of primary female orgasm disorder and has been used in individual, couples and group formats [20]. This treatment begins with patient education and an explanation of treatment rationale. Patients first learn to increase awareness of their body (especially genitals) and begin a series of visual and touching self-exploration exercises at home. These graduated exercises then focus on self-stimulation and exploration of what brings pleasure, with the ultimate goal of achieving orgasm. Patients are encouraged to explore with a variety of sexual stimuli including erotica and sexual toys. When orgasm can be reliably achieved by the patient, then these exercises incorporate a partner (if applicable) at home.

Special Populations

Relevant clinical guidelines, position statements, and standards of care for the populations discussed here are presented in the chapter addenda (see Addendum 6.1).

Postmenopausal Women

Genitourinary syndrome of menopause (GSM) is a collection of signs and symptoms associated with a decrease in sex steroids accompanying menopause that can include genital symptoms (irritation, burning and dryness), urinary symptoms (urgency, dysuria and urinary tract infections), and sexual symptoms (vaginal dryness, pain and discomfort) and affects approximately half of postmenopausal women in their lifetime. Symptoms do not improve without treatment, but treatment can improve sexual function. Thus, it may be particularly relevant to address symptoms of GSM in women presenting for infertility treatment due to premature or surgical menopause. Referral to a specialist with expertise in menopause who may be able to prescribe and manage treatment of GSM is likely warranted.

Cancer Patients

Some cancers and cancer treatments (i.e., radiation therapy, chemotherapy, surgery and endocrine treatments) may affect one's fertility and sexual functioning, either directly or indirectly, via their impact on psychological, interpersonal and physiological factors. Sexual dysfunction in cancer survivors is likely underestimated and undertreated. Physical impacts of cancer treatment can directly impact sexual function; for example, vulvectomy for the treatment of vulvar cancer can cause scarring of the perineum and pain in female patients. Chemotherapy or surgeries can result in infertility and early menopause and the associated loss of sex steroids described above (see "Postmenopausal Women"). Psychosocial concerns that may emerge following cancer diagnosis and/or treatment, such as anxiety, depression, and compromised self-esteem and body-image can contribute to disruptions in sexual functioning. Fertility counselors can work with patients to discuss decision-making regarding fertility preservation, and address potential or existing disruptions in sexual functioning associated with cancer and treatment. Treatment of sexual dysfunction in this population is best addressed in a multidisciplinary manner, and existing research evidences improvement in sexual function following couples-based psychotherapeutic and psychoeducational treatments.

Transgender and Gender Nonconforming Patients

Sexual functioning among transgender and gender nonconforming individuals is understudied. It was not that long ago that infertility was an inevitable cost in transitioning from one's sex assigned at birth. Transgender patients presenting for infertility treatment may experience sexual consequences from gender-affirming medical and surgical interventions (see Chapter 17). Moreover, transgender individuals are at higher risk for mental health conditions (due to discrimination) that may negatively affect sexual functioning. Transgender individuals should be counseled regarding the potential effects of gender-affirming medical or surgical treatments on fertility and sexual functioning.

Conclusion

In conclusion, sexual health is an important component of quality of life. Sexual function incorporates components of the sexual response cycle including desire, arousal/lubrication, orgasm/erection, as well as sexual pain and sexual satisfaction. It appears that rates of sexual dysfunction are higher among individuals diagnosed with infertility, and it is likely that the relationship between infertility and sexual dysfunction is complex and bidirectional. Assessment of sexual function is best conducted within a biopsychosocial framework, and screening for sexual problems should be conducted with every patient. The fertility counselor is well-suited to conduct a core level of sexual history taking and identification of a sexual problem within an individual or couple and to provide psychological approaches to the management of such sexual problems.

References

1. World Health Organization. Defining sexual health: report of a technical consultation on sexual health. 2006.

2. Masters WE, Johnson VE. *Human Sexual Response*. Boston, MA: Little, Brown & Co., 1966.

3. Kaplan HS. *Disorders of Sexual Desire and Other New Concepts and Techniques in Sex Therapy*. New York, NY: Brunner/Hazel, 1979.

4. Basson R, Leiblum S, Brotto L, et al. Definitions of women's sexual dysfunction reconsidered: advocating expansion and revision. *J Psychosom Obstet Gynaecol* 2003;**24**:221–229.

5. Kingsberg SA, Clayton AH, Pfaus JG. The female sexual response: current models, neurobiological underpinnings and agents currently approved or under investigation for the treatment of hypoactive sexual desire disorder. *CNS Drugs* 2015;**29**:915–933.

6. Perelman MA. Clinical application of CNS-acting agents in FSD. *J Sex Med* 2007;**4**(suppl):280–290.

7. Parish SJ, Goldstein AT, Goldstein SW, et al. Toward a more evidence-based nosology and nomenclature for female sexual dysfunctions: part II. *J Sex Med* 2016;**13**:1888–1906.

8. American Psychiatric Association. *Diagnostic and Statistical Manual of Mental Disorders: DSM-5*, 5th ed. Washington, DC: American Psychiatric Publishing, 2013.

9. McCabe MP, Sharlip ID, Atalla E, et al. Definitions of sexual dysfunctions in women and men: a consensus statement from the Fourth International Consultation on Sexual Medicine 2015. *J Sex Med* 2016;**13**:135–143.

10. Parish SJ, Hahn HR, Goldstein SW, et al. The International Society for the Study of Women's Sexual Health. Process of

care for the identification of sexual concerns and problems in women. *Mayo Clin Proc* 2019;**94**:842–856.

11. Lewis RW, Fugl-Meyer KS, Corona G, et al. Definitions/epidemiology/risk factors for sexual dysfunction. *J Sex Med* 2010;7:1598–1607.

12. Lotti F, Maggi M. Sexual dysfunction and male infertility. *Nature Rev Urol* 2018;**15**:187–307.

13. Rosen RC. Prevalence and risk factors of sexual dysfunction in men and women. *Curr Psychiatry Rep* 2000;**2**:189–195.

14. Shifren JL, Monz BU, Russo PA, Segreti A, Johannes CB. Sexual problems and distress in United States women: prevalence and correlates. *Obstet Gynecol* 2008;**112**:970–978.

15. Latthe P, Latthe M, Say L, et al. WHO systematic review of prevalence of chronic pain: a neglected reproductive health morbidity. *BMC Public Health* 2006;**6**:177.

16. Starc A, Trampus M, Jukic DP, et al. Infertility and sexual dysfunctions: a systematic literature review. *Acta Clin Croat* 2019;**58**:508–515.

17. Althof SE, Rosen RC, Perelman MA, Rubio-Aurioles E. Standard operating procedures for taking a sexual history. *J Sex Med* 2013;**10**:26–35.

18. Brotto LA, Basson R, Smith KB, Driscoll M, Sadownik L. Mindfulness-based group therapy for women with provoked vestibulodynia. *Mindfulness* 2015;**6**:417–432.

19. Weiner L, Avery-Clark C. *Sensate Focus in Sex Therapy: The Illustrated Manual.* New York, NY: Routledge, 2017.

20. Andersen BL. A comparison of systematic desensitization and directed masturbation in the treatment of primary orgasmic dysfunction in females. *J Consult Clin Psychol* 1981;**49**:568–570.

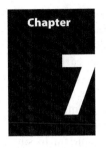

"It's Complicated": The Intersect Between Psychiatric Disorders and Infertility

Katherine Williams and Lauri Pasch

Introduction

Women and men are at an increased risk for new onset or recurrence of mood and anxiety disorders when they have trouble conceiving. Since the infertility evaluation process can be physically invasive and stressful, it can increase psychiatric symptoms in people with personality disorders as well. Furthermore, the fertility medications themselves may also have central nervous system effects. The goals of this chapter are to review the effects of the infertility evaluation and treatment process on mood, anxiety and personality disorders in women and men, including potential neuropsychiatric side effects of fertility medications. Risk factors for these psychiatric problems will be reviewed, and management methods introduced. Since to date, the majority of the psychological and psychiatric research has been in women, this chapter will mainly discuss findings in women. However, the impact of fertility stress in men is increasingly recognized, and discussion of men will be included, with gaps in the literature identified.

Mood and Anxiety Disorders in Infertility Patients

Prevalence and Risk Factors

Women undergoing infertility treatment have at least twice the rate of major depression (MDD) as women in the general population, 20–40% vs. 10–15% [1], and 30% of women with recurrent pregnancy loss meet MDD criteria [2]. There is also high prevalence of MDD in men whose partners are undergoing infertility treatment: 15% compared to 5% of men in the general population meet criteria for MDD in a variety of studies [1]. A previous history of MDD increases this risk in both women and men [1]. Certain conditions in women, such as endometriosis [3] and PCOS [4] increase risk for depression. In men with Klinefelter syndrome, (XXY), rates of major depression are high, ranging from 19–

24% of patients [5]. While anxiety symptoms are well documented in infertility patients, rates of actual anxiety disorders are not as well-known [6]. Patients with needle phobia would be expected to need special support if their treatment includes injectable medications. Despite these high rates of mood and anxiety symptoms and disorders, the majority of infertility patients do not receive mental health care [7].

Treatment Considerations: Antidepressants

Patients with a history of mood and/or anxiety disorders on antidepressants who are currently in remission and doing well despite the stress of infertility frequently seek counseling regarding whether to stay on or discontinue their psychotropic medication either while trying to conceive, or once pregnant. This decision is very individual and requires careful analysis of risks and benefits, with the guidance of the clinician who has been treating the patient for their psychiatric condition. While the role of MDD and anxiety disorders in decreasing natural conception rates remains controversial, the presence of current MDD does not appear to decrease the success of IVF or other non-IVF medication interventions, such as clomiphene citrate or gonadotropins [8]. However, women with untreated MDD during infertility evaluation and treatment are less likely to initiate fertility treatments [9] and more likely to discontinue treatment [10].

Major depression in men has the potential to decrease fertility. Women whose male partners meet criteria for MDD are less likely to conceive and decreased libido, fewer sexual interactions and for some men, erectile dysfunction are possible contributors to this finding [11]. MDD may have an effect on sperm production and function, as a history of major depression, and current major depression, has been associated with decreased sperm concentration [12]. The impact of psychiatric illness on fertility in men is an area in need of more research [13].

Treatment of new onset MDD, or continuation of serotonin reuptake inhibitor antidepressants (SSRIs) or buproprion (Wellbutrin) in patients with a history of MDD (recurrent) does not appear to be associated with a significantly increased risk of congenital malformations and they are not contraindicated in either pregnancy of lactation [14]. Very rarely, SSRIs have been associated with increased prolactin levels, which may be associated with menstrual cycle abnormalities [15]. No significant difference in quality of embryos, number of embryos transferred, pregnancy rate, spontaneous abortion rate or live birth rate have been found in IVF patients on SSRI antidepressants [16]. While some general population studies have reported an increased risk of spontaneous abortion in patients on antidepressants, there are many methodological problems in such studies. For instance, most studies do not control for important conditions independently associated with decreased fertility, such as body weight index (BMI), occult thyroid disease, ovarian reserve, or medical illnesses commonly associated with infertility. A recent systematic review reported that only paroxetine (Paxil) and venlafaxine (Effexor) are associated with increased rates of spontaneous abortion [17].

SSRIs have been associated with reversible effects on semen quality in men in some studies. While these studies have not been randomized, controlled trials, they have reported decreased sperm concentration, abnormal sperm morphology and increased DNA fragmentation; these effects increased over time and at higher doses [18].

Antidepressants and Perinatal Complications

The use of SSRIs after 20 weeks of pregnancy has been associated with an increase of persistent pulmonary hypertension (PPHN), a rare condition occurring in term or near-term newborns associated with severe respiratory failure. SSRIs in late pregnancy are associated with approximately twice the rate of PPHN in newborns, increasing the risk from 1/1,000 to 2/1,000 [19]. Some studies have reported higher rates of preterm delivery (delivery prior to 37 weeks) in women with depression on antidepressants in pregnancy compared to those who are not [20]. Maternal use of SSRIs in the third trimester of pregnancy has also been associated with neonatal adaptation syndrome (NAS) which has been reported in 20–30% of SSRI-exposed infants. The symptoms include restlessness, autonomic nervous system disturbances, respiratory distress, tremors, myoclonus and rarely seizures. NAS is not associated with long-term side effects in infants, or mortality [21].

The long-term neurodevelopmental effects of antidepressant exposure in utero remain unknown. Neurodevelopmental follow-up studies have many methodological problems. For instance, early studies reporting that children exposed to SSRIs in utero have higher rates of autism spectrum disorders (ASD) than nonexposed children did not control for family history of ASD, maternal or paternal psychiatric history or age, and later studies, which controlled for autism in siblings, failed to find this association [22].

Potential Risks of Major Depression in Pregnancy

Some patients choose to discontinue their antidepressants prior to or during pregnancy, and prospective studies have shown that four or more previous episodes of depression [23], poorly controlled anxiety, stressful life events, and poor social supports all increase the risk of recurrence of MDD during pregnancy [24]. The perinatal complications associated with MDD recurrence or relapse during pregnancy include increased risk of preterm birth, low birth weight, poor compliance with prenatal care, postpartum mood disorders, as well as potential adverse effects on mother–infant bonding and attachment and child development [25].

Bipolar Disorder: Prevalence and Risk Factors for Mood Instability

The life-time prevalence of bipolar disorder in both men and women in the general population is estimated to be 1% [26] and the prevalence in patients undergoing infertility treatment is currently unknown. Some women with bipolar disorder experience increased risk of mood disturbance at times of acute hormonal change, such as premenstrually or postpartum [27]. Consequently, ovarian stimulation protocols in which progesterone, and especially estrogen levels fluctuate dramatically, may be a time of increased risk for mood lability in these women. To date, the prevalence of this mood dysregulation is unknown, as no large prospective studies have been completed.

Bipolar Treatment Considerations: Mood Stabilizers

Women with bipolar disorder should be counseled extensively regarding the risks and benefits of continuing their mood stabilizers during pregnancy. Women with a history of recurrent severe manic or depressive episodes, including patients with a history of suicide attempts and/or hospitalization, should be counseled to continue their mood stabilizer or, in the case of valproic acid (Depakote) or carbamazepine (Tegretol), change to a nonteratogenic mood stabilizer, since these medications are associated with neural tube defects [28].

Lithium

Lithium is no longer considered contraindicated during pregnancy, and patients who have only been stable on lithium should be counseled that the risk of mood recurrence is high if the medication is discontinued [29]. Several recent studies do show an increased risk of congenital malformation in babies exposed to lithium in pregnancy, but the risk is not as high as once thought. A recent systemic review and meta-analysis of lithium exposure during pregnancy reported a 4.1% prevalence of any congenital anomaly in babies born to mothers who took lithium during pregnancy (odds ratio 1.81; 95% CI = 1.35–2.41) and of cardiac anomalies 1.2% (odds ratio 1.86; 95% CI = 1.16–2.96) [30]. The congenital malformation risk may be dose-related, and patients and their healthcare professionals should be encouraged to target treatment to the minimal effective dose, as doses above 900 mg/d are associated with the greatest risk [31]. All patients taking lithium in pregnancy should be encouraged to complete a high-level ultrasound at 16 weeks to evaluate the infant's cardiac function. Due to increased renal clearance in pregnancy, patients should be warned that many women require higher doses in the second and third trimester that need to be decreased back to pre-pregnancy levels immediately after delivery. Lithium levels and clinical status should be followed carefully postpartum [32].

Lamotrigine (Lamictal)

Lamotrigine has a favorable safety profile compared to other mood stabilizers, and studies do not report increased risk of congenital malformations or perinatal complications [32]. Due to increased metabolism, lamotrigine levels may need to be raised during the second and third trimester and should be decreased back to baseline levels postpartum [32].

Atypical Antipsychotics

Studies of atypical antipsychotics in pregnancy report no increased congenital malformations in general compared to control group [33]. However, atypical antipsychotics are associated with an increased risk of diabetes in the general population, and olanzapine and quietapine have been found to be associated with an increased risk of gestational diabetes in women who continue them [34]. Patients should be encouraged to discuss their risk of gestational diabetes with their physicians if they continue an atypical antipsychotic. More frequent weight, blood pressure and glucose monitoring may be indicated.

Posttraumatic Stress Disorder and Sexual Trauma

The prevalence of posttraumatic stress disorder (PTSD) in women undergoing infertility evaluation and treatment is unknown. Patients with a previous history of sexual trauma or reproductive system trauma (such as a previous traumatic birth) may be at an increased risk for reemergence of PTSD symptoms with invasive procedures, and staff are encouraged to take special care with these patients. Examples of interventions for these patients include trying to identify staff members they feel most comfortable with (i.e., male vs. female physicians) and limiting the number of observers/students/staff in the room. Consistent staff would be ideal, so that a trusting relationship can be built up. Extensive psychoeducation about what will be done regarding vaginal exams and ultrasounds may be needed, and all staff should proceed with extra patience and empathy.

Personality Disorders

Fertility treatment involves a roller coaster of emotions, loss of control and privacy, includes many appointments with a revolving team of healthcare professionals, and threatens one of the most important roles in many people's lives – parenthood. Further, the outcome is uncertain; it is often unsuccessful, and may ultimately fail completely. The stress is so great that the experience can be destabilizing for even the most resilient patient. For patients with personality disorders, the stress of fertility treatment can feel intolerable.

What sets personality disorders apart from other mental health conditions is that the pervasive issue is relational, that is, there is a relatively enduring pattern of inner experience and behavior that impedes most interpersonal functioning. Borderline personality disorder (BPD) is the most common and by far the most researched of the personality disorders and thus is the focus of our following discussion [35]. BPD is characterized by an amalgam of traits and symptoms including severely unstable mood, impulsive actions including substance use and risky behaviors, and a high tendency toward self-harm and suicidal ideation and behaviors. Although once believed to be lifelong and untreatable, recent evidence suggests that symptoms of BPD are the worst during young to middle adulthood (coincident with reproductive years) but that most people with BPD gradually improve, albeit with some residual dysfunction, and treatment can lead to substantial reduction in symptoms and improved life functioning [36].

In the fertility treatment setting, patients with BPD present major challenges for the treatment team. Patients with BPD have poor tolerance for physical or emotional distress. History of abuse is very common in patients with BPD and this may make fertility evaluation and treatment, which involves invasive and painful procedures, likely to trigger anxiety, intrusive memories and flashbacks. Patients with BPD are very sensitive to ordinary imperfections in communication and consistency in the IVF clinic that other patients reluctantly tolerate. Patients with BPD tend to exhibit disruptive rage reactions when they perceive their needs aren't being met. Whereas most fertility patients become upset and frustrated when a doctor rushes in and out of the room or when they receive unclear medication instructions or don't receive a timely return phone call, patients with BPD experience these relatively minor transgressions as rejection and abandonment. They often exhibit disruptive behaviors including yelling and making threats. These emotional outbursts can negatively impact staff well-being and sometimes, the care of other patients. Particularly when the IVF clinic is busy, understaffed, or disorganized, or when staff are feeling stretched to their limits, these patients can bring out the worst in everyone and make staff feel terrible.

One of the most challenging aspects of supporting patients with BPD is their tendency to use primitive defensive strategies [37]. While most patients manage the enormous stress of fertility treatment using healthy coping strategies like seeking support or focusing on the positive, patients with BPD generally use more ineffective and damaging defensive strategies including denial, splitting and projective identification. The consequences of these defensive strategies negatively impact the patient and the whole fertility treatment team. Clinic support staff, such as nurses, administrative staff and medical assistants often bear the brunt of patient angry outbursts. Very often when staff become angry, demoralized, and blame each other, the patient's role in the controversy is often not fully seen. See Table 7.1 for a summary of these defensive strategies and their operation and consequences in the IVF clinic.

Table 7.1 Primitive defenses operating in the IVF clinic (adapted from Stoudemire and Thompson, 1982)

Defensive strategy	Definition	Manifestation in the IVF clinic	Consequence
Denial	The tendency to not acknowledge foreboding or difficult information	Physicians and staff members share prognosis for IVF success, test results, protocols but patient does not take this in, continues to believe previous view and becomes irate if reminded of such	Patient has emotional outbursts when forced to face the truth, is nonadherent, makes illogical, uninformed treatment decisions Staff feel frustrated and threatened
Splitting	The tendency to see other people as either all good or all bad Splitters don't see middle ground and cannot tolerate ambiguity	Physicians and staff are divided by the patient into two opposing groups; the patient sees and interacts with one group as idealized and the other group as devalued, incompetent and punitive	Staff members respond to the patient depending on the group in which they have been placed Those perceived as good by the patient have positive interactions and develop a positive view of the patient while those perceived as bad will come to view the patient as ungrateful and demanding Staff disagree about how the patient should be managed Staff erupt into blaming and devaluing each other

Table 7.1 (cont.)

Defensive strategy	Definition	Manifestation in the IVF clinic	Consequence
			May develop between nurses and doctors, between nurses, between IVF clinics etc.
Projective identification	The tendency to place unwanted parts of the self onto others and then relate to that projected part through interaction with that person	Infertility is an intolerable blow to sense of self of someone whose sense of self is already fragile They feel bad and unworthy To try to keep this intolerably oppressive self-image from reaching awareness, they project or externalize this bad part of themselves onto medical staff They then direct the hate and rage they actually feel towards themselves outwardly onto the medical staff	Patient identifies with that person and acts to maintain an ongoing relationship in order to have an outlet for self-hatred These patients return regularly to demean their "bad" caregiver The caregiver is made to live with the projected negative part Very hard for healthcare professionals to escape falling into this trap Caregivers feel terrible, try to avoid the patient, express anger at the patient, all reflecting the misery of the patient (countertransference) Over time, chronic stress of working with patients like this hurts well-being and causes burn-out in staff

Frequently, the IVF team will request that the fertility counselor see the difficult patient with the hope that mental health treatment would "fix" the problem patient. Usually that is not practical or possible and runs the risk that the mental health professional would simply become drawn into the dysfunction, adopting a role as either the idealized helper or terrible interloper. However, the fertility counselor can effectively act as a consultant to help staff understand how the operation of primitive defenses affects them and how to develop effective management strategies. See Table 7.2 for basic clinic guidance in managing difficult patients.

At first, the IVF team will often be resistant to these suggestions and will make statements like "we cannot manage this patient," but with persistence, the fertility counselor can demonstrate their usefulness. Staff should be encouraged to express their feelings of frustration and hatred for the patient to the consultant, instead of at the patient. With relief and normalization of their feelings, staff are often ready to return to using their healthy coping strategies. It is extremely important that treatment staff are educated and given training in how to approach these situations to avoid splitting and further damage to the patient–treatment-team relationship. Angry rebuttals will only fuel the projective fires and lead to canceled or disrupted cycles and staff disturbances. Whenever possible,

Table 7.2 Checklist for management of difficult patients

1. Validate the stress of treatment
2. Keep staff emotions in check
3. Encourage frequent communication among the staff, including the physician, to develop a well-rounded view of the patient
4. Use firm, consistent and non-punitive limit setting
5. Pick your battles: ignore negative behaviors but clarify what is unacceptable (yelling, threats of violence)
6. Be proactive by checking in with the patient frequently, as opposed to responding each time the patient demands it

these patients will benefit from consistency in who is providing care as opposed to a revolving door of students or trainees, as this will heighten anxiety and threaten the fragile sense of bodily integrity that these patients have.

These patients desperately need clear, articulated boundaries. For example, they will keep calling after hours with questions that could have been addressed during the day. They need to be reminded in a calm caring way that the on-call staff is only for emergencies and criteria for emergencies should be reviewed. These boundaries will likely need to be stated repeatedly, in a consistent, nonemotional way.

While many therapists avoid working with patients with BPD because of the challenges, those who become knowledgeable and skilled in effective strategies for working with these patients will be highly valued and sought after as a consultant by the fertility treatment team.

Infertility Medication-emergent Side Effects

Oral Contraceptives

Oral contraceptives (OCPs) are a standard phase of early infertility treatment. Most women do not experience mood changes with OCPs [38]; however, women should be questioned about whether they have a history of mood problems with these medications, and if a specific OCP has been associated, then another OCP should be used, if possible.

Gonadotropin Releasing Hormone Agonists and Antagonists

Gonadotropin releasing hormone agonists (GnRHA), (for example leuprolide), and antagonists (for example ganirelix) are frequently used during initiation of fertility treatments with ovarian stimulation medications. Increased mood lability has been associated with GnRHA treatment [39]. If significant, distressing depression symptoms emerge, sertraline (Zoloft) has been found to be a useful treatment [40].

Clomiphene Citrate (Clomid)

Clomiphene citrate is a synthetic estrogen receptor modulator with mixed agonist–antagonist properties which women take orally days 3–7 of their menstrual cycle in order to increase the number of ovarian follicles. Many women report that clomiphene citrate is associated with mood lability, hot flushes and depressed mood [40]. Clomiphene is also used in men to increase sperm production [41]. In both sexes, it has even been associated with rare case reports of psychosis, occurring in patients with and without previous psychiatric history. In some of these case reports, there is a forewarning of sleeplessness and agitation progressing to auditory hallucinations, paranoia, delusions and ideas of reference. Notably, the onset of symptoms was within 48 hours of initiation of medication and neuroleptics and/or ECT resolved the symptoms [42].

Aromatase Inhibitors

Aromatase inhibition is a relatively recent addition to fertility treatment protocols, and it is increasingly used in women with unexplained infertility and polycystic ovarian syndrome (PCOS). Possible side effects include hot flushes, night sweats, insomnia and arthralgias, depression, anxiety and memory/concentration problems [43].

Human Menopausal Gonadotropins

Human menopausal gonadotropins (HMG) are injectable medications used to increase the number of ovarian follicles in either an IVF or IUI cycle, and they are associated with extremely high serum estradiol levels mid cycle. These medications are associated with mood lability, especially when transitioning from this estrogen-dominant phase to a progesterone-dominant late luteal phase [44]. Women with a previous diagnosis of anxiety or MDD have been reported to have greater shifts in mood symptoms than women without preexisting psychiatric diagnoses [45].

Progesterone

Progesterones are prescribed for a wide variety of fertility issues, including luteal phase deficiency, recurrent miscarriage and in most IVF cycles. Synthetic progesterones such as medroxyprogesterone have been associated with depressive symptoms in some women [46]. No large prospective comparative studies have been done to evaluate the risk of depressive symptoms with different preparations of progesterone. Micronized progesterone vaginally administered is commonly used in IVF cycles, and to date no studies have evaluated the prevalence of depression and anxiety symptoms with this more locally administered method. Table 7.3 identifies possible psychological effects of commonly used infertility medications.

When Should a Patient Be Counseled to "Wait" or Defer Fertility Treatments?

At times, fertility specialists need to recommend taking some time off from treatments, or waiting to begin treatment. It is crucial that all patients give informed consent about the potential psychological and psychiatric risks and benefits of infertility treatment on mood, anxiety and personality disorders. If a patient has active suicidal ideation, then deferring future treatments is indicated; and if

Table 7.3 Psychiatric effects of infertility medications

Drug	Use	Possible psychological effects
Aromatase inhibitors	PCOS, unexplained infertility	Hot flushes, insomnia,
Bromocriptine	Hyperprolactinemia	antidepressant effects, hypomania, psychosis
Clomiphene citrate	PCOS, unexplained infertility ovarian stimulation	Hot flushes, mood lability, "super PMS"
Gonadotropin releasing Hormone Agonists/ Antagonists	Hypothalamic "downregulation"	Depression, hot flushes, mood lability
Human menopausal gonadtropins	Ovarian stimulation (IVF)	Mood lability, insomnia
Progesterone	Endometrial support	Depression, decreased libido, irritability
Estradiol	Endometrial support	Antidepressant effects, induction of rapid cycling

they have severe depression associated with disabling vegetative symptoms such as lack of appetite with weight loss, severe insomnia, or ongoing substance abuse, these conditions should first be treated. Ovarian stimulation in a patient with an active, medically unstable eating disorder is contraindicated and these patients should be referred to an eating disorders specialist for treatment first. Other conditions that should be treated prior to infertility treatment include recurrent panic attacks, bipolar disorder with a recent manic or depressive episode and borderline personality disorder with poor self-regulation and recurrent suicidal gestures or attempts. Domestic violence should also be evaluated and the patient encouraged to work with a social worker and fertility treatments put on hold.

Please see the accompanying *Case Studies* Chapter 7 for a table on when to recommend delaying or discontinuing treatment.

Conclusion

Infertility evaluation and treatment are stressful and represent one of the most challenging phases of a woman and/or man's life. Patients with a history of mood and/or anxiety disorders and/or personality disorders are at significant risk for destabilization during this process due to either, or in combination of, the general psychological stress of the process or even due to the central nervous system side effects of the infertility medications. All women should be screened prior to and during the process for history of, or current symptoms of psychiatric illness, and provided with extra support and resources, such as can be found at mothertobaby.org and womensmentalhealth.org.

References

1. Holley SR, Pasch LA, Blei ME, Gregorich S, Katz PK, Adler NE. Prevalence and predictors of major depressive disorder for fertility treatment patients and their partners. *Fertil Steril* 2015;**103**(5):1332–1339.

2. Klock SC, Chang G, Hiley A, Hill J. Psychological distress among women with recurrent spontaneous abortion. *Psychosomatics* 1997;**38**(5):503–507.

3. Chen LC, Hsu JW, Huang KL, et al. Risk of developing major depression and anxiety disorders among women with endometriosis: a longitudinal follow-up study. *J Affect Disord* 2016;**190**:282–285.

4. Cooney LG, Lee I, Sammel MD, Dokras A. High prevalence of moderate and severe depressive and anxiety symptoms in polycystic ovary syndrome: a systematic review and meta-analysis. *Hum Reprod* 2017;**32**(5):1075–1091.

5. Skakkebæk A, Moore PJ, Pedersen AD, et al. Anxiety and depression in Klinefelter syndrome: the impact of personality and social engagement. *PloS One* 2018;**13**(11):53247532.

6. Chen TH, Chang SP, Tsai CF, et al. Prevalence of depressive and anxiety disorders in an assisted reproductive technique clinic. *Hum Reprod* 2004;**19**(10):2313–2318.

7. Pasch LA, Holley SR, Bleil ME, Shehab D, Katz P, Adler NE. Addressing the needs of fertility treatment patients and their partners: are they informed of and do they receive mental health services? *Fertil Steril* 2016;**106**(1):209–215 e2.

8. Evans-Hoeker EA, Eisenberg E, Diamond MP, et al. Major depression, antidepressant use, and male and female fertility. *Fertil Steril* 2018;**109**(5):879–887.

9. Crawford NM, Hoff HS, Mersereau JE. Infertile women who screen positive for depression are less likely to initiate fertility treatments. *Hum Reprod* 2017;**32**(3):582–587.

10. Pedro J, Sobral MP, Mesquita-Guimarães J. Couples' discontinuation of fertility treatments: a longitudinal study on demographic, biomedical, and psychosocial risk factors. *J Assist Reprod Genet* 2017;**34**(2):217–224.

11. Williams K, Reynolds MF. Sexual dysfunction in major depression. *CNS Spectr* 2006;**11**(8 Suppl. 9):19–23.

12. Yland JJ, Eisenberg ML, Hatch EE, et al. A North American prospective study of depression, psychotropic medication use, and semen quality. *Fertil Steril* 2021;**116**(3):833–842.

13. Evans-Hoeker EA, Eisenberg E, Diamond MP, et al. Reproductive Medicine Network. Major depression, antidepressant use, and male and female fertility. *Fertil Steril* 2018;**109**(5):879–887.

14. Payne JL. Psychopharmacology in pregnancy and breastfeeding. *Med Clin North Am* 2019;**103**(4):629–650.

15. Molitch ME. Medication-induced hyperprolactinemia. *Mayo Clin Proc* 2005;**80**(8):1050–1057.

16. Akioyamen LE, Holloway AC, Taylor V, et al. Effects of depression pharmacotherapy in fertility treatment on conception, birth, and neonatal health: a systematic review. *J Psychosom Res* 2016;**84**:69–80.

17. Broy P, Bérard A. Gestational exposure to antidepressants and the risk of spontaneous abortion: a review. *Curr Drug Deliv* 2010;**7**(1):76–92.

18. Beeder LA, Samplaski MK. Effect of antidepressant medications on semen parameters and male fertility. *Int J Urol* 2020;**27**(1):39–46.

19. Huybrechts KF, Bateman BT, Palmsten K, et al. Antidepressant use late in pregnancy and risk of persistent pulmonary hypertension of the newborn. *JAMA* 2015;**313**:2142–2151.

20. Bandoli G, Chambers C, Wells A, Palmsten K. Prenatal antidepressant use and risk of adverse neonatal outcomes. *Pediatrics* 2020;**146**(1):e20192493;

21. Levinson-Castiel R, Merlob P, Linder N, et al. Neonatal abstinence syndrome after in utero exposure to selective serotonin reuptake inhibitors in term infants. *Arch Pediatr Adolesc Med* 2006;**160**:173–176.

22. Sørensen MJ, Grønborg TK, Christensen J, et al. Antidepressant exposure in pregnancy and risk of autism spectrum disorders. *Clin Epidemiol* 2013;**5**:449–459.

23. Yonkers KA, Gotman N, Smith MV, et al. Does antidepressant use attenuate the risk of a major depressive episode in pregnancy? *Epidemiology* 2011;**22**(6):848–854.

24. Field T. Prenatal depression risk factors, developmental effects and interventions: a review. *J Pregnancy Child Health* 2017;**4**(1):301.

25. Szegda K, Markenson G, Bertone-Johnson ER, Chasan-Taber L. Depression during pregnancy: a risk factor for adverse neonatal outcomes? A critical review of the literature. *J Matern Fetal Neonatal Med* 2014;**27**(9):960–967.

26. Parial S. Bipolar disorder in women. *Indian J Psychiatry* 2015;**57**(Suppl.2):S252–S263.

27. Raffi ER, Nonacs R, Cohen LS. Safety of psychotropic medications during pregnancy. *Clin Perinatal* 2019;**46**:215–234.

28. Khan SJ, Fersh ME, Ernst C, Klipstein K, Albertini ES, Lusskin SI. Bipolar disorder in pregnancy and postpartum: principles of management. *Curr Psychiatry Rep* 2016;**8**(2):13.

29. Viguera AC, Nonacs R, Cohen LS, Tondo L, Murray A, Baldessarini RJ. Risk of recurrence of bipolar disorder in pregnant and nonpregnant women after discontinuing lithium maintenance. *Am J Psychiatry* 2000;**157**(2):179–184.

30. Fornaro M, Maritan E, Ferranti R, et al. Lithium exposure during pregnancy and the postpartum period: a systematic review and meta-analysis of safety and efficacy outcomes. *Am J Psychiatry* 2020;**177**(1):76–92.

31. Patorno E, Huybrechts KF, Bateman BT, et al. Lithium use in pregnancy and the risk of cardiac malformations. *N Engl J Med* 2017;**376**(23):2245–2254.

32. Khan SJ, Fersh ME, Ernst C, Klipstein K, Albertini ES, Lusskin SI. Bipolar disorder in pregnancy and postpartum: principles of management. *Curr Psychiatry Rep* 2016;**18**(2):13.

33. Cohen LS. Reproductive safety of second-generation antipsychotics: updated data from the Massachusetts General Hospital National Pregnancy Registry for Atypical Antipsychotics. *J Clin Psychiatry* 2021;**82**(4):20m13745.

34. Park Y, Hernandez-Diaz S, Bateman BT, et al. Continuation of atypical antipsychotic medication during early pregnancy and the risk of gestational diabetes. *Am J Psychiatry* 2018;**175**(6):564–574.

35. Paris J. *A Concise Guide to Personality Disorders*. Washington, DC: American Psychological Association, 2015.

36. Koerner K, Linehan MM. Research on dialectical behavior therapy for patients with borderline personality disorder. *Psychiatr Clin North Am* 2000;**23**(1):151–167.

37. Dubovsky AN, Kiefer M. Borderline personality disorder in the primary care setting. *Med Clin North Am* 2014;**98**(5):1049–1064.

38. Robakis T, Williams KE, Nutkiewicz L, Rasgon NL. Hormonal contraceptives and mood: review of the literature and implications for future research. *Curr Psychiatry Rep* 2019;**21**(7):57.

39. Gonzalez-Rodriguez A, Cobo J, Soria V, et al. Women *undergoing* hormonal treatments for infertility: a systematic review on *psychopathology* and newly diagnosed mood and psychotic disorders. *Front Psychiatry* 2020;**11**:479.

40. Warnock JK, Bundren JC, Morris DW. Sertraline in the treatment of depression associated with

gonadotropin-releasing hormone agonist therapy. *Biol Psychiatry* 1998;**43**(6):464–465.

41. Choi SH, Shapiro H, Robinson GE et al. Psychological side-effects of clomiphene citrate and human menopausal gonadotrophin. *J Psychosom Obstet Gynaecol* 2005;**26**(2):93–100.

41. Roth LW, Ryan AR, Meacham RB. Clomiphene citrate in the management of male infertility. *Semin Reprod Med* 2013;**31**(4):245–250.

42. Sinha GA. Could clomiphene kindle acute manic episode in a male patient? A case report. *Gen Hosp Psychiatry* 2014;**36**(5):549.e5–6.

43. Rosenfeld CS, Shay DA, Vieira-Potter VJ. Cognitive effects of aromatase and possible role in memory disorders. *Front Endocrinol* 2018 (online). https://doi.org/10.3389/fendo.2018.00610

44. Bloch M, Azem F, Aharonov I, et al. GnRH-agonist induced depressive and anxiety symptoms during in vitro fertilization-embryo transfer cycles. *Fertil Steril* 2011;**95**:307–309.

45. Zaig I, Azem F, Schreiber S, Amit A, Litvin YG, Bloch M. Psychological response and cortisol reactivity to in vitro fertilization treatment in women with a lifetime anxiety or unipolar mood disorder diagnosis. *J Clin Psychiatry* 2013;**74**(4):386–392.

46. Skovlund CW, Morch LS, Kessing LV. Association of hormonal contraception with depression. *JAMA Psych* 2016;**73**(11):1154–1162.

47. STOUDEMIRE A, THOMPSON TL. The borderline personality in the medical setting. Annals of Internal Medicine. 1982 Jan 1;96(1):76–9.

"Be Fruitful and Multiply": Addressing Spirituality in Fertility Counseling

Eileen Dombo and Megan Flood

The commandment to "be fruitful and multiply" is seen several times in the Old Testament. As part of the creation story in the Book of Genesis, God gives this commandment to both Adam and Eve, and Noah and his sons. This religious teaching informs much of Judeo-Christian messages on the subjects of marriage, childbirth and family. Also throughout the Old Testament are stories of infertility; of women like Rachel, Sarah and Hannah, who could not have children without God's intervention. The story of Hannah is a particularly powerful one, as she is the only wife of Elkanah who could not become pregnant. Her husband wants to see that Hannah can be happy just by being married to him; that should be enough for her, but it is not. Hannah prays to God time and again to allow her to bear a son, and promises to give that son to God. She does give birth to her son Samuel, and keeps her promise to God by turning him over to the temple to become a priest. Because she keeps her promise to God, she is rewarded with three more sons and two daughters. This story of prayer, perseverance and keeping promises made to God sends a powerful message to individuals and couples facing challenges to their own fertility [1,2].

As we see in the Old Testament as well as many other sacred texts, spirituality has been shown to be a source of comfort and support during times of distress. One's spiritual practices can help create meaning and bring strength to situations where it is normal to feel powerless and helpless, such as the struggle of infertility. Additionally, an individual's religious or spiritual traditions can influence the meaning they make of the experience of infertility, and the options they are willing to consider [3]. Given this, it is hard to believe that fertility counselors were not encouraged to discuss religion or spirituality with clients, nor did they receive proper training and education on how to do so [4]. Integrating the spiritual dimension of the person into treatment was thought to raise difficult ethical situations and blur boundaries between mental

The addenda referred to in this chapter are available for download at www.cambridge.org/covington-clinical-guide

health treatment and pastoral guidance [5]. Over the past three decades, we have seen an increased focus on the spiritual dimension in counseling, and many professionals are more aware of the need to discuss religion and spirituality with clients in an ethical manner [6].

This chapter will explore ways to address spirituality in fertility counseling, offer fertility counselors guidance on how to understand the degree of spirituality or religiosity in their clients' lives, and address how or if they are related to the challenges of infertility. For the purposes of this chapter, spirituality is defined as the search for meaning, purpose, and connection with self, others, the universe, or a higher power outside the self. This may or may not be expressed through religious practices or formal institutions. Religion, considered one expression of spirituality, is an organized, systematic set of beliefs, practices, and traditions related to spirituality, which is shared by a community or social institution [7]. These issues are explored in this chapter, and the reader is encouraged to consult Chapter 8 in the *Case Studies* text for examples of practice scenarios.

World Religions and Infertility

Most religious teachings speak to the significance of procreation, as well as the gender role expectations for men and women to become fathers and mothers. Through this lens, infertility can impact the self and relational identities of people wishing to become parents. Therefore, we see the risk for both a crisis of identity and of faith [8]. The relationship between religion and help-seeking for infertility is complicated [9], and continues to be a growing area for inquiry among doctors, fertility counselors and others in helping roles [10]. Fertility counselors treating individuals and couples grappling with the challenges of infertility are advised to approach this dynamic with an "informed not-knowing" stance, which will be explained later in this chapter.

The body of scholarly literature on the subject of infertility and the role religion plays in decisions regarding intervention is limited, and some significant scholarly works are quite dated [11]. Layne demonstrates that, regardless of faith tradition, people who experience infertility may feel a sense of shame rooted in specific religious teachings [12]. At the same time, religious practices can help to manage and alleviate that stigma. There are several important writings that shed light on the attitudes of specific faith communities with regard to infertility and its treatment. In some cultures, childlessness may be experienced as punishment for some previous transgression [11]. Exploring the lived experience of Orthodox Jews in New York, Kahn describes the current rabbinical debates about what interventions are and are not permitted [13]. Important considerations include evaluating the suffering of the couple as they grapple with the principle of family and Jewish integrity. Assisted reproductive technologies (ART) are viewed as aiding in fulfilling the commandment to be fruitful and multiply; therefore, Rabbis may permit many forms of ART with certain limitations or accommodations. This is consistent with previous research showing that people of Jewish faith tend to be more approving of the use of ART than those of the Christian faiths [14].

Exploring the tension between science and religion, Roberts investigates the ways Catholic physicians in Ecuador reconcile religious teachings with scientific endeavors. The Roman Catholic Church has long held clear prohibitions against ART. The Vatican asserts that it represents human intervention in a domain that belongs to God alone. As scientists in a predominately Catholic culture, these practitioners overcome this divide through their spirituality. Many hold beliefs that God "is in the laboratory" and "is taking direct action" through science ([15], p. 509). They pray during procedures, and believe that, ultimately, God decides which procedures are successful [15].

Moving beyond Judeo-Christian religions, Hindus in India have been grappling with the Western view of infertility. Here ART is employed to assist God, and outcomes from treatment are not guaranteed. Many couples interviewed in Bharadwaj's research speak of Hindu gods and goddesses they pray to for divine intervention. They recount being told by doctors and nurses to "leave things to God" after treatments ([16], p. 456). Many clinics have icons and pictures of patron saints, gods and goddesses, and some are even named for them. Pairing spiritual practices with science is seen as a form of *parallel sciences*. Like the Ecuadorian Catholic practitioners, Hindu practitioners in India speak of prayer as part of their scientific process. For those unable to conceive a child, the Hindu concept of *karma* can be a source of comfort; for example,

some women may see their childlessness as karma, or "destiny for a higher purpose in life" ([11], p. 751).

Islamic law prohibits ART that involves any third-party donation, as it violates teachings of the holy Q'uran related to adultery, incest and the integrity of biological descent. However, there are attempts to address this through legislation that would allow for embryo donation [17]. This has arisen through differences in beliefs between Sunni and Shi'ite Muslims in countries such as Iran, Egypt and Lebanon. Because of the cultural value placed on paternal lineage and property inheritance, there is less support for sperm donation than embryo or egg donation [18].

African traditional religion places a strong emphasis on interconnectedness. Infertility experienced by an individual or couple impacts the entire clan. Many believe that ancestors who are not properly respected through certain rituals are angered, and curse those family members with infertility. Therefore, there are important cultural and spiritual practices that must be carried out as part of any intervention for members of these cultures. As the majority of Africans report using traditional healing before approaching more conventional medical care, these practices should be explored when working with African clients in treatment for infertility [11,19].

It is vital for fertility counselors to be educated about the role of religion and spirituality in the lives of clients who are coping with infertility and considering seeking help to address it. Higher levels of religiosity have been found to be associated with lower levels of acceptance of childlessness, and higher levels of intent to seek assistance with solutions to infertility [9]. It is crucial that fertility counselors avoid making assumptions about infertility and spirituality that may or may not apply to their specific client system. A summary of the major world religions' positions on ART can be found in Table 8.1.

Understanding Your Client's Specific Ideology

Fertility counselors working with individuals and couples grappling with infertility should determine what, if any, spiritual or religious beliefs influence clients' decisions regarding medical intervention [20]. Social networks have been found to influence help-seeking behavior [21], and religion has been found to be both a resource and a burden when dealing with infertility [3]. Thus, it is useful to determine whether religious or spiritual communities are a part of the client's life, and in what way. Other variables that intersect with religion and spirituality should also be explored. For example, the role gender

Table 8.1 World religions and views on assisted reproductive technology

Religion	Permitted	Forbidden	Questionable
Anglican Church	Most forms of ART	None are strictly forbidden	MPR
Buddhism	Most forms of ART	MPR	SD related by blood ED SD
Eastern Orthodox	Only permits medicine and surgical interventions	All forms of ART	
Hinduism	Most forms of ART	MPR, SUR	
Islam	Any form of ART that does not include a third-party ED or SD	ED SD SUR	Embryo donation to infertile spouses.
Judaism	Most forms of ART that do not include a third-party ED or SD		ED, SD, MPR, ZIFT
Mormonism	AI and IVF that does not include a third-party ED or SD	ED SD SUR	No formal statements about other forms of ART
Protestantism*	AI, IVF	MPR	ED, SD, EMBD, GIFT and ZIFT
Roman Catholicism	GIFT	ED, EMB, IVF, MPR, SD, SUR, ZIFT	AI within married couples

* Includes Baptist, Methodist, Lutheran, Presbyterian, Episcopal, United Church of Christ, Christian Science, Jehovah's Witness and Mennonite denominations.

Abbreviations for ART used in Table 8.1 (assisted reproductive technologies)

AI = artificial insemination; ED = egg donation; EMBD = embryo donation; GIFT = gamete intrafallopian transfer; IVF = in vitro fertilization; MPR= multifetal pregnancy reduction; SD = sperm donation; SUR = surrogacy; ZIFT = zygote intrafallopian transfer

Sources: [10,14,25,26,27,28,29,30,31]

plays may also be a factor. For some, the pull to fulfil gender expectations of manhood and womanhood that relate to having children may override religious prohibitions against ART [22].

A thorough assessment of the significance of religion and spirituality for clients addressing infertility should include exploration of their use in making meaning, coping with psychosocial distress, and the presence of faith-based strengths to support them in the process [3]. Does the client experience their religious teaching, spiritual practices and community support as helping them to bear the unbearable, as a source of judgment and set of limitations on options, or both? Do conflicting religious beliefs and spiritual practices exist within a couple? If so, how does that impact decisions about ART? Not all spiritual people adhere to one specific religion or set of teachings, and individuals who identify with a specific religion may hold beliefs and engage in practices that differ from formal teachings [7]. The careful fertility counselor will assess for these beliefs and meanings and not make assumptions based on gender, religiosity or spirituality alone. Suggested assessment questions are presented in Addendum 8.1.

When assessing spirituality with clients, it is common for them to inquire about the fertility counselor's personal views and practices. Clients may seek out a particular fertility counselor because they assume shared religious traditions. Or, they may ask specifically about beliefs and practices if this has not been assumed. Fertility counselors should normalize wanting to know this information, as it is such an important part of life. Knowing how much of this personal information one is willing to disclose is helpful up front, to avoid awkward moments or sharing beyond what feels comfortable. This can also be a helpful moment in the engagement process, as the client is seen as unique, and the fertility counselor as wanting to understand more about what religion and spirituality means to them. Whether the fertility counselor and client are the "same" or "different," it is helpful to have a safe and confidential place to discuss the client's specific individual views and experiences. Some clients will feel more comfortable with someone who does not share the same religion because they will not judge them. Others will feel it is important that the fertility counselor understands their beliefs and practices. Either way, the fertility counselor can process the importance of religion and spirituality, thereby demonstrating openness to learning more from the client. In our experience, willingness to explore these themes outweighs the significance of the fertility counselor's personal beliefs.

Countertransference

Infertility is an experience fraught with complex emotions of grief, loss, anger, ambivalence, jealousy and more. Clients often present for treatment in the midst of a crisis, such as an unexpected diagnosis, a failed IVF cycle or a pregnancy loss. Fertility counselors working with these clients must have an awareness of how these powerful experiences can elicit a variety of emotional responses in themselves. If the fertility counselor is also undergoing infertility, or has a personal experience with infertility, as do many fertility counselors who choose this specialty, the potential for experiencing overwhelming countertransference is great. The subjects of spirituality and religion often are laden with myriad emotional material. Fertility counselors are not exempted from this. Fertility counselors working with these aspects of human experience simultaneously must be aware, as much as possible, of their own personal attitudes and unresolved feelings to understand the influence of these in the clinical work.

We have found that it is its critical to be aware of our own views about family building and spirituality or religion in providing fertility counseling. Our personal spiritual or religious ideologies, views of family, parenthood, and childfree lifestyles, attitudes towards ART, personal experience with infertility and loss, feelings towards authority (as may be represented by certain religious organizations or medical professionals, for instance) will surface when working with clients. It is imperative, though often very difficult, to keep in check our own desires and wishes for clients that are based in our own histories of family and spirituality, and to remain always in touch with what clients wish for themselves, which may be very different from choices we might make. We sometimes experience a sense of loss when clients choose options that we ourselves would not choose, or become invested in particular outcomes that may resonate with our own experiences. We have found that our own clinical supervision, peer support and personal therapy are essential to remaining aware of our countertransference and finding ways to use it to help us better understand our clients. For more on countertransference in this work, see Chapter 8 of the *Case Studies* text.

Spirituality and Spiritual Bypassing

In addition to determining the role that religiosity and spirituality play in decision-making, fertility counselors ought to be aware of the potential to use these resources as a means of avoiding deeper psychological work. The term *spiritual bypassing*, coined by John Welwood in 1984, refers to the use of spiritual ideas, practices and rituals to sidestep more psychologically painful work that may be necessary to face unresolved emotional issues [23]. When engaging in spiritual bypassing, people typically are defensive about their religious or spiritual practices, and not willing to explore them in depth. There is often an oversimplification of spiritual concepts, and an intellectualization of their spiritual practices. When clients are able to connect emotionally and spiritually to their struggles with infertility, they are not using spiritual bypassing. It is when these practices are used to remain emotionally numb and distant from the psychic pain that they are most likely attempting to sidestep the psychological distress.

It can be helpful to ask clients to explore the emotions that arise when praying or meditating, and how these practices help with their struggle. Clients who resist exploring the psychological dimensions of their spirituality may be engaging in spiritual bypassing. They may make statements such as "it's all in God's hands now, and there's nothing I can do" and "I'm giving it up to God." Further assessment must be done before making a determination, as clients who are not bypassing will make these types of statements as part of their acceptance of powerlessness over their fertility. This can be a good starting point for the fertility counselor to differentiate whether spiritual practices are being engaged as a support, or are being used to avoid difficult emotional experiences. For an example of how this can manifest with clients, see the case of Tran and Jake in Chapter 8 of the *Case Studies* text.

Spiritually-based Interventions for Infertility

For clients who are spiritually inclined, the crisis of infertility can ignite a simultaneous crisis of faith; others draw upon their spirituality as a source of strength; still others experience mixed feelings or confusion about previously unquestioned spiritual tenets. As each client experiences infertility idiosyncratically, so too is each client's understanding of the intersection of infertility and spirituality unique. Nevertheless, common themes surrounding spirituality may emerge in clinical work with patients experiencing challenges to family building.

As fertility counselors who are open to attending to spirituality in our work with clients experiencing obstacles to family building, we have identified the following intervention strategies to help clients navigate these two very profound and complex dimensions of the human experience. These include:

- informed not-knowing;
- telling the story;
- naming the losses;
- speaking the unspeakable;
- grieving the losses; and,
- identifying options.

These intervention strategies are not necessarily linear over the course of treatment. Instead, they are thematic and intended to provide the fertility counselor with a general guideline to treatment. In essence, they are tools to use in addition to an existing professional skill set. The client should set the pace of treatment, and feel free to return to earlier material, if necessary. The clinical vignettes presented in Chapter 8 of the *Case Studies* text show examples of application of these interventions.

Informed Not-knowing

Every fertility counselor brings his or her own professional training and personal experience to each client encounter, and, at times, the circumstances of clients' lives may seem all too familiar if the fertility counselor has a personal history of infertility or shares similar spiritual beliefs with his or her clients. By adopting a stance of informed not-knowing, fertility counselors are reminded that knowledge and training can provide an outline or rough draft out of which clients are able to tell their version of the story. The questions fertility counselors ask in assessment and throughout the treatment help bring diffuse feelings into sharper focus, and continue to challenge the fertility counselor's assumptions. The fertility counselor asks clients to define their experiences, rather than imposing the fertility counselor's own understandings upon clients. The questions the fertility counselor asks are informed by knowledge, training and personal experiences with spirituality and infertility, but clients are the experts on their own experiences, feelings and beliefs. The manner of the fertility counselor's questions and interventions communicates respect, curiosity and lack of judgment about clients. Fertility counselors are not afraid to ask for clarification if they do not understand what clients are telling them. This

attitude of informed not-knowing gives clients authority to help the fertility counselor understand their unique experiences of infertility and spirituality. Please refer to the case of Dav and Miriam, and their fertility counselor Melinda, in the *Case Studies* text for a clinical example.

Telling the Story

The experience of infertility can be an intensely personal and isolating one. Many clients have had few, if any, opportunities to tell the story of their family building journey to a supportive listener who is patient, concerned and familiar with matters related to infertility. Moreover, many clients are unaccustomed to considering the influence of the past on present events. Some clients, overwhelmed by intense feelings or single-minded in pursuit of medical treatments, haven't paused to think about the narrative of their experience. Additionally, if a client's spiritual community has an expressed position about expectations for family building or approved intervention options for treating infertility, he or she may feel hesitant to tell his or her story for fear of disapproval or pressure from the community to adhere to its guidelines. Therapy with a fertility counselor who is both experienced in working with infertility and open to understanding the client's spiritual orientation can provide an opportunity for the client to organize experiences, feelings and beliefs into his or her own unique story, without having to edit details for a particular audience.

Construction of a narrative can help the client understand his or her infertility as a story that has evolved over time, with characters that are influenced by a variety of life factors, including those of a spiritual nature. This is similar to Jaffe and Diamond's notion of the reproductive story [24]. Using this intervention, the fertility counselor helps the client surface unconscious or conscious narratives of family building and addresses how current challenges to fertility have interrupted those stories. Weaving in spirituality, the fertility counselor helps the client understand an additional, often powerful, dimension of the story. For a clinical example of this, see Eden's work with Saily in the *Case Studies* text.

Naming the Losses

Clients experiencing infertility, especially those who never have had a pregnancy, often feel an acute sense of grief, but have not labeled their experience as such, because of the intangibility of the losses. Previously held assumptions about fertility, good health, success, masculinity, femininity and the future, many of which are reinforced by faith communities, are no longer reliable. Because these losses are amorphous and invisible, clients often feel a sense of dissonance between their personal experience and the reactions of those around them. Well-meaning friends, family and faith community members can underscore this sense of confusion by encouraging clients to "hang in there" or "be grateful for all you have." Spiritual clients are sometimes told to think of their infertility as part of God's plan, which may invoke feelings of shame if they are angry or sad about their plight. In addition to the losses infertility brings, clients may also feel the loss of connection with those around them who are unable to understand their experience. Moreover, infertile clients may feel the loss of a previously unwavering faith in a loving higher power that now seems absent. The fertility counselor's task is to help their clients name these experiences as losses worthy of grieving, and validate the legitimacy of clients' feelings of loss where others are unable to do so. The focus of Wendy's work with Karim is a good example of naming the losses in the *Case Studies* text.

Speaking the Unspeakable

Some may consider the feelings evoked in clients by the experience of infertility unkind, inappropriate, and, even, blasphemous. Faith communities frequently discourage expressions of "negative" feelings such as envy, rage, hatred, frustration, fear and doubt, yet clients dealing with infertility commonly experience these feelings. Clients are often surprised when fertility counselors are interested in, and, even encourage them to speak about "unacceptable" thoughts and feelings out loud in sessions. The fertility counselor is tolerant, accepting and unafraid of hearing all of the client's thoughts, fears, fantasies and feelings about infertility, pregnancy, people with children, and, even, God. When these feelings are spoken in session and normalized by the fertility counselor, clients often are surprised to learn that they are not alone in their negative emotional responses to infertility. Often, clients feel relieved of the pressure they experience in many other settings to deny these feelings or pretend they feel otherwise. The fertility counselor may expect that, for some clients, speaking the unspeakable can feel alarming and shameful. It is important to allow the client to set the pace of expression of these feelings, and to attend to the experience of saying out loud and feeling in session frightening and forbidden material. The case of Richard's work with Leah in the *Case Studies* text highlights how powerful speaking the unspeakable truly is.

Grieving the Losses

As clients are able to identify their infertility-related losses, including those having to do with issues of faith, and articulate the unspeakable fears and feelings related to these losses, the task of treatment becomes helping clients engage in the grieving process. Clients are given space to express feelings of grief, and the fertility counselor assists in the mourning process by staying with the sadness in sessions. There is no rush to solve the problem, "look on the bright side," or deny any part of the reality of the experience for the patient. The fertility counselor allows the client to take the time he or she needs to feel feelings, without rushing to move away from the pain. Spiritually sensitive fertility counselors are attuned to ways in which clients' spirituality may serve as a source of support in the grieving process.

For some clients, part of the grief and healing process may include the practice of a ritual to formally acknowledge a loss. Rituals may be established practices through formal religions, such as funerals, burials or the Christian practice of Baptism of miscarried or stillborn babies. Clients may also choose to create their own ritual to remember the loss. In the *Case Studies* text, the ritual Melia and Lou use, after working through their grief with Nina, is a good example.

Identifying Options

Clients experiencing infertility usually are eager to identify solutions that will put an end to what is most always a very stressful and disappointing life chapter. Often, clients are better able to identify options and create plans after they have spent time in therapy exploring their feelings about infertility, parenthood, faith and their dreams of how their future family might look. Certain paths, such as ART, adoption, or living child-free, which once felt incomprehensible, may feel more viable after this exploration in therapy. If clients are spiritual, the fertility counselor can assist them in clarifying how spiritual beliefs may inform their decisions about parenthood moving forward. For some clients facing infertility, spiritual tenets provide guidelines that are reassuring and helpful in making choices about treatment. Making decisions that are consonant with their religious beliefs may mitigate, for these clients, accompanying feelings of loss or disappointment if parenthood is not the result of their treatment decisions. Other clients discover that they are willing to make choices that are not sanctioned by their faith communities. Sometimes clients are able to find a way to remain connected to their spiritual beliefs even if their choice departs from what is permissible by their religions. And, some clients choose to forsake their faith communities if they feel unsupported in their decisions about how to address their infertility. The process of identifying options is exemplified by the work Jessica does with her fertility counselor Pat. You will see in the *Case Studies* chapter how Jessica ultimately decides to adhere to the teachings of her Mormon Faith, and is able to feel at peace with it after exploring all options.

Spirituality as a Source of Strength

For many clients wrestling with infertility, spirituality is a main source of strength and healing from psychological distress caused by difficulty conceiving a child [32]. It is critical for fertility counselors to encourage clients to identify and draw upon this resource if it seems appropriate. Often, clients have built-in support systems in their faith communities and can call upon fellow believers or spiritual leaders for help. However, it is important to note that satisfaction with services and a sense of connectedness with providers is linked to including spirituality and religion in discussions about challenges with fertility [33]. It is also important to be aware of ways religious teachings assert patriarchal values that can be further shaming to women facing challenges conceiving [34].

Fertility counselors can help clients identify nontraditional expressions of spirituality in their lives that provide hope and strength while they are coping with infertility. Nonreligious clients may nevertheless engage in spiritual rituals that provide a sense of meaning and connection during the, often isolating, experience of infertility.

The fertility counselor may consider clients' search for meaning, purpose and connection to something greater than their own experiences in the same vein as other more traditional expressions of spirituality or religiosity. The experiences of Leslie and Jack, Lisa and Laura, and Julia in the *Case Studies* text demonstrate how spirituality can serve as a source of strength for clients.

Conclusion

Fertility counseling can be greatly enhanced by attending to the religious beliefs and spiritual practices of clients. A general understanding of the major religions of the world provides the fertility counselor with a good framework, but it is not adequate on its own. Practitioners who utilize an informed not-knowing stance can understand each client's unique experience of religious teachings and the influence those teachings may or may not have with

regards to what they are willing to do to have a child. In addition, working with spiritual practices and rituals to support clients in the midst of fertility counseling can greatly enhance the work and provide comfort and support for the clients. Along with supporting client strengths and resilience in the face of infertility, spirituality and religion can be used to avoid deeper psychological work. An ability to identify the signs of spiritual bypassing can help practitioners address this, or work collaboratively with a supportive person from within that spiritual community.

The interventions presented in this chapter are designed to give fertility counselors a sense of how themes of spirituality can be present with clients experiencing infertility, and to outline concrete interventions. For examples of how these interventions can be utilized, be sure to read the corresponding chapter in the *Case Studies* text. A thorough assessment of the client's spirituality can be vital to understanding the meaning made of infertility. It is also critical for the fertility counselor to pay attention to countertransference when providing counseling for infertility with clients who raise themes around spirituality. In order to meet clients where they are, and be most effective in helping them reach family building decisions that are best for them, fertility counselors must attend to the spiritual dimensions they present.

References

1. Dake CL. *Infertility: A Survival Guide for Couples and Those Who Love Them*. Birmingham, AL: New Hope Publishers, 2002.

2. Stein G. Hannah: a case of infertility and depression – psychiatry in the Old Testament. *Br J Psychiatry* 2010;**197** (6):492.

3. Roudsari RL, Allan HT. Women's experiences and preferences in relation to infertility counselling: a multifaith dialogue. *Int J Fertil Steril* 2011;5(3):158–167.

4. Magaldi-Dopman D. An "afterthought": counseling trainees' multicultural competence within the spiritual/religious domain. *J Multicult Couns Devel* 2014;**42** (4):194–204.

5. Gill CS, Freund RR. *Spirituality and Religion in Counseling: Competency-Based Strategies for Ethical Practice*. New York, NY: Routledge, 2018.

6. Hoge DR. Using spiritual interventions in practice: developing some guidelines from evidence-based practice. *Social Work* 2011;**56**(2):149–158.

7. Pargament KI. *Spiritually Integrated Psychotherapy: Understanding and Addressing the Sacred*. Hove: Guilford Press, 2011.

8. Klitzman R. How infertility patients and providers view and confront religious and spiritual issues. *J Relig Health* 2018;**57**:223–239.

9. Greil A, McQuillan J, Benjamins M, Johnson DR, Johnson KM, Heinz CR. Specifying the effects of religion on medical help-seeking. *Social Sci Med* 2010;**71**:734–742.

10. Sallam HN, Sallam NH. Religious aspects of assisted reproduction. *Facts Views Vis OBGYN* 2016;**8**(1):33–48.

11. Sewpaul V. Culture, religion, and infertility: a South African perspective. *Br J Social Work* 1999;**29**:741–754.

12. Layne LL. Pregnancy loss, stigma, irony, and masculinities: reflections on and future directions for research on religion in the global practice of IVF. *Cult Med Psychiatry* 2006;**30**:537–545.

13. Kahn SM. Making technology familiar: Orthodox Jews and infertility support, advice, and inspiration. *Cult Med Psychiatry* 2006;**30**:467–480.

14. Schenker JG. Assisted reproductive technology: perspectives in Halakha (Jewish religious law). *Reprod Biomed Online* 2008;**17**(3):17–24.

15. Roberts EF. God's laboratory: religious rationalities and modernity in Ecuadorian in vitro fertilization. *Cult Med Psychiatry* 2006;**30**:507–536.

16. Bharadwaj A. Sacred conceptions: clinical theodicies, uncertain science, and technologies of procreation in India. *Cult Med Psychiatry* 2006;**30**:451–465.

17. Al-Bar MA, Chamsi-Pasha H. *Contemporary Bioethics: Islamic Perspective*. London: Springer, 2015.

18. Inhorn MC. Making Muslim babies: IVF and gamete donation in Sunni versus Shi'a Islam. *Cult Med Psychiatry* 2006;**30**:427–450.

19. Seybold D. Choosing therapies: a Senegalese woman's experience with infertility. *Health Care Women Int* 2002;**23**:540–549.

20. Connor J, Sauer C, Doll K. Assisted reproductive technologies and world religions: implications for couples therapy. *J Fam Psychother* 2012;**23**:83–98.

21. White L, McQuillan J, Greil AL, Johnson DR. Infertility: testing a helpseeking model. *Soc Sci Med* 2006;**62**:1031–1041.

22. Jennnings PK. "God had something else in mind": family, religion, and infertility. *J Contemp Ethnogr* 2010;**39**(2):215–237.

23. Sheridan M. Addressing spiritual bypassing. In: Crisp BR, Ed. *The Routledge Handbook of Religion, Spirituality and Social Work*. New York, NY: Routledge, 2017, 358–368.

24. Jaffe J, Diamond MO. *Reproductive Trauma: Psychotherapy with Infertility and Pregnancy Loss Clients*. Washington, DC: American Psychological Association, 2011.

25. Alvare HM. Catholic teaching and the law concerning the new reproductive technologies. *Fordham Urban Law J* 2002;**30**:107–134.

26. Cohen C. Protestant perspectives on the uses of the new reproductive technologies. *Fordham Urban Law J* 2002;**30**:135–145.

27. Dutney A. Religion, infertility, and assisted reproductive technology. *Best Pract Res Clin Obstet Gynaecol* 2007;**21**(1):169–180.

28. Ott K. *A Time to Be Born: A Faith-based Guide to Assisted Reproductive Technologies*. Westport, CT: Religious Institute, 2009.

29. Schenker JG. Assisted reproductive practice: religious perspectives. *Reprod BioMed Online* 2005;**10**(3):310–319.

30. Simpson B. Managing potential in assisted reproductive technologies: reflections on gifts, kinship, and the process of vernacularization. *Curr Anthropol* 2013:**54**(7):87–96.

31. Proctor M. Bodies, babies, and birth control. *J Mormon Thought* 2003;**36**(3):159–176.

32. Ntiamoah D. The role of religiosity and spirituality in healing infertility and psychological distress. *J Philos Cult Relig* 2018;**38**:32–37.

33. Romeiro J, Caldeira S, Brady V, Hall J, Timmins F. The spiritual journey of infertile couples: discussing the opportunity for spiritual care. *Religions* 2017;**8**(4):76–90.

34. Göknar MD. *Achieving Procreation: Childlessness and IVF in Turkey*. Oxford: Berghahn Books, 2015.

Counseling Recipients of Nonidentified Donor Gametes

Patricia Sachs and Carol Toll

Where We Have Been, Where We Are, Where We Are Going

Introduction and Terminology

Since the first edition of this book, the terminology has changed in some areas related to recipient counseling, and reflects the continually evolving nature of the people and relationships linked through third-party reproduction. Donors who were selected from unidentified profiles in a database were referred to as "anonymous." However, with the rise of commercial genetic testing, anonymity can no longer be assured. Hence the change from " anonymous donor gamete" to "nonidentified"'; the implication being that one day, a nonidentified donor could most certainly become known to the recipient. The American Society of Reproductive Medicine (ASRM) has indicated that it is moving away from the use of "anonymous" [1] and will be continuing to update terminology to reflect this in the near future.

Furthermore, "donor siblings" are now referred to as "donor-linked individuals" to more accurately reflect that, unlike traditional siblings, they are not raised within the same family. We do not reference "donor moms" or "donor dads," as donors are simply "donors," since they do not parent the donor-conceived individual. Heterosexual couples may also be referred to as "opposite sex" couples, to move away from a heteronormative approach and acknowledge that we have seen an increase in many types of recipients using donor gametes: same sex couples, single women, single men and trans people. Recipient counseling has also grown to include people from a range of diverse backgrounds, cultures and countries, though travel restrictions due to the COVID-19 pandemic have placed limitations on cross-border reproductive care.

This chapter will focus on the many changes in the counseling of recipients that have evolved over the past

The addenda referred to in this chapter are available for download at www.cambridge.org/covington-clinical-guide

years, since the first edition of this book and over the 30 years we have each been practicing as fertility counselors. It will first address the history of donation, its uses today, and current research on the major issues relevant to donor recipient counseling at this time, and from an international perspective. The second part of the chapter will discuss practice implications for the counseling session today, and into the future.

History

The story of oocyte donation began in the 1980s, with the first egg donor pregnancy reported in Australia in 1984. Originally used for women with primary ovarian insufficiency (POI), egg donation evolved over the years to treat women who had survived cancer, experienced multiple pregnancy losses, carried genetic diseases, and had poor egg quality due to "advanced maternal age." Sperm donation, which had been utilized to treat men with severe male factor infertility, had been in existence for over 100 years and was the only option to achieve pregnancy in the female partners of men with no sperm or very low sperms counts. With the advent of ICSI in 1990, men with low sperm counts could still attempt pregnancy with surgical removal and injection of even one healthy sperm into the egg. A relatively new development is the creation of embryos through the use of donor egg and donor sperm. The resulting child, therefore, would be unrelated genetically to either parent. Due to these new developments, recipients may also find themselves with more embryos than they can use. They may then be in a position to consider becoming donors, themselves, of excess embryos (see Chapter 11 on embryo donation).

In the early days of sperm donation, secrecy was the primary approach recommended to couples by their physicians. Recipients were mainly heterosexual couples with male-factor infertility and following insemination they were told to basically "go home, have sex, and forget" what had happened. The husband's sperm was often mixed with the donor's sperm so that perhaps it might never be known which had actually led to conception. The approach was primarily for the protection of the husband from the shame and stigma of infertility, which was often associated with virility. Little thought was given to the longer-term implications of secrecy for the psychological well-being of the couple, let alone of a future child.

Today, due to many societal changes including the legalization of same sex marriages and greater acceptance/ normalization of single parenthood, the use of egg and sperm donation has broadened tremendously to now help form many different types of families: single women, same sex female couples, single men and same sex male couples, who utilize a gestational carrier in addition to an egg donor.

Psychosocial Impact

In the early days of recipient counseling of nonidentified donor gametes, we anticipated that it would involve dealing with much grief around the loss of the genetic connection to the potential child; fears about a lack of bonding and attachment during pregnancy; and later, rejection by the potential child of the parents, if their donor origins were ever discovered. Women needing a donated egg experienced feelings of being defective, damaged, and "less than," as their bodies did not work the way they were supposed to, and their husbands would feel helpless to ease their partner's pain. Men who required donor sperm would especially experience pain at their loss of a genetic tie to their child, as this was their only connection to a growing fetus; at least women who used an egg donor still had the opportunity to bond through the experience of pregnancy. Men also often experienced a greater sense of shock over their infertility, as, unlike with women and their eggs over time, the diminishing quality or quantity of sperm with aging is not a given. For those from cultures where the male "family line" was especially important, the use of donor sperm raised even greater issues of trauma and fear of rejection of themselves and a future child.

Making the Decision to Use a Donor

While of course some of those concerns still persist even today, donor conception has become so common and routinized that the starting point for recipient counseling now has become psychoeducation and implications, rather than counseling around grief and loss. The typical donor gamete recipients today seem overall accepting of the need for this type of treatment, often having exhausted other treatment attempts with their own

gametes, and even grateful for the opportunity that this medical advance provides them. Counseling therefore centers around a discussion of the issues most pertinent today: anonymity (or rather its nonexistence); disclosure; donor selection and social change; and more.

Issues Pertinent Today in Recipient Counseling (and into the Future)

Anonymity

As stated elsewhere in this book and chapter, the idea of an anonymous donor whose identity could almost assuredly remain secret forever, no longer exists; hence the change in language from "anonymous" to "nonidentified," implying that while unknown at present, the identity of the donor might well become known at some future time. In the past, recipients may have hoped for donor anonymity due perhaps to fears that if the donor became known to the child, they might want to pursue a relationship in the future or even reject the nongenetic parent in favor of the donor. For the donor's part, s/he might fear intrusion into their life in the future by a donor-conceived child, when their only intention had been to help the recipients to create *their* family, and perhaps s/he had never even told his/her spouse or their own children of the past donation.

Recipients and donors alike, today, must be counseled about the nonexistence of anonymity. For the most part, they realize that keeping the fact of donor conception secret from their offspring may be not only detrimental to the child's mental well-being, adjustment and relationship with their parents, but also impractical and impossible given the reality of genetic information that is available today. The psychoeducation of recipients, therefore, is and must continue to be about how they might prepare their potential child someday about what to expect if they wish to contact their donor. Would the child be looking primarily for updated or more extensive medical information? Or might they potentially be wanting some sort of relationship with the donor? Recipients should at least be made aware in the counseling session of this issue, and the fact that donors may react quite differently to requests for contact from a donor-conceived child. They should help prepare their child for what they might encounter, and the range of emotions that they might experience as a result.

One goal of recipient counseling, therefore, is to begin the discussion of creating a lifelong story that will "safeguard and promote the interests of donor-conceived offspring" ([2], p. 1135). Concurrently, donors should also be counseled about the likelihood that they may be contacted in the future by donor-conceived individuals, and the importance of sharing this information with their own offspring as well, as they too could be found through genetic registries. Since it is known that millions of people have now used genetic testing to find out information about their ancestry, the hope would be that this new genetic information is and will continue to be communicated to those involved in a way that protects privacy but also satisfies the need/right to know [2] (see also Chapter 13 on DNA and the end of anonymity).

Disclosure

The issue of whether, when and how to disclose to a potential child their donor origins was a significant component of recipients' counseling in the past. However, the appearance of wide-ranging genetic test kits with worldwide databases has made nondisclosure no longer an option. For parents who struggle to see the benefits of disclosure, the idea that their child might someday be contacted by a stranger claiming to be a relative who found them through DNA testing is most likely more distressing than deciding that they can reveal this information to their child in the way and at the time that feels best to them. Additionally, donor-conceived children may pick up on "hidden clues" [3], the fact that something feels different within the family, and if there is disclosure later on, this may cause damage to relationships and to the child's sense of trust and honesty. Rather than the shock, trauma and sense of betrayal that a child might feel towards their parents if this information is discovered accidentally, the "family story" can be revealed in a loving, age-appropriate way, and over time, adding more details and exploring deeper feelings as the child's interest and understanding grows.

It is, of course, important as a parent to pay close attention to how the child is reacting to and processing the information. If the child seems distressed or confused, then waiting for a better time when the child is more open and interested is appropriate. For example, a Swedish study of heterosexual parents with children aged 7–8 years sharing information about their identity-release sperm donors found that children act as "force or friction" in this process, and that recipient counseling can be a resource in assisting children with this information [4]. Helping recipients to see a potential child as a "whole person," with the fact that they are donor-conceived as just a "part" of who they are, not "only" who they are, is important in counseling, as other issues invariably will arise with their children (e.g.,

learning/social problems) which may take priority at any given time. The fertility counselor might give "permission" ahead of time for parents to put the issue of donor conception aside when needed and emphasize that "telling" is a process to be done over time rather than at a specific or one-time instance, depending always on the child's needs and best interests. It is important to note that families do best when children are told before the age of 7 [5]. In the sixth and final phase of this longitudinal study of families in the United Kingdom (UK) with donor-conceived children, adolescents were interviewed at age 14 and those who had been told at an early age were found to have more positive family relationships and higher levels of well-being.

In the past, recipients, also, struggled with the idea that even if they were to disclose their donor origins to a child, they would have little or no information about the donor to tell, thus causing only further distress. With the end of anonymity, the focus of counseling now shifts to helping recipients one day explore with their children the pros and cons of searching for and contacting their donor, and what to realistically expect. In another study looking at adolescents aged 14 who had all been told about their donor conception in early childhood, the findings showed that the majority felt "indifferent" about it, with a nearly equal number feeling either positive or ambivalent. Of the adolescents who had made contact with their donor, most felt positive about it, while the majority of those who had not been in contact remained interested in pursuing it [6]. Recipients can be counseled, therefore, that rather than fearing harm from possible future contact with a donor, they can feel encouraged that the evidence indicates that this can be a positive experience for the child and the family. (For more information see Chapter 14 on family life after donor-conception.)

Donor Selection/Social Change

In the past, when asked about what might be important to them in choosing a donor, recipients would commonly respond that they wished to find a donor who somewhat physically "looked like them," i.e., similar hair and eye color, body type and perhaps cultural background. Recipients tended to feel that if they had a child who physically resembled them and "fit in" with their extended family, the child and family both might have more privacy and face fewer potentially uncomfortable and invasive questions about "who they look like." A study by Becker on "resemblance talk," i.e., observations about a child's physical similarity to parents or other family members, found that parents of donor-conceived children felt quite vulnerable about this issue, in part because it embodied their sense of loss and was a reminder of their infertility [7]. Additionally, they wished to protect their children from the stigma and diminished sense of "legitimacy" that might come from a lack of family resemblance. Almost all parents had wished to find a donor that would help produce a child of the same race and who might look somewhat like them [7].

Recent societal changes and increased awareness of racial/ethnic disparities in the United States (US) have impacted recipients in a way not previously seen to this extent. Recipients now commonly state that they are open to donors from a variety of backgrounds. Recipients today may choose donors from different backgrounds, not only depending on availability, but also because of greater openness to creating diverse families. A recent change observed by fertility counselors is that of recipients seeming to consider as an option selecting a donor from a different background, though they might be concerned about not being "well-equipped" or sufficiently educated about the issues involved in raising a child of a different race/ethnicity/culture. They also worry about appearing culturally insensitive or even racist when considering selecting a donor.

The fertility counselor needs to recognize and address these feelings with recipients so as to be able to explore deeply what will be best for their individual family. For some, the choice of a donor of a different background would work perfectly well for them, their extended family and the child. For others, this might accentuate feelings of "different-ness" when a child may already feel this way due to their donor conception and may risk rejection from extended family who may see the child as not belonging. The goal, again, of counseling around this issue will be to try to understand and clarify the needs, expectations and reality of each particular recipient, rather than to make any assumptions based on recent societal changes and trends.

In looking at the research on donor selection by recipients, it becomes clear that little has been said about donors from different backgrounds. The questions of why this has not been addressed, as well as why there are fewer donors, remain. One study in the UK looking at egg and sperm donors from 2014–2018 showed fewer Asian donors compared to their percentage of the UK Asian population, perhaps due to cultural and religious factors that created stigma around donation [8]. The use of white donors in the UK, therefore, appears particularly high, perhaps due to the lack of availability of donors from certain ethnic groups.

In some countries, views are held that a child from a donor of a different race may be considered "other" and therefore not to be accepted by the family or culture, particularly if the child looks very different. In a study of cross-cultural reproduction, Swedish and Norwegian recipients were found to have travelled to Finland in search of donor eggs that would produce "a child of phenotypically plausible biological descent." The goal of recipients appeared to be achieving a child with a fair complexion, which, from the researchers' perspective seemed congruent with a larger history of racism in Europe [9]. Similarly, research on fertility clinics and egg donor agencies in South Africa revealed a matching process designed to maintain ""certain forms of whiteness" [10].

In other cultures, recipients of gamete donation may need additional support, as their communities may lack awareness of this type of treatment and the accompanying issues that arise over time. In Iran, for example, studies showed a reluctance by recipients to disclose the use of donor gametes for fear that a donor-conceived child would be ostracized in society and possibly harmed psychologically. Psychoeducation and support for these recipient couples as well as attempts to increase public awareness of reproductive donation could be helpful in decreasing stigma. Couples need not only support from family and friends in deciding to disclose, but also the availability of longer-term psychological counseling and support, as needed [11]. It is important to note that in some countries it may even be illegal for recipients to obtain donor gametes, and if they cross borders they may potentially face prosecution upon their return. Fertility counselors must therefore be aware of the risks and dilemmas recipients may face.

Identity-release Gamete Donation: The Future Is Here

There is little consensus about universal terminology for what are variously called "voluntarily registered donors," "identity-release donors," or "open-release donors." In many countries this option has become more popular as legislation has passed to enable and enforce this. For example, in Finland, prior to 2008, oocyte donors were only "nonidentified" but they could consent voluntarily to having their identifying information released to donor-conceived children; after 2008 donor-offspring could receive identifying information after the age of 18, if requested. A large Finnish survey revealed that a majority of both of these types of donors held positive (or neutral) feelings towards contact with donor offspring, with greater ambivalence expressed towards contact between their own children and donor offspring [12]. As one example in the US, "'open-release donors" now exist in the donor database of Donor Egg Bank USA (DEB USA). Open-release donors are those who consent to potential contact with a donor-conceived child, who can contact them, through the use of a third party, upon reaching the age of legal adulthood.

In the US, at least, nonidentified egg donation has historically been the choice (if not the only option) of most recipients. A recent study from an academic center for reproductive medicine in the US confirmed that anonymity continues to be the most common practice in gamete donation; however, there remains a conflict potentially between the donor-conceived child's "right to know" and protection of the donor's interests [13]. Counseling of recipients must include, therefore, a deep exploration of the meaning of anonymity, i.e., why anonymity may still be of such great importance to them, in order to help them make the best possible decisions for themselves and their future donor-conceived child.

With the decline of anonymity, it is likely that more and more fertility clinics will make open/identity-release donors an option for those going through a fresh donor cycle as well. It is important in recipient counseling, therefore, to explore and understand the reasons for reluctance to choose open or identity-release donors. If recipients are concerned about intrusion of the donor/donor's family into the donor-conceived child's life, this seems to be an unwarranted concern based at least on the Finnish study [9]. Similarly, for donors, fears about negative outcomes from being an identity-release donor also appear somewhat unfounded. (See Chapter 10 on counseling nonidentified gamete donors for more information.)

In sum, the ideas of the past about unknown donation are proving to be outdated, as the "stakeholder" parties increasingly are seeing the benefits of connecting. The use of donor gametes can no longer be seen just as a treatment option for infertility, but rather as a decision impacting family functioning into the future and should be addressed by the fertility counselor [14]. Recipient counseling should be seen as a potential resource to be returned to at different stages of the lifelong experience of being a donor-conceived family.

Recipient Counseling in Practice

The Role of the Fertility Counselor

Patients and those who provide medical care acknowledge the importance of emotional preparation before treatment through counseling. There is benefit not only at the time of treatment, but also it imparts a positive impact for the future of families created through egg donation, sperm donation and embryo donation.

There has been debate among mental health professionals and fertility counseling organizations over the role of the fertility counselor. Some believe that the counselor's role should have an evaluative component, a potential "gatekeeper." Others see it more as a matter of preparing the recipients for treatment, providing education on donor-related issues, discussing implications of donor conception, and offering support at the time of treatment and into the future.

It is important that the fertility counselor be clear with the recipients as to the nature of their role. When counseling is required as a part of the clinic's protocol, it is natural for them to experience some anxiety while wondering if they are being assessed or might possibly even be denied treatment. In the initial contact, the fertility counselor should inform the recipients of the purpose of and what can be expected from the session.

The goal of counseling and primary purpose of the interview is psychoeducational in nature, providing an opportunity to consider the implications of donor reproductive assistance, as well as to supply information and resources. The fertility counselor will ask about the recipient's journey to how they got to where they are today, including their reproductive history and decision to use donor gametes, while also exploring current thinking about major issues, and discussing how to handle these issues with others, as well as future children.

The general assumption is that most people seeking fertility treatment are emotionally healthy and not significantly different than others. These healthy individuals may find themselves faced with possibly unexpected and acutely stressful circumstances and are striving to cope, while making lifelong decisions. However, circumstances may come to light that indicate significant issues that need to be addressed before treatment is recommended. For couples, there may be significant disagreement about the desire to have a child, having a child through donor procedures, or about the impact of this decision on future family functioning. One partner may feel pressured or resistant to moving forward. Recipients may, also, exhibit significant relationship problems or find themselves at odds over life goals and financial choices. Communication may have become strained. Instead of being on their "best behavior" as is usually seen, patients may "fight" in front of the fertility counselor possibly as a way of expressing their distress. Untreated or unacknowledged mental health problems may impair their ability to complete treatment, make decisions or give consent. Changes in medications due to pregnancy may have emotional ramifications. Drug or alcohol abuse issues may surface and need to be addressed. Recipients may be reluctant to acknowledge their unique needs as a family created through donation. For example, they may be noncompliant with future children's rights to information where legally mandated. While it is expected that donor selection may be stressful and time-consuming for many, some recipients may have unusual difficulty in selecting a donor. Further, there are instances where no donor characteristics meet expectations. These difficulties may signal issues that need deeper exploration.

The role of the fertility counselor is, also, to bring appropriate concerns to the attention of the medical team and to work together with the recipients to find solutions to provide the best care possible. This might include making recommendations for referral to treatment, such as couple's counseling, drug/alcohol treatment or evaluation for psychiatric care/medication. The fertility counselor may also recommend to the medical team that treatment be deferred until the issues are resolved. By taking a ""defer not deny" attitude towards treatment, the fertility counselor is able to provide a valuable opportunity to think things through in a way that is supportive, rather than threatening, so as to help recipients make informed decisions about matters with lifelong implications.

The Recipient Interview

Historically, the recipient interview has been an in-person meeting interweaving topics in the broader areas of psychoeducation, preparation, assessment and support. Recipients entered the discussion at a challenging time, often considered a life crisis, with the choice to use a donor often offered as a "last option" after a long history of unsuccessful fertility treatment or an "only option" after less complicated treatment options were not deemed a possibility. The goal of the interview has been to establish a positive relationship between the fertility counselor and the recipients, providing a safe and confidential place to discuss their current situation as donor recipients, who now have an eye toward the future. Additionally, informing recipients of the availability and benefit of support groups, educational workshops, and online groups can reduce the perception that they are "the only ones" and help them to make connections with others who are walking the same path.

The fertility counselor's role today must also include an awareness of growth and change with regard to the issues discussed previously regarding anonymity, disclosure, donor selection, culture, diversity, cross-cultural influences and technology [1]. The worldwide pandemic of COVID-19 forced a crisis response, and fertility counseling rapidly moved out of the office and onto the computer screen. This change to virtual counseling has necessitated a reevaluation of licensing regulations as well. As the post-pandemic world emerges, no doubt there will continue to be some combination/hybrid practice of both telehealth and in-person counseling. (See Chapter 25 on telemental health in fertility counseling for more information.)

The recipient's interview can be organized into the following parts: administrative issues; the reproductive journey; donor selection; and disclosure/openness in donor conception.

Administrative Issues

Patient education is a vital part of the recipient's interview. Materials should be made available to the recipients prior to the meeting with the goal of providing information that can lead to a productive discussion of the issues, as well as for future use as resource information (see Addenda 9.1 and 9.2 for examples of helpful patient resource information).

As part of an informed consent process, the recipients should be provided with consent forms to be completed and returned to the fertility counselor prior to the counseling session (see Addendum 9.3 for an example). These consents should then be discussed verbally before the session begins. If the interview is to take place by telehealth/virtually, relevant consent forms should, also, be provided (see Addendum 9.4 for an example). The recipients should be made aware of how the information from the meeting will be used, i.e., what, if anything will be shared with the medical team, and should be given the opportunity to discuss any questions or concerns about this process. They should be informed about how any written notes/reports from the session will be retained or used. Recipients may also be encouraged to seek legal, ethical or religious counsel, if needed or desired.

The Reproductive Journey

The first step in the recipient's interview is to establish rapport between the fertility counselor and the recipients so that they feel open to sharing their reproductive history. Asking simply, "Tell me how you got to where you are today" can provide an opening for sharing the journey. This would include their story of how long they have been trying to become pregnant; what treatments they have tried; losses, disappointments, and history of counseling and medication, if relevant; and how they came to the decision to proceed with the use of donor gametes. The fertility counselor needs to understand the impact and meaning of their journey on their relationships, the stresses they have experienced, as well as the availability and use of social supports. What it means to use donor gametes, for each individual recipient, should be explored as well as any fears or concerns about bonding, sense of being a parent, and worries for the child-to-be. Using a donor to form a family and the meaning of the choice has unique ramifications. On the other hand, using a donor has evolved into a more mainstream approach, with families being formed in many ways. Helping recipients to frame their choices in a societal context as well as a personal one can relieve some stresses about family identity.

Donor Selection

When given the opportunity, most recipients are eager to discuss the topic of donor selection. Many may be inclined to choose a donor with physical characteristics, interests and talents that either are similar or complimentary to the recipients. There may be many choices before them: fresh vs. frozen eggs; eggs shared in a cycle with other recipients; clinic vs. private agency donors; nonidentified vs. known; or varying options for anonymity. Some recipients wish to know all they can about a donor, though the information available to them may be quite limited. Others may feel that personalizing the donor too much feels threatening to their legitimacy as a parent and prefer that a donor remain a distant figure. The role of the fertility counselor in donor selection may involve helping the recipients to grieve the loss of the genetic connection to a child, and to accept the limitations of the donor pool and the implications it has for the loss of their "fantasy" child. Discussing the donor screening process may help the recipients to feel more confident in their choice, while understanding that there is not just one "perfect" donor who can help them achieve the goal of a healthy baby.

Most recipients have little knowledge of and no experience in selecting a donor. It may appear a daunting task, made more intense by the very "deliberate" and "lifelong" nature of this decision. There is no right answer or only one ideal donor. Recipients may approach this with a combination of practical considerations (financial implications, desire for more than one child, availability of desired donor characteristics), age and time considerations, or consider broader issues (ethical, religious implications, where the child will be raised, age, being older parents, or using donor egg/sperm/embryo/egg and sperm). The fertility counselor can assist recipients in understanding their priorities and having realistic expectations that donors are "real people." This is especially important around anonymity issues and the prospect of a recipient's child becoming the young adult who may want to meet a donor or donor-linked individuals. Recipients often want to find a donor "they feel good about" and may include genetic and nongenetic donor characteristics. They often speak about the relief felt when they have selected a donor, after which the focus can return to the recipients.

Disclosure/Openness

The early days of sperm donation were shrouded in secrecy, and it was thought to be better that no one ever knew for sure whether the baby was conceived with the father's or the donor's sperm. This led to psychological confusion for all parties. Today, fertility counselors understand the problems that can occur around "family secrets" and generally agree it is best to be clear about the origin of the gametes. The language has also shifted from "secrecy" to "privacy," highlighting the idea that the use of donor gametes is not shameful, but rather a loving and positive choice.

In order to understand the thoughts, feelings and attitudes of the recipients about openness, the fertility counselor can ask questions that may lead to a discussion of how to handle this information with family, friends, and ultimately the child. Questions such as the following may be useful in exploring their concerns: How do they imagine their family might react to the knowledge that they had used a donor? Do they fear that the child might be rejected or not considered to be a member of the family? How important is resemblance in their family? This emphasis on genetic connection, or "resemblance talk" [7], is a way of "'reaffirming relationships" through focus on similarities between family members [15], and the lack thereof can potentially raise anxiety in parents. If recipients do disclose to family or friends, will they be able to respect their privacy? How might their future child feel upon learning that others knew of their donor history before they did? Through questions like these, the fertility counselor can also discover whether there are any moral, religious, cultural or ethical concerns. Recipients may find it beneficial to explore their current feelings, and although they have time to make decisions, it may be important for them to understand that choices they make right now may affect future options or cause regrets that information was shared too widely. Or, as has been said, "You can always tell, but you can't take it back!" Recipients may have reasons not to disclose to a child. The fertility counselor's role is to discuss the pros and cons while respecting the autonomy of the recipients to make their own decisions and suggest they may periodically reassess this decision.

It is important for the fertility counselor to remember that this may be the first time the recipients have considered disclosure issues. Periodically revisiting their thoughts and feelings about it provides an opportunity to keep current with the process of disclosure. Recipients may ask for guidance about who to tell, when to tell and how to tell about the use of a donor. Uncertainty about how to address these questions may present as a "'cloud of anxiety" over their heads as they enter into the role of recipients. It is beneficial to assess and to understand their specific concerns. It is helpful to empower the recipients by affirming that it is not a question of their *being* the parents, but rather *how* they *became* parents. The goal is to provide tools for their consideration, such as current thinking/research about openness and what to include in a family story. The story may begin with teaching about what makes a family, including the relationships in the family, the different ways families are configured, the desire to become parents and the need for help [15]. Table 9.1 provides a framework for the family story components.

Starting early (even while holding a baby in their arms) and choosing positive words, books for children, bedtime rituals or teachable moments with details appropriate to child developmental stages, helps to fill in the "whole story." Using a normal tone of voice, relaxed body language and empathetic responses to reactions from the child/ren allow them to see this information as something they have always known and part of the fabric of the family. Paying attention to technological and genetic advances helps prepare for possible links to other families in the future.

The Future

Changes in the field of reproductive medicine and technological advances almost certainly will have important implications for gamete donation and the role of the

Table 9.1 What to include in creating a family story

1. *What is a family?* Identify family members and how they came together.

2. *There are many kinds of families.* Describe the help needed for the creation of some families.

3. *Explain the desire to become parents and identify as one of the families that needed help.*

4. *Describe the help that was needed.* Use words, books for children, family story rituals and teachable moments.

5. *Relate the unique story throughout the developmental stages.* Use a normal tone of voice, relaxed body language and over time, include the details that tell the "whole story."

6. *Be open to listening with empathy to the varied responses of children as they learn about their stories.*

7. *Pay attention to technological advances that facilitate learning about genetic links to other families and what it might mean for possible future contact.*

fertility counselor. There is a growing trend toward openness with donor registries in use worldwide. Anonymity in general has nearly disappeared, replaced by a general understanding that it can no longer reasonably be guaranteed. With widespread use of low-cost genetic testing and data banks, and facial recognition software, social media and the like, the potential to be identified or even contacted in the future by a newly discovered donor-linked individual has increased. The fertility counselor must adapt to how these issues are addressed with potential donors and what it all means for the recipient's family. Advances in laboratory techniques in general, genetic screening of embryos prior to transfer, the possibility of sex selection of embryos, and options for donation of embryos to a donor embryo bank, impact choices available to donor recipients. The emphasis on lifelong psychoeducational support is a role that appears to be gaining greater importance. As we assist recipients to navigate and plan ahead, the ultimate goal remains as ever, past, present or future, to support the health and happiness of recipient families, however they were created.

References

1. Practice Committee of the American Society for Reproductive Medicine and the Practice Committee for the Society for Assisted Reproductive Technology. Guidance regarding gamete and embryo donation. *Fertil Steril* 2021;**115**(6):1395–1410.

2. Harper JC, Kennett D, Reisel D. The end of donor anonymity: how genetic testing is likely to drive anonymous donation out of business. *Hum Reprod* 2016;**31**(6):1135–1140.

3. Turner AJ, Coyle A. What does it mean to be a donor offspring? The identity experiences of adults conceived by donor insemination and the implications for counselling and therapy. *Hum Reprod* 2000;**15**(9):2041–2051.

4. Isaksson S, Skoog-Svanberg, A, Sydsio G, et al. It takes two to tango: information-sharing with offspring among heterosexual parents following identity-release sperm donation. *Hum Reprod* 2016; **31**(1):125–132.

5. Ilioi E, Blake L, Vasanti J, et al. The role of age of disclosure of biological origins in the psychological wellbeing of adolescents conceived by reproductive donation: a longitudinal study from age 1 to age 14. *J Child Psychol Psychiatry* 2017;**58**(3):315–324.

6. Zadeh S, Illioi EC, Jadva V, et al. The perspective of adolescents conceived using surrogacy, egg or sperm donation. *Hum Reprod* 2018; **33**(6):1099–1106.

7. Becker G, Butler A, Nachtigall RD. Resemblance talk: a challenge for parents whose children were conceived with donor gametes in the US. *Soc Sci Med* 2005;**61**:1300–1309.

8. Culley L, Hudson N, Rapport F. Assisted conception and South Asian Communities in the UK: public perceptions of the use of donor gametes in infertility treatment. *Hum Fertil* 2013;**16**(1):48–53.

9. Homanen R. Reproducing whiteness and enacting kin in the Nordic context of transnational egg donation: matching donors with cross-border traveller recipients in Finland. *Soc Sci Med* 2018;**203**:28–34.

10. Moll T. Making a match: curating race in South African gamete donation. *Med Anthropol* 2019;**38**(7):588–602.

11. Hadizadeh-Talasaz F, Simbar M, Latifnejad Roudsari R. Exploring infertile couples' decisions to disclose donor conception to the future child. *Int J Fertil Steril* 2020; **14**(3):240–246.

12. Miettinen A, Rotkirch A, Suikkari AM, et al. Attitudes of anonymous and identity-release oocyte donors towards future contact with donor offspring. *Hum Reprod* 2019;**34**(4):672–678.

13. De Melo-Martin I, Rubin LR, Cholst IN. "I want us to be a normal family": toward an understanding of the functions of anonymity among U.S. oocyte donors and recipients. *AJOB Empir Bioth* 2018;**9**(4):235–251.

14. Pasch LA. New realities for the practice of egg donation: a family-building perspective. *Fertil Steril* 2018;**110**(7):1194–1202.

15. Benward JM. Disclosure: helping families talk about assisted reproduction. In: Covington SN, Ed. *Fertility Counseling: Clinical Guide and Case Studies.* Cambridge: Cambridge University Press, 2015, 252–264.

Chapter 10

Counseling Nonidentified Gamete Donors

Uschi Van den Broeck and Laura Josephs

Introduction

> It's a very important decision in my life to donate sperm. It fits into my life and into my way of thinking. I'm a bone marrow donor, I'm registered as an organ donor in case I have an accident or something. I'm just saying, donating sperm is a very personal issue. It defines me.

The egg donor or sperm donor plays a very important role in the reproductive medicine practice. The donor is both a patient and not a patient. He or she is a patient in that he/she must be taken care of both physically and psychologically. He or she is not a patient, in that the donor is not presenting for his/her own treatment. When the gamete donor enters the consultation room, the fertility counselor will be challenged in his/her many different roles and responsibilities which we will identify and discuss in the following chapter. In addition, we will highlight key issues in how to prepare for and conduct the clinical interview, discuss the usefulness of psychological testing, demonstrate how to ensure that informed consent can be given, examine the short- and long-term implications of gamete donation and zoom in on the experience of the gamete donor.

This chapter focuses on nonidentified/unknown donors where no identifying information is provided on the donor and is not known to the recipients. At this point in time, there is consensus that anonymity is nonexistent (see Chapter 13 of this book). Donors as well as donor off-spring's right to information (identifiable or nonidentifiable) is dependent on the legal frameworks of the countries or institutions where gamete donation is practiced. (If the reader is interested in assessment and preparation in known donation and assisted reproduction, we refer the reader to the first edition of *Fertility Counseling*, Chapter 10.)

Nonidentified Gamete Donation: History and Current Practice

Though isolated cases of donor insemination were reported at various points in the early and mid-twentieth century, it was in the 1970s and 1980s that improved methods of sperm collection led to the creation of sperm banks. Oocyte donation requires the technology of in-vitro fertilization (IVF), which was pioneered in 1978. In 1983, oocyte donation was introduced when Australian physicians provided an egg from one patient to another fertility patient with ovarian failure [1].

Though sperm cryopreservation has been practiced for over 60 years, oocyte cryopreservation has been more challenging and was considered an experimental procedure by the American Society for Reproductive Medicine (ASRM) until 2012. Though egg donation with fresh oocytes (i.e., synchronization of donor egg recipient and donor in their cycles, retrieval of eggs from the donor, fertilization by the recipient's partner or sperm source, and consequent creation of an embryo or embryos which are then transferred into the uterus of the recipient) remains prevalent, egg "banks" of cryopreserved donor oocytes represent a growing trend in the world of egg donation.

Worldwide, gamete donation is by no means a homogenous entity. In some countries, gamete donation is legally prohibited. These prohibitions often stem from religious, moral and/or cultural traditions. The International Federation of Fertility Societies (IFFS) 2019 [2] survey found that sperm donation is allowed in 48 of 71 countries (68%), and is practiced in 41 of the 71 (58%). Oocyte donation is permitted in 43 of 69 (62%), but is performed in only 39 of 69 (56.5%). The majority of countries allowed compensation for sperm (67%) and oocyte donors (72%). The compensation usually included reimbursement for donors' time and expenses only (specifically for sperm donors 54% and oocyte donors 55%) though sometimes donors were compensated beyond their time and expenses (12% of sperm donors and up to 17% of oocyte donors). The practice of compensation beyond reimbursement was found in 11 countries which include the United States (US), Russian Federation, Argentina, Brazil, Bolivia, Colombia, Ecuador, Venezuela, Georgia, Greece and India.

Most of the surveyed countries [2] reported having regulations regarding anonymity of donors either by national or federal laws (57%), regional laws (9%), governmental agency overseeing these practices (15%) or professional organizations (35%). In addition, some countries (Cameroon, Colombia, Egypt, Germany, Greece, Jordan and Switzerland) regulated anonymity via what they called "cultural practice or a religious decree." Finally, 13% of surveyed countries did not report having any regulations.

Disclosure of information about gamete donors to the offspring varied widely according to the 2019 IFFS survey. Some countries, 22 of 46 (48%), allowed nonidentifying data to be provided by the donor to the offspring. Another 14 of 43 (30%) allowed identifying data to be disclosed, including Australia, Austria, Cameroon, Canada, Finland, Greece, Iceland, Kazakhstan, New Zealand, Nicaragua, Norway, Russian Federation, Switzerland and the US. However, these practices were only reported to be "customary" by a few of those countries.

Interestingly, the information from offspring to the donor is much less common practice: in only 40% of the countries surveyed could the donors obtain nonidentifying data from the offspring. Those countries include Australia, Barbados, Bolivia, Colombia, Finland, Greece, Hungary, Iceland, Kazakhstan, New Zealand, Russian Federation, Sri Lanka, Switzerland, Thailand, the US, United Kingdom (UK) and Uruguay. Australia, Cameroon, Kazakhstan, New Zealand, Russian Federation and the US allowed identifying information to be obtained by donors. Though available, disclosure practices were only observed in 53% of the countries regarding offspring to donor information and only in 33% of countries regarding donor to offspring information.

Gamete Donation and the Role of the Fertility Counselor

I think it's important to be able to see a professional counselor because, you know, it needs to be a conscious decision. You have to be sure you know what you're getting into.

The fertility counselor is a mental health professional with specialized training who, in the context of gamete donation, often serves multiple functions. One important function is consulting with the gamete donor for evaluation and counseling. Within this function the fertility counselor plays multiple critical roles, from "assessing the suitability of the donor, to facilitating the donor's understanding of the implications of donating one's genetic material to another person, and in providing long-term support and education" [1,3]. It is important that the fertility counselor recognizes the complex nuances of his/her clinical relationship with the donor.

A primary aim of the fertility counselor is to assess the donor in order to determine his/her suitability as a provider of gametes/genetic material to others (the recipients of the genetic material). But there are other goals as well. Specifically, the fertility counselor is addressing these broad questions:

1. Is there reasonable certainty that the donor is without significant psychological difficulties that could potentially indicate problematic genetic susceptibilities that could be passed on to prospective genetic offspring?
2. Is there reasonable certainty that the donor is being honest and forthright in the medical and psychosocial information given, as most of history taking is self-report?
3. Is there reasonable certainty that the donor can comply with donation requirements in a responsible manner and, for the egg donor, can psychologically withstand the physical burdens of oocyte donation in order to complete the donation process?
4. Is there reasonable certainty that the life experience of donating would be psychologically tolerable for the donor, that there are neither inherent psychological susceptibilities nor specific emotions/psychological conflicts about donating gametes which could render the experience of donation emotionally harmful or destabilizing for the donor?

It is important for the fertility counselor to recognize the nature of his/her clinical relationship with the donor, and gamete donor candidates need to be made aware that the fertility counselor is meeting with them for assessment rather than therapeutic purposes. At the same time, the fertility counselor must prioritize the psychological well-being of the egg or sperm donor in the fertility counselor's dealings with the donor and with the medical team.

In their Practice Committee opinion in 2021 [4], the American Society of Reproductive Medicine (ASRM) strongly recommends psychological evaluation and counseling by a qualified mental health professional of oocyte and sperm donors. In addition, the European

Society of Human Reproduction and Embryology (ESHRE) has issued a wide array of Task Force reports including one on gamete donation [5]. Included in the ESHRE guidelines are recommendations that the psychological evaluation include an assessment "of the general abilities and intellectual capacity of the donor candidates." More specifically, the Psychological Special Interest Group (SIG) of ESHRE published Guidelines for Counselling Infertility, a comprehensive document outlining infertility counseling issues with specific clinical recommendations on sperm and oocyte donation [6]. In addition, many countries have professional (in)fertility counseling organizations that offer practice guidelines for gamete donation such as Germany (Beratungsnetzwerk für Kinderwunsch Deutschland, (BKID)), the UK (British Infertility Counseling Association, (BICA)), Canada (Canadian Fertility and Andrology Society – Counselling Special Interest Group) and The Australian and New Zealand Infertility Counsellors Association (ANZICA).

Over the years, worldwide, fresh egg donation cycles have generally taken place within a reproductive medicine practice or program where egg donors are evaluated by a fertility counselor, as per ASRM recommendations [4], frequently one who practices within the reproductive medicine program or has an ongoing affiliation with the program. In contrast, sperm donors were historically not offered fertility counseling for gamete donation. Donation cycles generally take place in physicians' offices and reproductive medicine programs, with sperm banks supplying the frozen sperm and, while sperm donors are evaluated medically by the banks, they rarely met with a mental health professional for fertility counseling or assessment. However, in recent years there has been growing pressure to include counseling and, as a result, sperm banks in the US and worldwide are increasingly including psychological evaluation as part of their donor assessment process.

Assessment of the Gamete Donor

The psychological evaluation of the gamete donor and the attention to the donor's well-being go hand in hand in the fertility counselor's interactions with the donor. The fertility counselor will need to draw on and explicate his/her different roles – as an evaluator, supportive counselor and implications counselor – so as to be able to approach the counseling session in a transparent way [3]. It's recommended that fertility counselors address these multiple roles and purposes of the assessment at the start of the consultation. In addition, information about confidentiality and if, how, and when information from the consultation and psychological testing can be shared with the medical team, as well as the potential recipient of the gametes, should be discussed with the potential gamete donor.

Evaluation of the donor involves a psychological assessment that includes a clinical interview that can be complemented by standardized psychological testing. Some professional organizations (such as the ASRM) have recommendations about the use of psychological testing, though the practice seems to vary internationally. Often, either the Minnesota Multiphasic Personality Inventory-2 (MMPI-2) or the Personality Assessment Inventory (PAI) is used for gamete donation assessment. (The accompanying *Case Studies*, Chapter 10 on gamete donation provides insight in how psychological testing can be used clinically in gamete donation assessment.)

Furthermore, topics of interest in the clinical interview of gamete donors can consist of exploring the donor's childhood and life history, his/her psychological functioning both as a child and as an adult, and the assessment of any psychopathology, including possible mental health and substance abuse issues. Table 10.1 contains a detailed list of areas to be addressed in the psychological assessment of the gamete donor.

Psychological assessment of the donor also includes a detailed effort to understand the donor's relationship to his/her donation: motivation for and feelings about donating gametes; feelings about the prospective genetic offspring; implications of the donation in terms of anonymity vs. identity-release; and implications of the donation in light of the impossibility of assuring permanent anonymity for the donor, regardless of intended anonymity status. Table 10.2 details important areas to cover in speaking with donors about the psychological meaning of and implications of donating one's gametes.

During the course of the psychological assessment process and when taking into account the donor's well-being, the fertility counselor may uncover aspects of the donor's emotional status, which could indicate that either: (1) s/he might not be suitable as a provider of gametes/genetic material; or (2) s/he might be adversely impacted by serving as a gamete donor – or both. Psychological indicators for acceptance or rejection of gamete donors have been described by several authors [1, 4]. Donors should be without significant psychopathology and without significant current stress, including significant economic instability. They should be able to

Table 10.1 Donor interview: psychological assessment

(A) Current/Adult Life Situation

1. Job/career
2. Educational background
3. Relative stability of life situation vs. current/ongoing stresses
4. Marital/relationship status and relationship history
5. Interpersonal/social relationships
6. High and low points of donor's adult life

(B) Childhood/Family History

1. Family constellation/family life
2. Donor's personality/experience of self as a child
3. Donor's experience of parents
4. Parents' relationship with each other
5. Donor's experience of siblings
6. Significant family problems – physical or mental illness of parent or other family member, alcoholism/substance abuse in family member, abuse within or outside family, sexual abuse within or outside the family
7. High and low points of donor's childhood

(C) Psychological Assessment

1. Mood and affect of donor
2. Content and process of thought
3. Donor's communication with interviewer
4. Assessment of possible mood disorder
5. Assessment of possible anxiety disorder
6. Assessment of possible eating disorder
7. Assessment of possible alcohol/substance use/abuse
8. Assessment of psychosis

(D) Psychological History

1. History of psychological difficulties
2. History of psychotherapy
3. Psychiatric medication usage past or present
4. Alcohol/substance abuse history
5. Family history of psychological and/or substance problems

Table 10.2 Donor interview: implications of donation

(A) Motivation

1. Stated motivation for donating eggs or sperm
2. Altruistic and/or economic motives, or other motives (personal/psychological motives)
3. Need for money, plan for using money earned through donating
4. Any coercion/pressure from others (e.g., for financial reasons)
5. History of reproductive/pregnancy loss or pregnancy termination
6. Donor's relationship to his/her own children

(B) Donation of Genes/Genetic Connection with Prospective Child

1. Perceived connection to recipient(s); feelings about person(s) receiving gametes
2. Relinquishment of control/dominion over gametes
3. Feelings about genetic connection with child "out there" who is not one's own
4. Thinking about prospective genetic connection in the shorter and longer term
5. Relationship to/feelings about own's own gametes/DNA

(C) Anonymity vs. Identity Release Issues

1. Clarity of donor regarding anonymous vs. nonanonymous nature of gamete donation
2. Comfort of donor with anonymity (or nonanonymity) plan
3. Limits of anonymity
4. Implications of anonymity or identity release over the long-term
5. Willingness to be contacted in the future if there is medical need of donor-conceived offspring

(D) Physical/Medical Aspects

1. Comfort with medical setting
2. For egg donors, comfort with medical procedures and medications
3. For egg donors, appreciation of risks of donation process
4. Restrictive aspects of serving as a gamete donor

(E) Social Support

1. If donor has an intimate partner, has he/she discussed the donation with the partner?
2. Is donating likely to introduce any difficulties into the donor's primary relationship?
3. Has donor discussed prospective donation with others in social network?
4. Does donor have good sources of social support?

provide informed consent. Their standardized psychological testing should be within normal limits. Positive history of major psychiatric disorders or substance use disorders, or history of legal problems/sociopathy would warrant exclusion of the prospective donor. Family history of psychiatric disorders or substance abuse would also potentially rule out the prospective donor. Though historically the active use of psychotropic medications was found to be an excluding factor, nowadays the use of psychotropic medications is more frequent and commonly prescribed for a range of psychological symptoms and complaints. Therefore, the active use of psychotropic medication is not an excluding factor per se but needs to be evaluated in light of the possibility of passing on significant psychological or psychiatric problems to genetic offspring, as well as the impact of the donation procedure on the emotional stability of the prospective donor. In this situation the prospective donation may conflict with the donor's own interest. In contrast, there are prospective gamete donation cases that are halted due to program/recipient interests, as opposed to the donor's interests. A case where the donor herself is without significant psychological problems, yet has a family member with psychological and/or substance abuse problems, would be an example of the latter.

Assessment of Donor Motivations

It is important for fertility counselors to discuss with the prospective donor his or her motivations as well as his or her sense of the implications, now and in the future, of making a donation. For donors who are compensated monetarily, it is to be expected that economic motives will be present. However, if the fertility counselor perceives that the donor desperately needs money, this will compromise the prospective donor's ability to evaluate his/her comfort with donation with reasonable objectivity. For donors who are donating in a system/country without monetary compensation, it is to be expected that more altruistic motives, as well as more personal and psychological motives, may play an important role in the decision to donate. In these cases, the fertility counselor should ascertain if these motives are balanced in a healthy way and that the prospective donor is aware of the short- and long-term implications of donating gametes. In addition, the fertility counselor needs to be aware of and able to explore and make explicit the multifactorial aspects of gamete donation. The different aspects of a prospective donor's motivation can then be addressed in implications counseling and integrated into a balanced decision [7].

Evaluating Informed Consent

The process of obtaining informed consent from a prospective donor may not be straightforward because of the multilayered nature of the donor's motivation. Skillern and colleagues point out that, for the egg donor, financial compensation "may limit information seeking and impair decision-making" ([8], p. 1737). Beyond an appreciation of the physical risks, it is vital that the fertility counselor ascertain that the gamete donor understands as much as possible about the short-term and long-term emotional implications of donation [7]. Skillern and associates have developed the Egg Donor Informed Consent Tool (EDICT) in order to better assess prospective donors' understanding of the process of egg donation and its risks, especially the physical risks. Parallel to this there may be factors and pressures that hinder the fertility team or program in providing adequate informed consent and taking into account the multilayered donor motivation. For example, as Skillern and associates describe, the physician or donor recruiter "may be eager to have a potential donor agree to proceed" ([8], p. 1737).

Weighing Conflicts around Donor Autonomy

In certain cases, a donor's autonomy needs to be balanced against the potential negative or detrimental impact on the donor's current (committed) relationship. If the donor is married, or has a significant other, and the partner opposes the donation, the fertility counselor should consider excluding the donor, given the weight of foreseeable harm to the donor's committed relationship and thus to his/her day-to-day life and future. However, many gamete donors evince a less clear-cut version of this dynamic, as the prospective donation is not always openly discussed in the relationship. The fertility counselor should then address the reasoning or motivation behind this lack of transparency. For a prospective donor who is not at all certain about the future of his/her current intimate relationship and who makes life decisions very independently of the partner, donation might proceed so long as the donor understands the potential implications and emotional risks of the planned donation. Worldwide, practices vary in their requirement to include a donor's significant other in the assessment and/or informed consent process. Though the impact of gamete donation on the partner's current and future relationship is equally important for sperm donors as for egg donors, this is usually not reflected in clinical practice. In the case of sperm donors, many fertility centers or sperm banks don't even offer psychological counseling for the donor himself, nor do they seek the input of a current partner or spouse. In contrast, in the case of oocyte donors, the practice to offer counseling for both the prospective donor and her partner is more commonplace.

Addressing Limits to Anonymity and Access to Information

Importantly, a gamete donor assessment should include an in-depth discussion of issues regarding the possibility of discovery of personal and identifying information of the donor, even regardless of the legal system and secure and confidential recordkeeping of the gamete donor program [7]. In the recent decade, there has been a rapid increase and growth in the possibility and use of direct-to-consumer genetic testing in addition to other diagnostic tools available on the Internet. Most importantly, direct-to-consumer genetic testing protocols, such as 23andMe and Ancestry DNA, are available to the public and arguably will only become more widely used over time. These protocols can potentially link up individuals, with their agreement, who are genetically related to each other. A donor-conceived individual could be linked to a close relative of the donor, even if the donor him/herself did not participate in such testing. In fact, cases have already been reported where individuals have learned through direct-to-consumer genetic testing that they have been conceived via sperm donation, or who their donor is, prompting the conclusion that "there is no such thing as anonymity" [9,10] when it comes to sperm donation. As individuals conceived with egg donation (a newer technology) grow up, this can be applied to donor-egg-conceived individuals as well [7]. In addition, other noncommercial initiatives have created registries to facilitate and provide opportunities to access information both for donor-conceived offspring, their parents as well as donors. Some of these registries are founded by donor-conceived offspring such as the Donor Sibling Registry in the US. Others are government funded such as the Donor Conceived Register in the UK.

Even in countries still offering an anonymous system in gamete donation, there should be an appreciation and acceptance of the gamete donor of the various ways in which such anonymity is limited by current and future genetic testing [10]. In addition to societal changes and technological advances, gamete donors should also be aware of the possibility of future legal changes that may affect donor anonymity. In light of all these changes and future challenges, the fertility counselor should be aware of the implications for all stakeholders, not only donors but also recipients and donor offspring as well as the fertility center offering gamete donation. (See Chapters 13 and 14 for more information.)

Experience of the Gamete Donor

As with many things in life, practice makes perfect. Fertility counselors performing assessments and providing counseling for prospective gamete donors learn best about the specifics and pitfalls of gamete donation by seeing as many different donors as they possibly can. However, today a growing body of evidence in the literature [7,11,12] can help us gain insight into donor characteristics and experiences that we should take into account when meeting with a prospective egg or sperm donor.

Motivation of Gamete Donors

In general, studies have distinguished between four different types of motivation: altruism, financial compensation, procreation or genetic fatherhood, and finally questions or concerns about the donor's own fertility. It seems evident that a gamete donor's motivation is multifaceted. However, in practice, the focus is mostly on either financial or altruistic motives and these are frequently thought of as being diametrically opposed to one another. Other factors, such as legal and institutional aspects (e.g., the system a country or center uses to recruit donors), or the way in which the donor is asked about his/her motivation can influence what a donor will reveal about his/her primary incentive (e.g., the donor knows about laws against financial compensation). Though financial or altruistic motives may be seen as primary motives, a number of secondary motives may be just as, or even more, important to potential donors as they are of a more intrinsic nature but perhaps not perceived by the donor as socially acceptable. Secondary motives frequently mentioned in studies include procreation, passing on their own genes and investigating their own fertility status. Interestingly, egg and sperm donors' primary motivations seem similar. Sperm donors seem to indicate more secondary motivations (such as procreating and investigating their fertility status in their decision to donate sperm), but these motivations are, also, evident among egg donors.

Recruitment Strategies

Interestingly, the way in which donors are recruited can influence the type of donor a center may attract. The literature clearly shows that the media, advertisements and word-of-mouth advertising are good ways to inform and attract potential donors. The role of relational factors and donors' perceptions of the views of the wider social network should be taken into account when recruiting donors [7,13,14]. An anonymous questionnaire study [14] among a large sample of students showed that those not interested in donating sperm stated that the genetic link to the offspring was of major importance to them. The researchers concluded that for nondonors the meaning of having a child with a genetic link of one's own is valued so highly that it can only be linked to the self and not to donated gamete offspring. By contrast, altruism seemed more important to doubtful donors whereas potential donors reported passing on one's genes and enhancing one's self-worth as more important than doubtful donors.

Attitude of Donors with Regard to Donor Offspring

Recent literature shows that a large proportion of donors seem to support disclosure to children conceived by their gametes [15]. Furthermore, many oocyte and sperm donors seem willing to donate in an (more) identifiable system and are open to revealing nonidentifying information to offspring [16,17]. However, attitudes towards disclosure and anonymity appear complex and more well-designed studies are needed to inform legislation and clinical practice about donors' preferences and experiences which can then allow adequate counseling for potential donors.

There is some evidence to show that the demographic profile of recruited sperm donors, in particular their marital status and age, can have a profound impact on their attitude towards anonymity and contact with offspring, though results remain inconsistent [11,14]. Younger, single donors are often students largely motivated by financial gains and compensation, are less likely to continue donating without the guarantee of anonymity, and are less likely to want or seek contact with offspring. They are, however, open to revealing nonidentifying information to offspring. It has been suggested (both by researchers and actual donors) that donors of this type may benefit from implications counseling, as they may not fully be aware of the future implications of their current sperm donation.

On the other hand, older, married donors who often have children of their own are largely motivated by altruism related to the positive experience of fathering a child. Most of them would continue donating even when anonymity could not be guaranteed. This type of donor feels comfortable disclosing nonidentifying information, but the point of view on contact and disclosure to offspring varies: some of these donors are more open to contact with offspring because they take into account offspring's feelings and curiosity about their conception; others do not wish contact with offspring.

The literature reveals an important distinction between potential donors' openness towards anonymity and the release of nonidentifying information, and their openness towards providing the recipients and offspring with identifying information. Though there seems to be willingness to provide and exchange information with offspring, there was also uncertainty about negative consequences (for the donor and his/her family) and a certain amount of ambiguity [17]. More pre- and postcounseling may help to reduce some of the donor's uncertainties and make more explicit the possible impact on the donor and his/her children. Though few studies have investigated the impact of donor counseling on donor attitudes, there is some evidence to suggest that attitudes towards disclosure changed after a counseling session [18].

Research seems to indicate that donors often think about donor offspring. Specifically, they have thoughts and even worry about donor offspring's well-being. Some egg donors report feeling somewhat responsible for the donor offspring and are worried about donor recipients' parenting style. The same concern for donor offspring's well-being was consistently reported in several studies investigating sperm donors [13]. Even more so, some gamete donors feel morally obliged to help resulting donor offspring, if this were ever necessary [13]. The interest of gamete donors in having information about the result of their donation and moreover in the well-being of resulting children might be explained by the fact that these donors helped create the child and share some of their genes.

Impact of Legislation on Gamete Donors

As the 2019 IFFS survey [2] clearly demonstrates, legislation, as well as regulation of gamete donation, differs considerably across different regions in the world and countries. There is some indication that country of residence (and regulations and laws that are country-specific) may influence the type of motivation in gamete donors. Countries or centers with commercial systems (such as the US) often report higher percentages of donors with a financial motivation, whereas countries or centers (such as Sweden, Australia) without financial compensation report higher percentages of altruistic motivation [11]. Several countries have recently made changes in their legislation regarding donor anonymity (State of Victoria in Australia in 2016, Finland in 2007, UK in 2005, the Netherlands in 2004). A frequently cited concern from medical professionals providing assisted reproductive treatments is that the number of donors will decrease without an anonymous system. However, in those countries such as Sweden and the UK where donor-conceived offspring have the right to access information about their origins, no long-term decrease in donations has been found. Interestingly, studies did show a change in the donor profile and a shift towards a donor that is older and well-informed about the decision to donate gametes [20].

Psychosocial Needs of the Donor

Whatever the motivation a potential egg or sperm donor may have in starting the donation process, it is clear that some of the donor's attitudes (e.g., anonymity, donor payment, contact with offspring) may shift during the donation process. For example, potential donors are often more unclear about anonymity and disclosure to offspring compared with actual donors. However, a considerable number of donors feel very uncertain and undecided about both anonymity and future contact with offspring. This implies that counseling pre- and postdonation might be beneficial to donors, especially considering the cultural shift towards more openness and the limits of anonymity in third-party reproduction.

Gamete donation programs should ensure adequate follow up of prospective donors [3,4,7]. Particularly in the case where a prospective donor has been rejected, the fertility counselor should address the reason for exclusion from the program and, whether it be medical or psychological, should attempt to ensure that the exclusion does not destabilize the donor's (current and future) emotional health. In these cases, the rejected donor's self-esteem may be affected and/or s/he may have questions regarding the impact on his/her own current or future children. The fertility counselor can provide reassurance in terms of the very strict guidelines for gamete donors and offer a platform for the rejected donor to discuss the implications of his/her exclusion from the program.

Sometimes egg donors are excluded due to results of psychological testing, such as the MMPI-2 or the PAI. Psychological testing in screening gamete donors is useful in that such testing may reveal the possibility of hidden psychopathology. If testing indicates the presence of significant psychopathology such as a substance use disorder, psychosis, mood or anxiety disorder, or a personality disorder, then the candidate would not be allowed to proceed as a donor. Psychological testing can also indicate if the donor is approaching the process in an open, forthright manner. Both the MMPI-2 and PAI contain validity scales, which reflect subjects' defensiveness. It is expected that donor applicants, who are being evaluated, will attempt to present well, and will therefore show a degree of defensiveness. However, significant defensiveness will diminish the validity of a test's clinical scales.

Screening out the possibility of psychopathology is an important goal for a gamete donation program. However, for the individual donor candidate herself, psychological testing is but one important piece of data. Should a prospective donor be excluded due to psychological testing results, it is important to clarify with the candidate that no single psychological test is diagnostic, and the testing should not be taken by her as definitive evidence of a particular pathology. After discussing with the candidate, the need for the donor egg program to "err on the side of caution" in not accepting donors who may have underlying psychological problems, the meaning and possible implications of her test results, for her personally, should be discussed. If she identifies at all with the problems that the testing shows, then referral for appropriate treatment is indicated. Finally, though psychological testing is routine and often mandatory in egg donation programs throughout the US, this practice is not applied globally. Many countries and centers prefer relying on the clinical impression and experience of the fertility counselor and the self-report of the donor candidate in screening for psychopathology. These clinical issues will be discussed more in depth in the *Case Studies*, Chapter 10.

Impact of Gamete Donation on the Donor

On the whole, there is consistent evidence demonstrating that the oocyte donation procedure is well tolerated and most donors of all donation types report high levels of satisfaction with the quality of medical care [12,16]. An important feature in a donor's experiences of donation was the opportunity to meet with the fertility counselor. Studies have found that the majority of donors of all donor groups questioned found counseling invaluable and helpful [18] though there was often not much interest in follow-up counseling [15]. Recent years have seen an increase in studies [15,16,19] focusing on and documenting the experience of sperm donors that go beyond a technical "means to an end" and that start to consider the donor as an important "party" in third-party reproduction.

In this way, there can be more room for and attention to the inherent complexities, interests and resulting ambiguities of all stakeholders in gamete donation: *the donor* in terms of his/her rights, responsibilities, motives and attitudes; *the intended parents* and their rights, responsibilities, opportunity for access to information, social parenthood vs. genetic parenthood; *the child* and his/her right and access to information about his/her origin; *the professionals* in terms of their (legal and/or medical) responsibility in screening potential donors and parents, their responsibilities towards the resulting child; and finally *society* with its legal, religious, cultural, and ethical frameworks that guides third-party reproduction practices.

References

1. Applegarth LD, Kingsberg SA. The donor as patient: assessment and support. In: Covington SN, Burns LH, Eds. *Infertility Counseling: A Handbook for Clinicians*, 2nd ed. New York, NY: Cambridge University Press, 2006, 339–355.

2. International Federation of Fertility Societies' Surveillance (IFFS) 2019: Global Trends in Reproductive Policy and Practice, 8th ed. *Global Reprod Health* 2019;**4**(1):29.

3. Braverman AM. Mental health counseling in third-party reproduction in the United States: evaluation, psychoeducation, or ethical gatekeeping? *Fertil Steril* 2015;**104**(3):501–506.

4. Practice Committee of the American Society for Reproductive Medicine and the Practice Committee of the Society for Assisted Reproductive Technology: Guidance regarding gamete and embryo donation. *Fertil Steril* 2021;**115**(6):1395–1410.

5. ESHRE: Task Force on Ethics and Law. Gamete and embryo donation. *Hum Reprod* 2002;**17**:1407–1408.

6. Guidelines for counseling in infertility [Online]. Available from: www.eshre.eu

7. Pasch LA. New realities for the practice of egg donation: a family-building perspective. *Fertil Steril* 2018;**110**(7):1194–1202.

8. Skillern A, Cedars M, Huddleston H. Egg donor informed consent tool (EDICT): development and validation of a new informed consent tool for oocyte donors. *Fertil Steril* 2013;**99**:1733–1738.

9. Samplaski M, Klipstein S. There is no such thing as anonymity: loss of donor sperm anonymity in the era of direct to consumer (DTC) genetic testing. *Fertility and Sterility*, Editorial Office, American Society for Reproductive Medicine. Available from: www.fertstertdialog.com/posts/there-is-no-such-thing-as-anonymity-loss-of-donor-sperm-anonymity-in-the-era-of-direct-to-consumer-dtc-genetic-testing [last accessed June 16, 2022].

10. Harper JC, Kennett D, Reisel D. The end of donor anonymity: how genetic testing is likely to drive anonymous gamete donation out of business. *Hum Reprod* 2016;**31**(6):1135–1140.

11. Van den Broeck U, Vandermeeren M, Vanderschueren D, Enzlin P, Demyttenaere K, D'Hooghe T. A systematic review of sperm donors: demographic characteristics, attitudes, motives and experiences of the process of sperm donation. *Hum Reprod Update* 2013;**19**(1):1–15.

12. Purewal S, van den Akker OBA. Systematic review of oocyte donation: investigating attitudes, motivations and experiences. *Hum Reprod Update* 2009;**15**:499–515.

13. Jadva V, Freeman T, Kramer W, Golombok S. Sperm and oocyte donors' experiences of anonymous donation and subsequent contact with donor offspring. *Hum Reprod* 2011;**26**:638–646.

14. Provoost V, Van Rompuy F, Pennings G. Non-donors' attitudes towards sperm donation and their willingness to donate. *J Assist Reprod Genet* 2018;**35**(1):107–118.

15. Lampic C, Skoog Svanberg A, Sydsjö G. Attitudes towards disclosure and relationship to donor offspring among a national cohort of identity-release oocyte and sperm donors. *Hum Reprod* 2014;**29**(9):1978–1986.

16. Bracewell-Milnes T, Saso S, Bora S, et al. Investigating psychosocial attitudes, motivations and experiences of oocyte donors, recipients and egg sharers: a systematic review. *Hum Reprod Update* 2016;**22**(4):450–465.

17. Kirkman M, Bourne K, Fisher J, Johnson L, Hammarberg K. Gamete donors' expectations and experiences of contact with their donor offspring. *Hum Reprod* 2014;**29**(4):731–738.

18. Hammarburg K, Carmichael M, Tinney L, Mulder A. Gamete donors' and recipients' evaluation of donor counseling: a prospective longitudinal cohort study. *Aust N Z J Gynaecol* 2008;**48**:601–606.

19. Miettinen A, Rotkirch A, Suikkari AM, Söderström-Anttila V. Attitudes of anonymous and identity-release oocyte donors towards future contact with donor offspring. *Hum Reprod* 2019;**34**(4):672–678.

20. Daniels K, Lalos O. The Swedish Insemination Act and the availability of donors. *Hum Reprod* 1995;**7**:1871–1874.

Counseling Embryo Donors and Recipients

Elaine Gordon and Maya Grobel

Introduction

Over the past 50 years, technological advances in reproductive medicine, particularly in in vitro fertilization (IVF), have provided opportunities for patients who would not be able to conceive otherwise. Refinement of embryo cryopreservation techniques allows patients to store unused embryos for future use, and fertility patients commonly seek to create as many potentially viable embryos as possible in order to increase their chances for success. Unfortunately, they seldom consider the disposition of remaining embryos at the outset of this process. Once family-building is complete, they are faced with a dilemma.

Nevertheless, these patients are required to select a disposition option for any remaining embryos at the outset, a most inopportune time, because their focus is on procreation [1,2]. Disposition options include: (1) Store for future family-building; (2) discard; (3) donate to science; (4) compassionate transfer; and (5) donate to another for family-building. Consequently, a disposition choice is often duly selected with little thought given to the implications of it. There is no option to delay the decision for a time when the patient would be better equipped to consider the implications of these choices. Patients frequently experience emotional distress around decision-making, as many feel none of the options are acceptable and thus enter a state of paralysis and continue to store indefinitely or as long as possible [3].

While the number of donated embryo cycles remains low, the demand for donated embryos is increasing. As an ever-growing number of people struggle with fertility challenges and the cost of third-party reproduction rises, embryo donation could be a viable option for many patients who would otherwise not have many family-building options.

The number of cryopreserved embryos worldwide now far exceeds one million and this number is increasing exponentially. This surplus of embryos is scattered across the globe, with no comprehensive strategy to address decision-making for both embryo donors and recipients. Religious biases, cultural values, and the policies and regulations that grow out of them vary from country to country and within countries, making it challenging for embryo donation to be widely accessible as a disposition choice and family-building option.

With more in-depth education and psychosocial supports, patients could better explore their options and make decisions that constitute true informed consent in a more timely manner. Allowing for patients to select "conditional" or known/open/directed donation could increase the acceptability of embryo donation for potential donors [4].

Embryo donation is fraught with pragmatic and emotional roadblocks for both recipients and donors. Donors and recipients have separate, often overlapping and sometimes conflicting needs when it comes to the donation arrangement. Current embryo donation protocols are confusing and haphazard, and there is little consistency across programs within the United States (US) and in other countries.

Of all the third-party family-building options, embryo donation is also the most complex and least utilized. The consequences of embarking on an embryo donation arrangement are not the same as those for sperm or egg donation. Unlike in sperm and egg donations, there are far greater implications for the relationship one family has with another, as all of the children that are born of these embryos are full genetic siblings, and often embryo donors did not intend to be donors in the same way egg or sperm donors do.

There is much to learn and determine about how to effectively counsel potential donors and recipients and how to create an embryo donation program that honors the needs of the three major stakeholders – donor, recipients and offspring. A successful protocol would not dictate what a donor or recipient must do. Instead, it would provide all the pertinent information necessary to make a deliberate decision, offer the opportunity to explore what each stakeholder is feeling about the various disposition choices, and attempt to meet those expressed

The addenda referred to in this chapter are available for download at www.cambridge.org/covington-clinical-guide

needs and concerns. When counseling patients, it is essential for the fertility counselor to be well versed in the nuances of these complex relationships in order to help the stakeholders navigate these muddy waters and support adaptive changes in current embryo donation practices.

Historical Overview of Embryo Donation

Early Embryo Donations

In the early days of embryo donation (the mid-1980s), the decision to donate remaining embryos to another for their family-building was made informally within the confines of the medical practice, with no guidelines or established protocol in place. Some arrangements were made between relatives, friends and acquaintances. Others were physician-driven and usually done under the cover of anonymity, as donors relinquished custody of their remaining embryos to their doctors, giving them full control. The exchange of information was controlled and directed by the doctor. These donations were not commonplace or formalized and only served a small cohort of the infertile community.

There were few formalized embryo donation programs, and those that existed treated embryo donation as "embryo adoption," and were conservative in their policies of who could participate. However, as the demand for more inclusive practices increased, many of these programs have shifted their policies, resulting in greater access, though there are still not many programs available. In addition, there has been an increase in fertility programs that create embryos with egg and sperm donors; these donor–donor embryos, while often referred to as donated embryos, are not what is typically identified as embryo donation, as they are in fact embryos created for treatment by practices rather than patients.

Embryo Donation Versus Embryo Adoption

Because embryo donation shares similarities with both donor conception and adoption, patients often use the terms embryo donation and embryo adoption interchangeably. However, the American Society for Reproductive Medicine (ASRM) states the use of the term "adoption" is misleading [5]. ASRM states that while embryos have special status due to their potential for personhood, they should not be offered the same legal or moral status as persons. Adoption requires a legal set of procedures determined by judicial law [6]. Embryo adoption often follows similar protocols as those used in traditional adoption arrangements, which ASRM notes are "not appropriate and unjustly burden recipients" [5].

Embryo Donation Around the World

Policies regarding embryo donation grow out of personal bias, individual value systems, ethics, religious leanings, regional customs, and the broad influence of a socio-political climate. The variation in embryo donation protocols throughout the world makes it challenging to identify best practices. In some countries, embryo donation is forbidden. Other countries impose strict regulatory guidelines. Some have lax policies or none at all, leaving medical facilities to manage embryo donation as they see fit.

The global trend for countries allowing embryo donation is steadily rising. According to a 2019 survey conducted by the International Federation of Fertility Societies' Surveillance (IFFS), 58% of the countries surveyed allowed embryo donation, however, of those countries only 47% actually practiced embryo donation [7]. In countries allowing embryo donation, the regulations and practices in use vary widely in cost, number of offspring permitted, and allowances for genetic screening, anonymity, and rights to identifying and nonidentifying information. These policies are constantly changing, making it difficult to provide up-to-date information on embryo donation policies worldwide.

Some embryo recipients engage in "reproductive tourism" and cross-border care, traveling to countries where the laws and policies are more conducive to their reproductive needs. These variations compound the challenges for embryo recipients, as there are different implications for fertility counselors to discuss with patients, including potential language barriers, and cultural differences between donors and recipients that can impact the child's narrative and experience if they wish to connect to genetic relatives.

Theoretical Frameworks

Theoretical frameworks can help counselors interpret a client's actions, thoughts and feelings. It is the context used to offer guidance to clients navigating their fertility journey.

One framework for patients making disposition decisions for their remaining embryos resulted from a study conducted by Nachtigall et al. in 2005 [8]. The study suggested that the disposition decision-making process for potential donors roughly follows four sequential stages:

Stage 1: Reassurance – While undergoing IVF treatment, couples are reassured by having large numbers of surplus embryos.

Stage 2: Avoidance – Once their childbearing is completed, most couples spend little time thinking about their frozen embryos.

Stage 3: Confrontation – When couples actually begin to confront the disposition decision, their reaction is frequently one of discomfort and uncertainty. Several identifiable elements contribute to the difficulty of coming to a disposition decision.

Stage 4: Resolution – Those couples who were able to come to an agreement frequently expressed a profound sense of completeness and resolution.

When patients reach the confrontation stage, fertility counselors have the opportunity to help them explore various disposition options in depth. One useful tool for patients in this stage is the Victorian Assisted Reproductive Treatment Authority (VARTA) Unused Embryos Decision Tool (see Addendum 11.1).

There are a number of conceptual frameworks that are applicable to understanding the complexities of an embryo donation arrangement (see Table 11.1). Because embryo donation is such a fluid process, where feelings and thoughts change over the course of time, it may be helpful to utilize different frameworks at different crossroads in this journey.

The Emotional Landscape of Embryo Donation

The emotional trajectory for fertility patients is often in flux, as they move toward making a decision to either donate or receive embryos. Individuals and couples come to embryo donation with unique backgrounds, experiences and perspectives that shape how they approach embryo donation. While the ability to gather insight into each patient's particular experience is imperative, there are emotional considerations that patients often share, which must be factored into the therapeutic process.

The Embryo Donor

While cryopreservation of remaining embryos may initially be reassuring for patients, decision-making around remaining embryos can cause significant distress [3]. The majority of patients delay decision-making by 5 years or

Table 11.1 Theoretical frameworks applicable to embryo donation counseling

Crisis intervention

Crisis intervention is a process by which a mental health worker identifies, assesses and intervenes with an individual in crisis so as to restore balance and reduce the effects of the crisis in his/her life. The individual is then connected with a resource network to reinforce the change. Bruce Baldwin

Solution-focused therapy

Solution-focused therapy is a modality in which mental health workers collaborate with clients to identify the problems the clients are facing and work in a goal-directed way to find feasible solutions. Steve De Shazer, Insoo Kim Berg

Family systems therapy

Family systems therapy is a modality working under the theory that human behavior is defined by an individual's early experiences in their family unit. The interconnected social system of the family and the way the members interact with and influence each other creates an individual's habitual model for behavior in broader society. Murray Bowen

Social exchange theory

Social exchange theory proposes that all social behavior is a process of exchange. Each individual chooses to exchange in order to maximize their benefits and minimize their costs. According to this theory, people are always weighing the potential costs and benefits of social relationships. When the risks outweigh the rewards, people terminate or abandon relationships. George Homans

Stigma therapy

Stigma therapy attempts to directly target a client's notion that having a particular attribute will tarnish their reputation or social status and help them navigate the challenges that may arise if they experience rejection within their community for their identity and/or choices. Erving Goffman

Attachment theory

Attachment theory, taken from developmental psychology, states that humans are born with a need to form a close emotional bond with a primary caregiver and that such a bond will develop during the first 6 months of a child's life if the caregiver engages in appropriate bonding behaviors. The type of bond that a child makes with this caregiver, often their parent(s), becomes the model for how that child will approach attachment to others throughout life. John Bowlby, Mary Ainsworth

Psychosocial theory

Psychosocial theory explains the changes in self-understanding, social relationships and one's relationship to larger society individuals. The theory proposes that the eight stages of development are universal, and that within each stage, there is a conflict to be resolved. Identity formation is said to occur at stage four. Erik Erickson

more post-treatment [9]. This indicates the uncertainty that many experience towards the end of their fertility journey.

Various disposition options offered (or not offered) at fertility clinics can exacerbate decision-making dilemmas.

Patients are increasingly interested in open donation and want the option of being able to choose their recipients [4]. Patients at clinics that don't offer embryo donation, or only offer unknown/closed or nonidentified arrangements, may be additionally tasked with the logistics of finding suitable recipients. Additionally, embryo donors with a large number of remaining embryos may struggle with how to disperse those embryos. This could potentially be a time-consuming process that takes years to complete. The donor can opt for a sequential donation where all the remaining embryos are relinquished to a selected recipient, and when that recipient completes their family, they donate the remaining embryos to another recipient. Or the original donors can disperse the embryos as they see fit.

Embryo Conceptualization

How patients conceptualize their cryopreserved embryos plays a key role in their posttreatment decision-making. While some patients see them as little more than biological matter [8], research in the US has begun to show that 5 years after IVF treatment, patients with cryopreserved embryos perceive these embryos as siblings to their existing children [10], and that patients' disposition decisions correlate to the perceived moral status of their embryos [3]. While some patients may feel a moral or religious obligation to their embryos, viewing them unequivocally as future human beings, others may find their view changes throughout the journey. For those who establish that their family is complete at the end of IVF treatment, feelings of connection to the remaining embryos become complex. Further, the increasing popularity of preimplantation genetic testing (PGT), which provides insight into the chromosome health and sex of embryos, may solidify the conceptualization of embryos as future children or siblings to the children of embryo donors.

It is not uncommon for partners to disagree on disposition or have different feelings about embryo donation. This can create relational stress and add to their decision-making paralysis. Those with remaining embryos that were created by donated gametes may face more complications. When one member of a couple is genetically related to the embryo and the other is not, disparities may arise in terms of the level of attachment or connection felt to those remaining embryos.

The Embryo Recipient

For individuals and couples considering family-building through embryo donation, there is often a past history of unexpected life events, reproductive challenges and trauma. While one individual may come to embryo donation as a first choice for family-building, for example, a single woman of advanced maternal age, another might come to the process after prior treatments have been unsuccessful. How patients make sense of their history and envision their future family through embryo donation can ignite a myriad of emotions – from grief around the concept of genetic loss to gratitude for the opportunity to have a child. Recipients may be apprehensive about this unique family-building option; giving birth to a nongenetic child is often hard to comprehend. As part of this process, recipients must grapple with and ultimately make peace with the idea of parenting a nongenetic child. With the guidance of a fertility counselor, they can explore ways to embrace the genetics of other individuals, know what resources are available to find suitable embryos and figure out how to best pursue embryo donation.

Family Conceptualization

An important part of the recipient's emotional journey is the ability to embrace nongenetic parenting and to develop a coherent family narrative for themselves and their future child. As part of their sensemaking, recipients must reflect on what it means to raise a child that does not share their genetics and how their future child may feel about it. Some recipients connect to an adoption narrative, though embryo donation and traditional adoption are quite different.

Fertility counselors can point to research showing the absence of a genetic link in gamete donation families does not have an adverse effect on relationships or children's psychological well-being [11,12], and that, for most recipients, attachment anxieties and other fears often dissipate once they have been successful through childbirth and established confidence in themselves as parents. Understanding the potential for an evolution in their emotions may better prepare them to forecast possible needs and interests for themselves and their children as it relates to embryo donation.

Feelings Experienced in Donor and Recipient Families

Once patients decide to donate their remaining embryos, they may experience joy in helping others who have struggled with fertility and gratitude towards their recipients, who can give their embryo a chance to be born. At the same time, they may face anxiety, fear and even grief as they relinquish control of embryos that share the same genetic makeup as their own children. Patients may also grapple with how their own children will feel about genetic siblings who are being raised in other homes with other parents.

Recipients who have limited information about their donors and the potential child's genetic history may worry about how their child will experience life without access to genetic relatives. With the emergence of direct-to-consumer genetic testing and relative-finding services, recipients must also make meaning of the likelihood that their future child(ren) will know – or want to know – the identity of their genetic relatives (see Chapter 13 for further information).

Recipients who are considering a known/open/directed donation process, when they know their donor, often struggle with how and where to find a suitable match and how much to invest in the relationship before knowing the outcome. Many also worry about the role their donor will play in their child's life and may be fearful about the impact that genetic relatives will have on their ability to bond with their child. They may also worry about being rejected by their children once the children learn they are genetically unrelated to their parent(s) [19]. However, in her most recent book *We Are Family*, Susan Golombok sums up her research on donor-conceived families stating, "genetic relatedness is less important than previously thought for raising happy and well-adjusted children" [3,11].

Equity and Access Considerations for Donors and Recipients

It is important for fertility counselors to understand the limits of access and availability for different populations as it relates to embryo donation. As donors and recipients navigate embryo donation as a disposition and family-building option, they may face disparities that impact their decision-making. Despite the global trend toward antidiscrimination legislation that broadens access to assisted reproductive technologies (ART) [13], inequities remain. This is especially true in countries where lack of insurance coverage renders fertility treatment cost prohibitive for the majority of individuals. In the US, less than one quarter of those who need fertility treatment have access to care [14]. Those who do have access are predominantly white, high-earning individuals with postsecondary degrees [15]. Further, a longitudinal study in the United Kingdom (UK) found that all ethnic groups utilized white egg donors most commonly, which points to a lack of availability of nonwhite donors and to potential challenges for recipients of color in finding donors who are an ethnic match [16].

Another arena where inequality disproportionately exists is for individuals who identify with nontraditional family structures, such as singles and same-sex couples, and LGBTQIA+ individuals. There are some embryo donation agencies that limit access to heterosexual married couples. Working to support inclusivity and providing resources for patients is important, as is being conscious of inequities and how they impact specific patient populations.

Embryo Donation Arrangement Options

There is a spectrum of relationship arrangement options for donors, recipients and their families to consider. At one end of the spectrum, donors and recipients can opt to have no contact with one another in what is considered an unknown/closed or nonidentified arrangement. Alternatively, donors and recipients can choose to match with each other via an open/known or directed arrangement and work toward ongoing contact. Semi-known arrangements are also an option and involve matches wherein donors and recipients are open to contact in the future, particularly if it is the desire of the children.

Unknown/Closed/Nonidentified Arrangements

Unknown/closed/nonidentified arrangements, in which donors and recipients do not know each other, matches are most often facilitated by a third-party coordinator at a medical clinic or by agency personnel. In some cases, ownership of the embryos has been relinquished to the clinic and, subsequently, matches are made as per clinic policies. Typically, information about the embryo(s) and donors is limited, and donors and recipients are not provided with identifying information about one another. It is feasible that large sets of remaining embryos may be divided among multiple recipients, and patients may be unaware if a pregnancy occurred or a child was born.

Donors drawn to an unknown arrangement may want to help other fertility patients or give their remaining embryo(s) a chance at life with limited emotional labor and involvement. For recipients, this type of arrangement may allow for more choice in embryo selection without the stress of being chosen or matching with a donor. It is often an easier process with fewer logistical complications. Furthermore, some recipients feel more secure in knowing there will be no interference from genetic contributors and will afford them the space to embrace parenthood.

What may appear to be a simple relationship choice initially may become more complicated later on. Both parties may face challenges navigating what to do if children become interested in connecting with genetic relatives in the future. It is important for patients to explore their own assumptions and fears, as well as the potential future needs of the children created through embryo donation when assessing the options available to them.

Known/Open/Directed Arrangements

In known/open/directed donation arrangements, in which third-party decision-makers are absent, donors and recipients have autonomy in selecting and matching with each other. These matches are usually established through a matching service or agency, or independently through friends, family or social media. Donors and recipients commonly discuss and determine the terms of their relationship. While some prefer infrequent communication and interaction, others favor more frequent contact, even viewing one another as extended family.

While most known/open/directed arrangements are protected by legal contracts, the expectations and conditions of their arrangement will likely evolve over time, and participants need to be prepared to explore changes in feelings and preferences throughout the years. Fertility counselors and legal professionals are often called upon to help resolve emerging issues or complexities along the way, such as when one party does not uphold the contact parameters originally agreed upon or when there is a misalignment in parenting practices between parties. More serious challenges can occur when a child conceived through embryo donation is born with unexpected medical or health-related issues.

Semi-known Arrangements

In semi-known relationships, donors and recipients may feel some uncertainty about the level of contact desired. They are generally open to contact, but not sure when that should be, and want the option of seeing how things go before making any promises about how the families will relate. Oftentimes, donors and recipients want to postpone contact until they are able to determine what might be in the best interest of their child.

Logistical Considerations

Embryo donation is not merely a disposition option, it is a life choice and an understandably difficult one for potential donors and recipients to navigate. Organizations such

Table 11.2 Example framework to support patients in understanding the embryo donation process: EM·POWER*

Education provided for patients on family-building options and medical eligibility to increase decision-making confidence.

Mental health consultations provided for donors and recipients, individually and jointly if feasible, to foster psychosocial well-being and to inform relational considerations.

Preferences for matching determined by donors and recipients, that informatively factor in the logistical, legal and relational considerations of their preferred arrangement, from known to unknown.

Obligatory medical clearance obtained for both donors and recipients with possible support from genetic counselors to understand the genetic considerations and risk factors involved in embryo donation.

Written contracts developed that outline the logistical and relational decisions of the match, with support from separate legal professionals for donors and recipients who have experience in assisted reproductive technology and third-party family building.

Embryo transfer logistics implemented by donors and recipients based on the written contract.

Relationship expectations managed after the transfer, with ongoing support from counselors to foster long-term family functioning and to prioritize the needs of the children.

*Adapted with permission from EM·POWER donation LLC

as the European Society for Human Reproduction and Embryology (ESHRE) and the ASRM offer guidelines addressing the information to be provided for fertility patients as part of embryo donation, from the legal and medical requirements, to education options that patients should be informed about. Education initiatives like EM·POWER [17] also provide frameworks that clinic staff can use to support patients in understanding the various components of the embryo donation process, as exemplified in Table 11.2.

As patients move through the logistical journey of embryo donation, it is helpful to develop a team of legal, mental health and medical professionals. Furthermore, genetic counselors can be instrumental in supporting patients around the genetic considerations and risk factors involved in embryo donation, and how the accessibility of direct-to-consumer genetic testing may impact their family and their relationship decisions in the future.

The Role of the Fertility Counselor

Fertility counseling is a developing professional specialty that combines mental health, reproductive medicine, genetic counseling, bioethics and reproductive law [18]. It has become more encompassing as an overall discipline due to the ever-increasing number of family-building options available to patients. Embryo donation, in particular, provides the counselor with challenges that the other third-party arrangements do not have to face. The process of one family having to engage with another can be exciting, yet overwhelming. As reproductive technology progresses rapidly, greater demands are continuously being made, and counseling these patients requires a specialized skill-set, including familiarity with the various family-building options and reproductive medical protocols.

Psychoeducation/Emotional Support

An important role of the fertility counselor is to provide psychoeducation, as patients weigh the implications of their choices for both themselves and their children/potential children (see Addendum 11.2 for additional educational resources).

For potential embryo donors, decision-making regarding disposition is complicated and dependent on many factors [4,19]. Sheryl de Lacey, in her work on embryo disposition, states that the role of moral reasoning, dilemma, conflict, and culturally embedded beliefs and values impact decisions about remaining embryos [20]. There is a growing need for skilled psychological practitioners to work with donors who are in a state of paralysis to hopefully resolve their dilemma in making an appropriate choice. If the decision is to donate embryos to another, continued exploration of the feelings, process, logistics, desires and expectations must be explored.

For potential embryo recipients, fertility counselors provide much needed support to discuss past fertility history and the transition to embryo donation, the process and meaning of becoming a parent through embryo donation, and specifically the implications for children conceived via embryo donation. The counselor assists patients in processing their fertility journey and genetic loss, working through the trauma and associated pain of that loss and exploring suitable resolutions utilizing an appropriate therapeutic approach. They are trained to educate patients and dispel myths and misconceptions, the goal being to guide potential donors and recipients toward making the personal decision that will be right for them, based on their desires, relationship expectations, cultural influences, religious beliefs and moral and ethical stances.

Consultations

Psychological counseling is recommended or required by most reproductive medicine societies and governing bodies that provide guidance on ART. Fertility counselors are usually called upon to provide consultations to donors and recipients individually, and to the match in a joint session. See Addendum 11.3 for a list of topics to be included in embryo donation consultations.

Long-term Family Support

The counselor's job does not end once a successful transfer and birth occur, but will continue as needed by the donor, recipient and their families. During pregnancy, birth and postbirth, new feelings may emerge regarding bonding, disclosure, regrets and other unresolved issues. It is a long-term process in which thoughts and feelings emerge about how to make sense of these new family configurations and relationships. Additionally, counselors may be called upon to support patients in grief work if a transfer has been unsuccessful or if there is conflict within the match. After children are born, fertility counselors can provide much needed education and support with the goal of promoting healthy family functioning.

Best Practices in Talking to Children

The consensus among child developmental experts is that children do have a right to know about their genetic origins [21]. Arguments against disclosing often have more to do with the parents' sense of shame about their infertility or fear that their child(ren) will reject them or be ostracized [11]. Helping parents work through any feelings of shame or fear early on will help them move to a place of confidence in sharing their child's conception narrative, and will better serve the long-term functioning of the family.

Technology, social media, biometric recognition techniques and DNA testing have eliminated the concept of anonymity in the world of reproductive medicine. Any promises of anonymity are misleading and unfair to reproductive consumers. From a psychological perspective, the professional community has shifted its opinion and now claims that anonymity is no longer in the best interests of these children [11].

Also relevant is the understanding of identity formation for not only the donor-conceived children but for their full genetic siblings. Erik Erikson, a leading theorist in identity formation, proposed eight stages of psychosocial development [22]. It is in the third stage, during the tumultuous adolescent years, that they are charged with the task of integrating their life experiences, family dynamics, socio-cultural exposures, environment and relationships into a stable and predictable identity. It is not a stretch to imagine how ambiguity about their genetic origins might negatively impact a donor-conceived child's sense of self (see also Chapter 14 for further information).

It is for this reason that it is a best practice to share truths about a child's genetic origins when the child is young, prior to age seven [11], and to continue the discussion over time in age-appropriate ways, as early disclosure creates fewer problematic repercussions.

Disclosure in Known/Open/Directed Embryo Donation Arrangements

Since disclosure is important for both the children of embryo recipients and the children of embryo donors, both the donor and receiving family need to collaborate in how and when this information will be shared and discussed with their respective children. How the children will come to know and refer to each other is important to discuss as well. Though it is likely that disclosure parameters were discussed and agreed upon at the beginning of the process, it is important for both families to make room for subsequent changes of opinion and the needs and desires of the children. Respecting everyone's perspective in how they see their connectedness may be a challenge, but it is one that holds significant benefits and opportunities for personal growth.

Disclosure in Unknown/Closed/Nonidentified Embryo Donation Arrangements

Families formed through unknown/closed/nonidentified embryo donation may not have much information about the donors. In these cases, parents may feel confused about how or what to disclose to their children. Fertility counselors can help parents become more comfortable and confident about sharing their conception narrative with their children, even when they have a lack of information. Counselors can support parents in validating their child's feelings and curiosities while providing whatever information is available and acknowledging what is lacking.

Embryo donors who have donated in an unknown/closed/nonidentified way will need to share their decision to donate with their family and the possible outcomes of their donation, which they may not know. Encouraging parents to be open and honest with their children will best serve the family unit and allow children to ask questions

and explore their feelings, as they construct their own narrative.

Outcomes for Children in Donor Conception and Embryo Donation

The body of research done by Susan Golombok supports the claim that children from alternative families are considered to be no different than those from traditional family formations [11]. The relationship between children and parents is seemingly healthy, showing no detrimental consequences regarding their relationship and psychological health. Additionally, when parents talk to their children about their conception story from an early age, it appears they are better able to integrate this information into their identity [11]. Providing parents with research that validates positive outcomes for donor-conceived families may decrease feelings of fear and insecurity. Fertility counselors may be asked to provide guidance and support for families who are wanting to disclose to older children. While it is never too late to disclose, talking to older children about genetic truths they may not be expecting can be more complicated, and parents should be prepared for a myriad of potential emotions from older children and donor-conceived adults. Helping the family unit work through this can be challenging but rewarding work.

What the Future Holds

Because of the novel nature of families connected through embryo donation, conceptualization of the relationships and language to describe the relationships are still being constructed. While there is an exceedingly low percentage of embryo donation cycles as a percentage of all ART cycles globally, interest in this field has been on the rise. And as the number of cryopreserved embryos continues to increase, patients will need more tailored education and counseling support around disposition choices, including embryo donation. The future of embryo donation is exciting, but will certainly continue to be complex.

Increasing numbers of frozen embryos combined with limited storage space and the liability involved in abandoned embryos may encourage fertility clinics to increase patient education around embryo disposition. An understanding of the emotional challenges disposition decisions can cause for patients may justify an increase in psychosocial support for patients to make informed decisions and to navigate the emotional and logistical elements of embryo donation. There is a current lack of education for embryo donation patients and low satisfaction with support services.

Due to increasing interest of patients in open/known donation, combined with the influences of social media, consumer DNA testing and ancestry finding services, more clinics may be motivated to support patients in open/known/directed donation arrangements. Additionally, policies may eventually shift anonymity legislation around the world to more closely mirror that of Australia, New Zealand, the UK and several other countries where anonymous donations are no longer legal.

The ongoing advances in genetic technology will continue to provide patients with more information about their embryos, which may also impact patients' conceptualization of remaining embryos, decisional conflict in disposition choice and emotional well-being post-IVF.

Social media and other channels like podcasts, films and print media that highlight the voices of donor-conceived people may significantly impact decision-making around donor conception. All stakeholders will likely need psychological support to process feelings and make sense and meaning of engaging in embryo donation, with important consideration paid to the future needs of children.

Fertility counselors have an opportunity to make the embryo donation landscape more inclusive, better understood, and more accessible for patients, through education and counseling support. Embryo donation can and does bring hope and joy to many patients and their families, many of whom, on both the donor and recipient side, are able to finally resolve their fertility journey. Counselors can continue this important work in helping to normalize and advocate for diversity in families and new family forms.

References

1. Lyerly AD, Steinhauser K, Namey E, et al. Factors that affect infertility patients' decisions about disposition of frozen embryos. *Fertil Steril* 2006;**85**:1623–1630.

2. Deniz S, Hughes E, Neal M, Faghih M, Amin S, Karnis M. Are health care providers adequately educating couples for embryo disposition decisions? *Fertil Steril* 2016;**105**(3):684–689.

3. Lyerly AD, Steinhauser K, Voils C, et al. Fertility patients' views about frozen embryo disposition: results of a multi-institutional U.S. survey. *Fertil Steril* 2008;**93**(2):499–509.

4. McMahon C, Saunders D. Attitudes of couples with stored frozen embryos toward conditional embryo donation. *Fertil Steril* 2009;**91**(1):140–147.

5. Ethics Committee of the American Society for Reproductive Medicine. Defining embryo donation: an Ethics Committee opinion. *Fertil Steril* 2016;**106**(1):15–282.

6. ASRM Ethics Committee Opinion Fertility and Sterility. Interest, obligation and rights in gamete and embryo donation. *Fertil Steril* 2019;**111**(4):15–282.

7. Global Reproductive Health. International Federation of Fertility Societies' Surveillance (IFFS) 2019: Global Trends in Reproductive Policy and Practice. 2019.

8. Nachtigall RD, Becker G, Friese C, Butler A, MacDougall K. Parents' conceptualization of their frozen embryos complicates the disposition decision. *Fertil Steril* 2005;**84**(2):431–434.

9. McMahon C, Gibson F, Cohen J, Leslie G, Tennant C, Saunders D. Mothers conceiving through in vitro fertilization: siblings, setbacks, and embryo dilemmas. *Reprod Technol* 2000;**10**:131–135.

10. Stiel M, McMahon C, Elwyn G, Boivin J. Pre-birth characteristics and 5-year follow-up of women with cryopreserved embryos after successful in vitro fertilisation treatment. *J Psychosom Obstet Gynaecol* 2010;**31**(1):32–39.

11. Golombok S. *We Are Family: The Modern Transformation of Parents and Children*. New York, NY: Public Affairs, 2020.

12. Golombok S. *Modern Families: Parents and Children in New Family Forms*. Cambridge: Cambridge University Press, 2015.

13. International Federation of Fertility Societies' Surveillance (IFFS) 2019: Global Trends in Reproductive Policy and Practice. *Global Reprod Health* 2019;**4**(1):29.

14. American Society for Reproductive Medicine. White Paper: Access to Care Summit. 2015. Available from: www .asrm.org/globalassets/asrm/asrm-content/news-and-publications/news-and-research/press-releases-and-bulletins /pdf/atcwhitepaper.pdf [last accessed June 16, 2022].

15. Quinn M, Fujimoto V. Racial and ethnic disparities in assisted reproductive technology access and outcomes. *Fertil Steril* 2016;**105**:1119–1123.

16. Human Fertilization & Embryology Authority. Ethnic Diversity in Fertility Treatment 2018: UK Ethnicity Statistics for IVF and DI Fertility Treatment. 2021. Available from: www.hfea.gov.uk/about-us/publications/r esearch-and-data/ethnic-diversity-in-fertility-treatment-2 018/ [last accessed June 16, 2022].

17. EMPOWER with Moxi. Video 4: The Empower Method (Video Series]). 2019. Available from: www.youtube.com/ watch?v=AYujv07ELxY [last accessed June 16, 2022].

18. Feingold ML. Infertility, Reproductive Medicine, and the Role of the Psychologist. 2007. Available from: www .madelinefeingoldphd.com/infertility-reproductive-medicine-and-the-role-of-the-psychologist/ [last accessed June 16, 2022].

19. Klock SC, Sheinin S, Kazer RR. The disposition of unused frozen embryos [letter]. *N Engl J Med* 2001;**345**:69–70.

20. de Lacey S. Parent identity and 'virtual' children: why patients discard rather than donate unused embryos. *Hum Reprod* 2005;**20**(6):1661–1669. https://doi.org/10.1093/humrep/deh831

21. Baran A, Pannor R. *Lethal Secrets: The Psychology of Donor Insemination: Problems and Solutions*. Las Vegas, NV: Triadoption Publications, 2008.

22. Erikson EH. *Identity and the Life Cycle: Selected Papers*. New York, NY: International Universities Press, 1959.

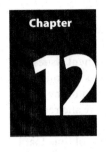

Special Considerations in Gestational Surrogacy Assessments and Arrangements

Tara Simpson and Mary Riddle

Introduction

Although traditional surrogacy has been documented since at least biblical times, more recent technological advances in assisted reproductive technologies (ART) have made it possible for a woman, referred to as a gestational carrier (GC), to gestate and give birth to a child that is not genetically related to her on the behalf of intended parents (IP) who are to be the legal, rearing parent(s) [1]. Since the first contemporary legally and medically mediated gestational surrogacy cycle in the 1970s, the use of such an arrangement to achieve a pregnancy has increased over time. In 1999, there were 727 cases of in vitro fertilization (IVF) with gestational surrogacy arrangements (GSA) reported, representing 1% of all ART cycles for that year. Most recent data demonstrates that there were 5,526 GC carrier cycles for 2016 which accounted for almost 4% of all transfers [2]. In addition, there were 9,029 GC carrier cycles listed for 2019 in preliminary data [3].

Gestational surrogacy differs from traditional surrogacy (TS), in which a woman both supplies her eggs and gestates the pregnancy and is therefore the biological mother of the child. As Kim [4] highlights that, due to legal and ethical difficulties resulting from the genetic link between the surrogate and the child(ren), TS is discouraged and is no longer offered by most programs in the United States (US). This chapter will focus on special considerations for the fertility counselor in GSAs and will not address issues related to TS.

Gestational surrogacy allows for broader opportunity of parentage for women who are unable to carry a pregnancy themselves, as well as for single men and male couples. An increasing number of GCs conceive with both sperm donor and/or egg donor gametes for IPs. Some women are even repeat carriers and serve in the role multiple times for the same IPs or for a different match. Women acting as a GC may be commercially recruited through an agency or

attorney and are paid for their service, or may be altruistic or compassionate, as when a family member or friend volunteers pro bono. At times, IPs may try to find a GC on their own, either online or by word of mouth. At one end of the spectrum, the GC may be a person with whom the IPs have had a long-term relationship with, such as a relative or best friend. At the other end of the extreme, the GC and IPs may not meet in person until the birth. In some countries, the GC and the IPs may never meet [4].

The US has no national policy on reproductive technologies like surrogacy and gestational parenting. Issues of family law are routinely decided by individual states and are constantly evolving. Some states ban surrogacy outright, some ban paid surrogacy but allow a woman to offer her services as a volunteer, while others are permissive of paid arrangements.

International cross-border surrogacy arrangements have proliferated due to a number of factors. Countries that have strong religious or cultural influences in their governing bodies prohibit surrogacy on the basis of religious tenets. Some countries may lack expertise, affordable, safe and private treatment, or have a low supply of donor gametes and surrogates. For other countries, the service may not be available for certain categories of individuals on the basis of age, marital status or sexual orientation. Finally, services may simply be less expensive in other countries. It is important to note that some countries which once hosted the majority of GSA have made sudden and restrictive changes to the availability of such services due to concerns over the exploitation of women. The laws and policies around GSA are constantly changing and evolving in particular countries [5].

The involvement of physicians, nurses, attorneys and fertility counselors make GC cases particularly resource intensive [6]. Due to all of the participants and the competing vulnerabilities and needs of each, there is a vital role for the fertility counselor in surrogacy arrangements. The goals of treatment with a GC are the birth of a healthy baby for the IPs, while maintaining the medical and psychological well-being of the GC [4]. Like legal

The addenda referred to in this chapter are available for download at www.cambridge.org/covington-clinical-guide

consultation, the surrogacy assessment with a fertility counselor will help all participants make sound decisions, provide accurate information to all parties, and create a basis for an informed consent. Thus, how these arrangements and relationships are facilitated become crucial in their success.

This chapter is on "special considerations" in gestational surrogacy. It is not a "how to" in regard to conducting a surrogacy arrangement assessment, which has been well documented in other literature [5]. Rather, this chapter goes beyond "how to" and considers the complexity of these arrangements, from competency of the fertility counselor to the delicate balance of the multitude of psychological factors the fertility counselor must consider for all parties involved.

The Role and Competence of the Fertility Counselor in Gestational Surrogacy Arrangements

The role of the fertility counselor in consideration of a GSA has evolved over time and, in the US, is fairly well defined. One of the most significant roles that the fertility counselor plays in a GC arrangement is to complete a psychological assessment of the entire arrangement. The Practice Committee of the American Society of Reproductive Medicine (ASRM) [7] released recommendations for practices utilizing GCs as an effort to address, among several other topics, the complex psychological issues that confront all involved parties as well as to make screening procedures more consistent across professionals who conduct these assessments. The Practice Committee document states that treating physicians should strongly recommend that qualified fertility counselors provide psychosocial counseling and psychoeducation to all parties involved in a GSA (IPs, potential GCs and their partners). We want to stress as authors that, while the Practice Committee recommends psychosocial counseling and education, we feel this should be *required*. We also feel that there are no shortcuts in this process and that cutting corners in this practice is both unethical and potentially dangerous for those involved in the arrangement.

It is the responsibility of the qualified fertility counselor to follow guidelines and recommendations and adhere to the suggested number/types of appointments. The fertility counselor must allow for adequate time for consultation and assessment with each party and then facilitate thorough exploration of all topics/information in suggested best practice guidelines. Established practice

in the US typically involves a fertility counselor providing psychological screening of a GC candidate and her partner (if she has one), a psychoeducational meeting with the IPs, and then a group consult where pertinent issues are addressed all together to minimize the risks of miscommunication. Addendum 12.1 identifies each of the counseling components with the specific purpose and required participants for the session.

Although there is no prescribed amount of time that it might take to complete an assessment for a GSA, we (the authors) have conducted hundreds of these types of evaluations and can offer some parameters on time needed to complete these assessments competently and ethically. The average duration of the three components typically required for the complete assessment is 2 hours for the IP interview, 2.5–3.5 hours for the psychological evaluation and testing of the GC, and 1.5 hours for the group meeting.

Countries vary in their specific approaches and guidelines in regard to presurrogacy counseling and the role of the fertility counselor in GSAs. Generally speaking, providing education and counseling to all parties involved in GSAs has been a primary role of the fertility counselor around the globe [7,8]. Additionally, and perhaps because of the proliferation of commercial arrangements in the US, the expectation of stakeholders and referral sources is that the fertility counselor will provide "clearance" of a GC, which drives the use of psychological tests in the assessment and screening of GCs. In the US, ASRM Practice Committee Guidelines [7] recommend referrals to a qualified mental health professional or any member of a GSA (IPs, GCs, or GC partner/spouse) who appears to warrant further psychological evaluation and/or counseling. The Ethics Committee of ASRM [1] recommends that GCs should have access to and receive psychological evaluation and counseling before, during and after participation in such an arrangement. These two opinions lay an aspirational framework for fertility counselors as they attempt to assist GCs and/or IPs in their psychosocial evaluations before proceeding forward.

At last count, the membership of the Mental Health Professional Group (MHPG) of ASRM was over 600. The combination of an explosion of gestational surrogacy arrangements in the US and an ever-growing number of fertility counselors conducting psychological evaluations for GC candidates has led to increased awareness of the importance of competency in the role of the fertility counselor in this process, which is clearly an evaluative one.

In the US, referral sources (clinics, lawyers, agencies) expect that a fertility counselor acts as a "gatekeeper" [9] who provides a "bottom line" or "clearance" of a surrogate to move forward in the process. These referral sources also have an implicit expectation that the fertility counselor has the training and competence to provide this clearance that they are seeking. However, the increased awareness of the psychosocial complexities inherent in surrogacy highlights the importance to consider the responsibility placed on the fertility counselor to extend beyond clearance, and truly consider how to best counsel and prepare GCs and their families so that their psychological well-being is a primary consideration. Furthermore, each arrangement is unique and there is no "one size fits all" approach to consideration of the appropriateness of any given arrangement. Each new arrangement will require thought and sensitivity towards all parties and considerations that are unique to each arrangement. Sometimes there can be a tendency towards an idealized vision of surrogacy by all members of an arrangement and this highlights the responsibility of the fertility counselor to carefully consider all aspects of this potential arrangement.

In addition, referral sources usually do not challenge results and trust that the person completing the assessment of an arrangement is well qualified to do so. Identifying and clarifying who is qualified to conduct such an evaluation has been debated, but recently published qualifications for fertility counselors, in particular qualifications of those who wish to use psychological testing as part of their assessment, have recently been developed by the Practice Committee of ASRM [10]. These should be carefully reviewed by a fertility counselor who wishes to move into this area of work, to ensure the competence necessary to conduct ethical evaluations. It is also important to note that these evaluations present the greatest legal risk for a fertility counselor and thus competency and practicing with standards will be crucial in the event of any legal defense. They are, in effect, forensic evaluations and fertility counselors should always be very conscious of the fact that they could be called in to testify in defense of their evaluation in the case that a GSA would be litigated. Everyone is invested in a positive outcome, therefore there should be no shortcuts at the start of this process in regard to the multiple psychological factors that must be considered.

From the beginning of commercial arrangements, the unknown psychological toll of bearing a baby with the intent to relinquish it for monetary gain raised concerns by critics of the practice that the process was unnatural and that there would be long-term psychological consequences [11,12]. And although there were psychologists who were "screening" potential surrogates using standardized psychological measures, there was no formal process or protocol, nor literature detailing the referral questions to be answered. Public concerns were only magnified by the controversy surrounding the Baby M case, when, in 1986, traditional surrogate Mary Beth Whitehead contracted with a couple to bear a child for them, but then changed her mind. Whitehead had undergone a psychological evaluation, later introduced as evidence in court, in which the psychologist had documented that Whitehead expressed strong feelings about relinquishing a baby [13]. The controversy over the case highlighted the need to identify the factors that should be assessed in a presurrogacy evaluation.

Early considerations placed emphasis on screening potential surrogates for psychopathology and making sure they would be able to relinquish a child in the end [11]. However, current guidelines and referral questions are far more detailed, including 35 counseling topics, nine exclusion criteria, and eight relative exclusion criteria [7]. Fertility counselors use these topics and criteria in their assessment of a GC candidate. Some of the primary considerations in the assessment of a GC are presence/absence of psychopathology, personality characteristics of GCs that could potentially impact the arrangement, and a GC's capacity to provide informed consent. Additionally, interpersonal relationships, motivations, life stressors and an appraisal of her primary support system are important to assess. It is also important to help a potential GC reflect on her expectations of the process and how surrogacy may impact both her life and the lives of her family members [5,7,12,14,15]. Addendum 12.2 identifies positive indications for GC participation in a GSA arrangement.

Competency and the Role of Psychological Testing

It is standard practice in the US that the fertility counselor, as part of the GC evaluation, will administer standardized psychological tests to aid in their decision-making regarding the arrangement. The most commonly used psychological tests in the US are the Minnesota Multiphasic Personality Inventory – 2 (MMPI-2) and the Personality Assessment Inventory (PAI). These are primarily because the instruments are often used in forensic settings and both tests have been studied in this population. Although, historically, the use of psychological tests was to screen for psychopathology among GC candidates, the rationale for the use of testing has evolved over time and can potentially address several aspects of the psychological consideration of a GC arrangement. Although screening for significant psychopathology is still important when evaluating a GC candidate, careful interpretation of test data can also identify personality factors that could potentially impact outcomes (such as compliance with medical regimens) and interpretation of data might also be useful in identifying psychological vulnerabilities in the GC as well as interpersonal dynamics that might impact a GC arrangement [16].

There is much to be gained by the competent and ethical use of psychological testing in the surrogacy process. The use of psychological tests can both validate findings on clinical interview and potentially enhance the evaluation process. Unfortunately, there may be a lack of awareness that the use of testing can contribute to the psychological protection of all parties by identifying the interpersonal vulnerabilities and potential dynamics that can influence the course of any given arrangement. The administration and interpretation by untrained, inexperienced clinicians raises liability issues for all involved [17]. There is a misperception by some that a psychological test is like a blood test, where definitive results are obtained that do not require the subtle interpretations to be conducted by an experienced and competent clinician [17]. Utilizing psychological tests simply because it is something to be "checked off a list" is unethical and the misinterpretation of data can have significant consequences, not the least of which are lawsuits. It cannot be overstated how important it is to use these tests as they have been designed and only by those with the credentials to do so.

Common Challenges in Gestational Surrogacy Arrangement Participant Management

Despite widely accepted published professional guidelines, it is not uncommon for patients, doctors, fertility centers and/or agencies to question the recommended components of a GSA evaluation. This may be related to several factors. Due to the number of participants and the different types of appointments needed to proceed with the assisted reproductive treatment, the timelines for GSA are complex and patients will often convey a sense of time urgency in completing the psychological component. A consequence of the number of participants and the time intensiveness of the entire GSA process may put pressure on the fertility counselor by the patients to "cut

corners" of the assessment to save time. Participants may have been told of the requirement without explanation or rationale provided. Referral sources should ideally be well-informed on the recommendations for these evaluations, but this may not be consistent across all referring parties. This can create confusion amongst the parties and increases the risk that the assessment becomes an item on a checklist. There may also be a pressure by the patients to modify or omit recommended components of the GSA to save money in what is an expensive process. It is also common for patients to state that they believe that the evaluation is unnecessary or unimportant. It is the job of the fertility counselor to uphold the recommendations and demonstrate that the GSA evaluation and assessment is to protect all parties, as well as the children not born yet, involved in the arrangement. It is also the job of the fertility counselor to educate referral sources and point them towards the relevant resources in their country. Ultimately, everyone involved in these arrangements will benefit from a uniform understanding of the assessment process and the goal of protecting all parties.

There are several challenges to completing a thorough mental health screening for any surrogacy arrangement. The sheer number of different people who need to coordinate multiple appointments at different times with a fertility counselor make this task arduous. The realities of scheduling and coordinating all of these moving pieces requiring appointments can be daunting for a practitioner. A unique aspect of the gestational surrogacy assessment is that there are very few therapeutic relationships in which a fertility counselor may find themselves with competing roles/responsibilities to protect divergent parties. It is not uncommon for one practitioner to conduct all of the necessary psychosocial counseling sessions for all parties. In these types of assessments, being able to conduct all components of a GSA is not typically seen as a conflict of interest. This is because there are advantages to being able to get to know all parties and being able to facilitate conversations between parties. Ultimately, the fertility counselor is being asked to comment on the arrangement as a whole. Only doing one piece of the assessment can, in some ways, put the fertility counselor at a disadvantage and it is critical that, if this is the case, that all professionals are in close contact throughout the assessment process.

Another significant factor that contributes to the complexity of the GSA are the geographical locations of the GC and the IP. Scheduling can still be a challenge when all parties are local to each other, but when they are not, it is even more complicated. Historically, it is common for the

GC to travel to the IP's fertility center for a series of appointments, often with small windows of time to fit them in, including the counseling components. Due to the location of each party, there may be situations in which two fertility counselors in different countries or different states/provinces from one another are meeting with one of the interested parties and having to coordinate the case.

Historically, all the components of a GSA were conducted in person. In the past it was considered poor practice to evaluate GCs via videoconference, often seeming to be a shortcoming or a shortcut to the assessment process. With the onset of the COVID-19 pandemic, telehealth options for the GSA evaluation and psychosocial consult have become more common practice. In the early aftermath of shutdowns across the country, many rules and restrictions were relaxed within the mental health field so as to maximize patient access to care. In the world of gestational surrogacy assessments, this created significant changes to previously well-accepted standards. Conducting evaluations remotely became more common and, initially, restrictions on state licensing standards were less rigid.

It is inherently important to review and understand the available tele-mental health guidelines (see also Chapter 25) regarding competent and ethical use of videoconference platforms, particularly in the complicated and high liability application to GSA. In addition, the utilization of videoconference results is a challenge for the fertility counselor's professional license and ability to provide clinical services across national or international jurisdictions. The fertility counselor bears the burden of understanding their state/province and national professional licensing laws (as well as the exceptions during state of emergency for waivers and the time limits of treating clients in other jurisdictions). It is important to increase access to care for such assessment, while at the same time appreciating the data we get from in-person assessments versus videoconference platforms. The fertility counselor must weigh the advantages and liabilities of conducting GSA evaluations in each of those modalities, and do so ethically and competently. It is also important to recognize the limitations of tele-mental health. These limitations should be both articulated to referring agencies and well-documented in the report.

Relationships, Expectations, Vulnerabilities

There is almost an endless list of potential pitfalls in any given surrogacy arrangement. This is because of both the psychological characteristics of the players and the ways in which these arrangements play out. Although referral sources may be looking for "bottom-line clearance," fertility counselors are also tasked with psychoeducation and counseling. This requires moving beyond a cookie-cutter checklist and being able to recognize and work with the dynamic subtleties in each unique arrangement. In order to fully consider the myriad of psychological complexities inherent in any GSA, we must first consider what we know about the parties involved. These factors and vulnerabilities will inform relationships and expectations throughout a pregnancy and beyond. This section will give an overview of what we know about the primary participants in a GSA and how the intricate dynamics of this relationship can be impacted by expectations on both sides, as well as a discussion on the inherent vulnerabilities of both parties (GCs and IPs).

Gestational Carriers

There are a number of vulnerabilities associated with being a surrogate that are moderated by psychological factors common to women who desire to become surrogates. Understanding and considering a potential GC's psychological vulnerabilities is important in both the psychological assessment of the surrogate and in considering how surrogates are matched and to whom. These vulnerabilities can also inform counseling of a potential GC and provide guidance for the fertility counselor in helping her consider the potential impact of a surrogate pregnancy, both on herself and on her family members. A number of studies have been conducted over the years on both gestational and traditional surrogates, which has resulted in a "typical" psychological presentation of GCs in the US: they are thought to be women who love and feel contented with pregnancy, but who also may seek a sense of achievement and feelings of "specialness" and self-worth [18,19,20,21]; and may also be women who are somewhat unorthodox and unconventional in their lives and expression of feminine roles [22].

One of the most critical dynamics in a GSA is the relationship between GC and IP(s). It is often this relationship that is most important to a GC. In fact, research has shown that the importance of this relationship might be a significant vulnerability, in that GCs often feel a special attachment to IPs [23]. Therefore, there is increased risk for negative feelings to develop in cases where GCs may have experienced loss of the special attention they may have received, or disappointment because things did not work out the way they had envisioned [23].

Other risks that pose psychological vulnerabilities are risks that are inherent in any pregnancy. A GC may have an idealized vision of what surrogacy will be and may even be naïve to the risks inherent in this endeavor [16]. Although GCs do not share a genetic connection with the baby they are carrying for the IP, they accept the risks of pregnancy, including the potential for reproductive losses as well as the ultimate risk of her own life. In order to be considered for surrogacy, GCs in the US must have previously given birth and therefore have a proven obstetrical history of fertility. When a GC experiences reproductive loss within surrogacy, there may be increased vulnerability to feelings of failure because of both inexperience with reproductive loss and the attachment they may feel to their IPs [23].

Gestational Carriers' Families

Although most GCs do not suffer negative psychological outcomes [24], little is known about the families of surrogates. Early studies devoted to the psychological issues inherent in surrogacy [11], current ASRM guidelines [7], and literature devoted to the psychological assessment of gestational carrier candidates [5] recommend both counseling and consideration of a surrogate's family. But only recently has a handful of studies been conducted to examine their well-being and the impact of surrogacy on the families of surrogates [15,25,26].

There have been two studies that focused on the children of surrogates and only one study has examined the impact of surrogacy on the entire family system. Jadva and Imrie [25] collected data from 23 families (36 children aged 12–25 years) in the UK and compared the children of genetic and gestational surrogates on measures of psychological well-being and family relationships. The children in this study reported that the overall experience of surrogacy had been positive and particularly focused on the relationships that grew out of the surrogacy arrangement (GC family, IPs, and children born of surrogacy). A smaller study conducted in the US with younger children (aged 7–17) [26] found that children fell within normal limits on standardized measures of psychological well-being, but also that some younger children endorsed negative feelings about the experience as well as anxiety over their mother's health and well-being. A more recent study by Riddle [15] found that overall, families are functioning well and family members report surrogacy as having been a positive influence on the family. However, mothers may overestimate how positively their children actually felt about having a mother who had been a surrogate.

Given the importance of including family members in both assessment and counseling of GSAs, more research is needed into the impact of surrogacy on the family system. Understanding the potential impact of surrogacy on surrogates and their family members is important for fertility counselors to consider in how they work to prepare GCs for the process of surrogacy.

Intended Parents

The emotional well-being of IPs varies greatly at the outset of a GSA. The grief and loss that is common in opposite-sex IPs who come to surrogacy after a multitude of heartbreaking losses can color the arrangement, as it is natural for IPs to perhaps be slow to warm up out of fear of more loss. This is a different dynamic than that of a same-sex gay couple who come to the arrangement happy and excited because they may never have anticipated the chance of having a child.

Other challenges can emerge because of the make-up of the arrangement or how it came to be. For example, there are differences in an arrangement between strangers brokered by an agency and a sister agreeing to carry for a family member. Other considerations include the way in which a match occurred and fertility counselors should be cautious in considering this as a factor. Some IPs and GCs meet through Facebook groups and it creates challenges for fertility counselors who walk into the assessment process with parties already strongly bonded. Any concerns raised by the fertility counselor during the counseling can be difficult. Nonetheless, the nature of the match should not influence recommendations made through an assessment. There can be any number of challenges created by the nature of the match. Boundary issues in family arrangements can be especially difficult to discern, with emotional, financial and perhaps even elements of coercion, an exclusionary factor which should be assessed very carefully.

Intended parents often come to the evaluation process skeptical about the need or value of such an encounter, and this might be influenced by the nature of the match. For an agency match, all parties likely walk into the evaluation understanding it is a necessary part of the process, although agencies can vary in their requirements. For arrangements that match online, often the "horse is out of the barn" and parties can become very attached, which adds a layer of complexity to the assessment process. For international arrangements, managing expectations is key, as it known that many GCs are invested in having IPs who are active participants in a pregnancy and who want to keep in touch afterwards. Language barriers and cultural differences need to be acknowledged. These are important discussions to have prior to a pregnancy so that unrealistic expectations can be addressed ahead of time and lines of communication can remain open.

Gestational Surrogacy Arrangements: Specific Dilemmas

Some of the most complicated discussions in the psychosocial consults of parties in a GSA arrangement lie in the "what ifs" and in the potential for negative outcomes. Participants often become uncomfortable with considering the challenges that a GSA arrangement afford and may deflect, downplay or deny that any adverse events or interpersonal conflicts may arise. GCs and IPs, in the excitement to finally have found a match, may not attend to vulnerabilities in either party's mental health history or current stressors/contraindications to proceeding. In addition, participants may have a difficult time conceptualizing the end of the GSA before it even begins. If the individual or couple IP has had a history of infertility and/or loss, a reluctance to discuss the actuality of a baby

or child from the arrangement, including the disclosure to the child of their origin as well as the type of relationship they would want for their offspring with the GC, may seem too abstract.

For all of these reasons, a thorough exploration of each person's preferences and beliefs regarding: specific potential medical decisions; preferences for privacy vs. transparency for each stakeholder throughout the entire relationship; problem solving and anticipating miscommunication and conflict resolution; as well as envisioning the future management of the relationship following delivery are essential. A discussion about each participant's beliefs and willingness to terminate a pregnancy; preferences of who will be in attendance at the birth; plans of disclosure of the arrangement to the child and others; and the future visions of the relationship after the delivery are the most essential topics to explore. As shown in Table 12.1, a skilled fertility counselor should facilitate a discussion of each of these decisions and dilemmas, with each participant separately and as a group, as each person considers the potential complexities prior to, during and after the GSA arrangement has ended.

Table 12.1 Gestational surrogacy arrangement specific decisions and dilemmas

Decision and dilemma	Things to consider
Medical: 1. PGT (pre-genetic testing) of embryos 2. Medication (including psychiatric) considerations 3. Number of embryos to be transferred 4. Selective reduction/pregnancy termination 5. Exposure to viruses 6. Fertility and pregnancy concerns	1. Availability of data regarding genetic makeup of embryos for greater chance of healthy live birth. 2. Decision to taper/wean off medications vs. remain on them during pregnancy. Weigh cost/benefits to GC and fetus. 3. Desire for/willingness to carry multiple pregnancy. 4. Willingness of/for GC to terminate a pregnancy due to multifetal and/or genetic anomaly. 5. Risks of infection/mortality for GC and fetus exposed to viruses and preferences regarding vaccinations and testing. 6. Prepare parties for unsuccessful/cancelled ART cycles, miscarriage/pregnancy loss, bed rest/pregnancy complications, labor and delivery complications.
Preferences regarding privacy vs. transparency of stakeholders:	1. Use of donated gametes/whose gametes to use to conceive. 2. Previous reproductive history and sexual history (including HIV status). 3. Medical results regarding fetus vs. GC 4. Identifying info permissible for IP(s)/GC to share about the other participants. 5. Attendance/presence at fertility treatments, obstetric appointments and the birth. 6. Intention to disclose to offspring about conception and role/identity of GC.
Miscommunication and conflict resolution:	1. Preferences and identification of all parties' communication styles. 2. Explore how participants have handled previous interpersonal conflict with others or each other. 3. Anticipate potential conflict to occur before, during and after the GSA and problem solve how such issues could/would be addressed.
The end of the GSA arrangement:	1. Expectations of when, how and where will say goodbye to each other and the baby. 2. Concerns about relinquishment of the baby. 3. Expectations of each participant regarding the short-term and long-term future management and maintenance of the relationships between all parties following the birth of the baby.

Conclusion

Each GSA is unique and the fertility counselor wears many hats in their role. These include the fertility counselor as evaluator, gatekeeper, educator and facilitator. It is important to remember that people come into an arrangement with their own history (perhaps one of grief and loss) and psychological needs (perhaps feeling a need for achievement). The overarching common goal is a positive outcome for all parties.

The fertility counselor must treat these dynamics with sensitivity, because they often reflect psychological history/needs that may be out of the conscious awareness of the individuals involved. It can also not be understated that, in order to ensure the psychological protection of all parties and with the goal of a harmonious experience and positive outcome, the responsibility placed on the shoulders of the fertility counselor is significant. Appropriate training and expertise is critical for legal and ethical practice. In addition, the role of peer consultation, supervision and attention to self-care is imperative. A fertility counselor is not immune to feelings of countertransference that may arise from the difficult dilemmas that the patient is grappling with as well as that the fertility counselor may have in their own background. Being a fertility counselor in the field of reproductive health is very rewarding but also can be very stressful and taxing.

References

1. American Society for Reproductive Medicine Ethics Committee. Considerations of the gestational carrier: an Ethics Committee Opinion. *Fertil Steril* 2018;**110** (6):1017–1021.

2. Centers for Disease Control and Prevention. Assisted reproductive technology national summary report. 2019. Available at: www.cdc.gov/art/pdf/2016-national-summary-slides/ART_2016_graphs_and_charts.pdf [last accessed June 16, 2022].

3. Society for Assisted Reproductive Technology. IVF Success: 2019 preliminary national data. 2019. Available at: www.sartcorsonline.com/rptCSR_PublicMultYear.aspx?reportingYear=2019 [last accessed June 16, 2022].

4. Kim HH. Selecting the optimal gestational carrier: medical, reproductive, and ethical considerations. *Fertil Steril* 2020;**113**(5):892–896.

5. Simpson TH, Hanafin H. Counseling surrogate carrier participants. In: Covington SN, Ed. *Fertility Counseling: Clinical Guide and Case Studies.* Cambridge: Cambridge University Press, 2015, 122–135.

6. Klock SC, Lindheim SR. Gestational surrogacy: medical, psychosocial, and legal considerations. *Fertil Steril* 2020;**113** (5):889–891.

7. American Society for Reproductive Medicine Practice Committee. Recommendations for practices utilizing gestational carriers: an ASRM Practice Committee guideline. *Fertil Steril* 2017;**107**:e3–e10.

8. Shenfield F, Pennings G, Cohen J, Devroey P, de Wert G, Tarlatzis B. ESHRE Task Force on Ethics and Law: Surrogacy. *Hum Reprod* 2005;**20**(10):2705–2707.

9. Braverman AM. Mental health counseling in third-party reproduction in the United States: evaluation, psychoeducation, or ethical gatekeeping? *Fertil Steril* 2015;**104**:501–506.

10. Practice Committee and the Mental Health Professional Group of the American Society for Reproductive Medicine. Guidance on qualifications for fertility counselors: a committee opinion. *Fertil Steril* 2021;**115**(6):1411–1415.

11. Schwartz LL. Psychological and legal perspectives on surrogate motherhood. *Am J Fam Ther* 1991;**19**:363–366.

12. Hanafin H. Surrogacy and gestational carrier participants. In: Covington SN, Hammer-Burns L., Eds. *Infertility Counseling: A Comprehensive Handbook for Clinicians*, 2nd ed. Cambridge: Cambridge University Press, 2006, 370–386.

13. Hanley R. Father of Baby M thought mother had been screened. *New York Times* [Internet]. January 14, 1987 [cited January 15, 2020]: B1. Available from: www.nytimes.com/1987/01/14/nyregion/father-of-baby-m-thought-mother-had-been-screened.html [last accessed June 16, 2022].

14. Riddle MP. Psychological assessment of gestational carrier candidates: current approaches, challenges, and future considerations. *Fertil Steril* 2020a;**113**(5):897–902.

15. Riddle MP. The psychological impact of surrogacy on the families of gestational surrogates: implications for clinical practice. *J Psychosom Obstet Gynaecol* 2020b (online). https://doi.org/10.1080/0167482X.2020.1814729

16. Riddle MP, Jenkins SR. Clinical considerations in the psychological assessment of gestational surrogates: uses of narrative assessment. *Hum Fertil* 2020 (online). https://doi.org/10.1080/14647273.2020.1778802

17. Butcher JN, Ed. *Clinical Personality Assessment: Practical Approaches.* New York, NY: Oxford University Press, 1995.

18. Blyth E. "I wanted to be interesting. I wanted to be able to say that 'I've done something interesting in my life'": interviews with surrogate mothers in Britain. *J Reprod Infant Psychol* 1994;**12**:189–198.

19. Ciccarelli JC, Beckman LI. Navigating rough waters: an overview of psychological aspects of surrogacy. *J Soc Issues* 2005;**61**:21–43.

20. Jadva V, Murray C, Lycette E, MacCallum F, Golombok S. Surrogacy: the experiences of surrogate mothers. *Hum Reprod* 2003;**18**:2196–2204.

21. Van den Akker O. Genetic and gestational surrogate mothers' experience of surrogacy. *J Reprod Infant Psychol* 2003;**21**:145–161.

22. Klock SC, Covington SN. Results of the Minnesota Multiphasic Personality Inventory-2 among gestational surrogacy candidates. *Int J Gynecol Obstet* 2015;**130**:257–260.

23. Berend Z. Surrogate losses: failed conception and pregnancy loss among American surrogate mothers. In Komaromy C, Ed. *Understanding Reproductive Loss: Perspectives on Life, Death, and Fertility.* Abingdon: Taylor and Francis, 2012, 93–104.

24. Soderstrom-Antilla V, Wennerholm UB, Loft A, et al. Surrogacy: outcomes for surrogate mothers, children, and the resulting families – a systematic review. *Hum Reprod Update* 2016;**22**:260–276.

25. Jadva V, Imrie S. Children of surrogate mothers: psychological well-being, family relationships and experiences of surrogacy. *Hum Reprod* 2014;**29**:90–96.

26. Riddle M. An investigation into the psychological well-being of the biological children of surrogates. *Cogent Psychology* 2017;**4**:1305035.

Chapter 13

DNA and the End of Anonymity: Disclosure, Donor-Linkage and Fertility Counseling

Kate Bourne

Introduction

In the first edition of this book, a chapter about DNA testing and the impact on donor anonymity wasn't included, as the issue was only just emerging [1]. The impact of direct-to-consumer (DTC) DNA testing is now significant. DTC DNA testing has serious implications for all aspects of donor conception. People are discovering they are donor-conceived as a result of taking a test and are using the technology to connect with donor relatives. It is now impossible for donors to remain anonymous. Parents need to be aware that it is unfeasible to keep their child's donor conception a secret as the risk of discovering this is so high.

Consequently, there are substantial implications for fertility counselors and health professionals working in this field. All those working with clients considering using a donor, recipient parents, for people who are considering donating, and for those who have donated in the past, need to be familiar with these repercussions. Donor-conceived people (DCP), especially those who were raised at a time when parents were encouraged to keep their conception status secret and are now finding out as adults, are also likely to need and to seek support from fertility counselors to process this new information and possibly may wish to seek information about and contact with their donor and donor siblings.

Background

It is estimated that as many people had purchased a DTC DNA kit in 2018 as in all the previous years combined and, at the start of 2019, more than 26 million people had taken a DNA test [2]. At the time of publication, this number is likely to be exponentially higher. People take DNA tests due to curiosity, interest in their heritage, or to determine if they have a medical risk of inheriting certain conditions, to specifically seek connection with genetic

The addenda referred to in this chapter are available for download at www.cambridge.org/covington-clinical-guide

family members, or because they have been given a test as a gift. Unexpected results may occur. The largest DTC testing company, Ancestry, advises, "You may discover unexpected facts about yourself, your family, or your health when using our services. Once discoveries are made, we can't undo them" [3]. Testing recipients may discover their mother or father isn't their biological parent and they have been created with the help of a donor. They may also unexpectedly be informed of other people who have been conceived by the same donor (i.e., donor siblings).

DNA Testing: How Does It Work?

DNA companies advertise their services, primarily online, and regularly offer discounts at particular times of the year, such as Christmas. These kits are now very affordable and are often given as gifts. They are also of great appeal to anyone interested in genealogy, finding out the possible risk of inherited medical conditions or people seeking genetic relatives such as adoptees, DCPs or donors.

The kit is ordered online and sent to the purchaser, who provides a sample in the form of a cheek swab or saliva. The company then analyses the sample (commonly called "fingerprinting") and provides information about the person's heritage or ethnic background based on their DNA profile. They may also notify them of anyone who has also submitted DNA and has a similar genetic profile, together with an estimate of how close the relationship is. Parents and full siblings share approximately 50% of the DNA, whilst half genetic siblings, grandparents, aunts/uncles and nieces/nephews share 25%. More distant relatives share less DNA. It is possible to send messages to other people registered with the same company, depending on the privacy settings they set.

People can also upload their results to other DNA companies. This can increase the chances of matching with genetic relatives. It is important to note that a person needn't have taken a test themselves to be identified. Even if a distant relative has been tested, it is possible to be identified from this information. Nonidentifying donor profile information can also assist in helping to identify who the donor is, when triangulated with social media information which is publicly available.

Direct to consumer DNA testing can also be used to identify the donor and donor siblings and so it is possible to then contact them. Consequently, many donor-conceived people, their donors and donor siblings are making contact independently of the clinic/bank their parent(s) used; either intentionally or because of unexpected match/es. This was not anticipated when donor conception treatment was first practiced. Then, donors and patients were assured of anonymity and parents were encouraged to not inform their children.

What People Need to Consider before Testing

People considering having a DNA test should be aware that there is currently very little regulation of DTC DNA companies, and it is also unclear who "owns" the data. Their confidential information is also at risk if the company is sold, goes bankrupt or is hacked.

It is important for potential DTC DNA consumers to consider:

- What do they want to achieve from the test?
- Have they thought about possible unexpected outcomes?
- How might they respond to an outreach from a genetic relative they don't know or if the genetic relative doesn't know how they are related to them?
- It can be difficult to interpret the results of the DNA test. They may need to enlist some help from someone who is knowledgeable [4].
- What privacy settings they use.

DNA Testing Implications

Unexpected Results

People are regularly discovering unexpected ethnicity information or a match on a DNA database, with a person to whom they didn't know they were genetically connected. For DCPs, this could be a person conceived by the same donor, their donor or a relative of either of these. They may receive a friend request on Facebook from someone they don't know. Donors (or their extended family or children) who donated decades ago

are receiving messages on ancestry websites from people they helped create, wondering how they share 50% of their DNA. DCPs can be put in the very difficult situation of connecting with a donor sibling who isn't aware they are donor conceived. This scenario can lead to very difficult conversations to understand how they could possibly be related.

Family Secrets Are Being Revealed

For the DCP, they may then come to realize that their social parent is not their biological parent, as they presumed; however, they may not know the circumstances. They may assume their mother had an affair rather than having had donor treatment. This is not an easy subject to discuss with parents, so some DCPs may not talk to them. Sometimes, even when they do broach this sensitive subject with their parents, they may not be told the truth, as the parents may deny they had treatment. This can intensify the DCPs confusion and possibly lead to incorrect conclusions.

Processing finding out as an adult you are conceived by a donor can be overwhelming, with feelings of shock, disbelief, confusion, bewilderment and grief. It can be an extremely disorienting and distressing experience as it involves rethinking one's identity. Trust in parents may also be affected, as a DCP can feel they have been lied to and betrayed, as the truth has been withheld. This experience was eloquently described by Dani Shapiro in her memoir, *Inheritance* [5]. Finding out may also help to explain some perceived anomalies, for example, lack of physical resemblance or a feeling of being different from other members of their family.

Donor conceived people may describe this discovery as changing *everything and nothing*. They may attempt to review their life, relationships and identity to date. What does it mean for their relationship with their nonbiological parent and their extended family? While they may feel their bond remains very secure, and consider their Dad is still their Dad or their Mum is still their Mum; where does the donor fit in? If their family relationships are insecure or dysfunctional, this new information can be even more challenging to deal with. However, in such cases, the information may assist in perhaps understanding a possible cause for the longstanding issues or potentially providing some relief that they are not genetically related, if that relationship has caused pain.

The DCP may also discover that their siblings (if they have them) may not have been conceived from the same donor; so, they are in fact half genetic siblings rather than the full genetic siblings they assumed they were.

This can also lead to a questioning of the relationship. How much is based on shared genetics and how much because of a shared upbringing? Again, this may also explain physical and/or personality differences between siblings.

Discovering this new status is likely to also lead to questions about nature vs. nurture. What do I inherit from my parent/s and my donor? What influence has my nonbiological parent had on me? Who do I look like? Many DCPs describe looking into the mirror for hours, in the days following the new discovery. The DCP may have children of their own and may have concerns about their genetic medical history and what possible medical risks they may have inadvertently passed onto their children. How do they explain donor conception to their children?

To add to the complexity, one parent or both parents, or the donor may have died or have dementia, so the DCP may never be able to find answers to the important questions they may have about their parent's treatment and their donor. Some of the secrets may quite literally have been taken to the grave, as occurred for Shapiro [5].

New Family Secrets: Donor Conceived People Not Telling Parents or Siblings

Just as recipient parents have faced the dilemma of whether to tell their donor-conceived children, now DCPs are facing a similar dilemma. This situation is frequently reported in the peer support group I run. It is often a source of anguish and anxiety. Some DCPs may delay telling their parents for months or years, or decide never to tell them, as they think informing them may cause too much distress. This can result in the DCP putting aside their own needs and wishes and instead prioritizing the perceived needs of their parents. Ironically, a new kind of family secret is then consequently perpetuated.

Even if a DCP does tell their parent they know, the parents may not then tell their other children they are donor-conceived, and ask that the sibling who knows not to tell them. This can result in one or more siblings knowing they were conceived by a donor and the other siblings not being informed. This can be an excruciating secret for the DCP/s to keep. Nonetheless, they may feel it is not their business to reveal the truth. This situation may go on for months or even years. Other DCPs may feel that their sibling should know and tell them regardless.

Family Secrets Revealed: Implications for Parents

Parents who used a donor to become a family a generation ago were usually encouraged to keep this a secret. Consequently, most haven't told their adult children and are usually shocked and unprepared when their child discovers this without the parents informing them themselves. It may trigger complex emotions relating to their infertility and treatment. Couples may not have discussed using a donor with anyone else. They might also feel they were misinformed by the clinic professionals who encouraged them not to tell and assured them the information would never be revealed. Sometimes one parent may have tried to persuade the other parent to tell their child earlier, and may regret that they didn't try harder to persuade them to tell. Couples may have separated since treatment and may not be in contact with each other or communicate well together.

Counseling Newly Informed Donor Conceived People

Historically, fertility counselors have primarily only counseled clients who were considering donor treatment or potential donors. It is important to broaden our expertise to counsel the people who were created from this treatment, as they grapple with the implications of being created from donor treatment. DCPs who find out as teenagers or adults are likely to benefit from counseling support as they process this new information. It may also be beneficial to include their parents if the DCP wants them to be included.

Supporting a DCP client who has recently discovered they are donor-conceived is similar to counseling any client who experiences disenfranchised grief, and has parallels to counseling someone who has recently discovered they are adopted. The experience will mean different things to different people. It can take months or years to come to terms with and incorporate the new reality and navigate rebuilding their family relationships, if they have been damaged.

DNA Discovery: Disclosure Implications for Fertility Counselors and Health Professionals

The increasing use of DTC DNA testing and resulting discoveries have enormous ramifications for all people considering donor treatment and recipient parents.

Fertility counselors and the treating doctors need to inform their clients that disclosure about donor conception should no longer be considered a choice. It is now imperative that parents tell their children about how their family was formed, as the risk of not doing so is now untenable and impractical. There are now many children's books, resources, and parent seminars to assist parents in discussing how they became a family with their children. Past and present donors should also be advised to tell their children, partner and extended family, as they may well be contacted by donor offspring directly. There are fewer resources available to assist donors to talk to others than for recipient parents, however they are growing [6,7,8]. Whilst ideally disclosure occurs when the child is young, it is never too late for parents to talk to their child.

Disclosure Counseling

Whether counseling new parents, parents of adults, donors or DCPs who plan to talk to their parents, preparations are very similar. It is important to assist them to feel proud of their story and to explore any anxieties that may be preventing them from initiating the discussion, to provide them with resources, help them to formulate a "telling script," and a plan of action including the timing and setting. The language used is of course vital, for example, referring to the donor as the "donor" rather than the "real parent." Coming up with words can be challenging for clients and it can be helpful to role play what they might say, trying different scripts to find what is most comfortable for them, and to give feedback.

It is common for there to be a difference of opinion between parents about whether to tell. The nonbiological parent may fear rejection or may feel particularly vulnerable. They need to be sensitively supported and reassured that this will not occur. It may trigger some of the feelings they experienced when they were diagnosed with infertility or having treatment that they may have thought they had dealt with.

For clients who will be informing their adult children, it can be helpful for the fertility counselor to assist the client to write a letter. This can be given prior to or after the telling conversation and may, also, be used instead when a face-to-face conversation isn't possible. The writing itself can be an effective tool, as it helps the client process their feelings. Naturally, telling a teenager or an adult son or daughter is likely to be more challenging, so

Table 13.1 Key messages for any "telling event"

The person is loved; they are part of a family
The facts of the situation – what, when, why, how
The reason for delaying telling (if this has occurred) and apologizing for this
Reiterate the person is loved
Let's talk again

preparing their parents for the likely reactions and responses is crucial. Maintaining support for the parents as they manage the emotional implications of telling and then supporting their child/ren is essential (see also Chapter 14).

I feel particularly for DCPs grappling with how to tell their parents that they know of their conception story. Of course, their parents already know they used a donor; they just don't know their adult child knows. It is unfortunate that DCPs feel the burden of carrying this knowledge and supporting their parents when usually it is the role of the parent to do this. They may require sensitive counseling support to not only come to terms with discovering they are donor-conceived but, also, how to relay their newfound knowledge to their parents. Likewise, their parents may also require support and counseling when they have been informed that their secret has been revealed unexpectedly. Table 13.1 identifies key messages in any "telling event."

After telling, clients may benefit from debriefing. They and their family members may also benefit from counseling support to assist in processing the possible immediate ramifications, particularly if teenagers or adults have been informed. It is also important that the client is encouraged to keep conversation going after the telling event, with the offer of any questions to be answered and ongoing support given to all affected family members.

Broader DNA Discovery Implications for Health Professionals

Given DTC DNA testing and discoveries renders it impossible for donors to be anonymous, it is desirable that all clinics offering donor treatment modify their donor programs accordingly. It is important that all prospective donors are recruited on the condition of identity-release only, and that all prospective recipient parents are advised of this.

As it is highly probable that donor offspring may wish to have contact with their donor and/or donor siblings, it is, also, imperative (though currently not happening in many countries) that the use of the donation is limited to a workable family limit. This is crucial for DCP, so they do not have large numbers of donor siblings. This is important not only for concerns about consanguinity but, also, the potential difficulty in managing a large number of potential contacts or relationships. This is equally vital for donors who are likely to need to manage potential interactions with donor offspring without the process become overwhelming for them or their family, and so their offspring have a better chance of being well received.

Past donors should ideally be contacted by the clinic/donor bank and informed that they can no longer be considered anonymous and may be contacted by their offspring or parents who have used their donation. It is also important for donors to realize that people don't need to have had testing themselves in order to be identified, a fact that is commonly misunderstood. This should be of particular concern to donors if the donations have been used to help create large numbers of people. Preferably, the clinic/bank should offer counseling support both prior to and if/when the donor is contacted, to prepare them and their family and to help them consider how they may respond.

Parents who have previously used a donor should also be advised of the implications of DNA testing, not just regarding the implications for disclosure but also that their child/ren may contact the donor and/or donor siblings and may do this independently. They may find this potentially challenging and may need counseling assistance to learn to understand their child's motivation and to be able to support them in their quest for information and/or potential contact.

Fertility counselors may also find their client-base broadening to include donor-conceived people and if so, need to become proficient in counseling them. This includes those DCPs who discover their status as teenagers and adults and who may wish to seek information and/or contact with their donor and donor relatives.

Donor-Linking

Donor-Conceived People Using DNA to Seek Donor Information

Donor conceived people are utilizing this new technology to contact their donor. Common reasons for DCPs wanting information include interest in medical information; to understand motivations of the donor to donate; their appearance, hobbies, interests, personality, cultural and ethnic heritage; or as Susan Golombok writes, "to gain a better understanding of who they are, where they came from and where they fit in" [9].

There are few options for DCPs to help them find donor information or to connect with donor siblings, other than to use DNA testing, as there are currently very few donor registers, support services or resources to assist them. This contrasts with support services and resources available in the adoption reunion field. Few clinics or donor banks will assist DCPs, donor siblings and donors to connect. Voluntary Registers, which do exist, include the voluntary DNA registers Donor Sibling Registry (international); The Sperm Bank of California (TSPC) Family Contact list; Donor Conceived Register and Donor Sibling Link managed by the HEFA (UK); several in various states of Australia (Victoria, Western Australia, New South Wales); and the FIOM KID-DNA database (The Netherlands). For matches to occur on a Voluntary Register, other genetic relatives need to have registered also, so many applicants wait without matches occurring.

The Central Register managed by The Victorian Assisted Reproductive Treatment Authority (VARTA) in Victoria, Australia is one of the few organizations which provides an outreach service to donors on the DCP's behalf. It includes professional counseling support, advice and intermediary services, to DCPs, donors and their respective families. Donor identity-release programs, such as The Sperm Bank of California (TSBC) and donor identity-release to be enacted by legislation in the UK in 2023, will provide information and services to DCPs as they come of age.

Consequently, with few support services available, many DCPs seek information using DTC DNA information. They may be assisted to find their genetic relative by a "DNA Detective" or "Search Angel," as they are commonly referred to. These DNA detectives are skilled in interpreting DNA results and may help either voluntarily or for a fee. They may be motivated purely by altruism or because they are themselves donor-conceived or adopted. Assistance can be readily found on social media sites. At the time of writing, the Facebook group, DNA Detectives, had 155,322 members [10].

Outreaching to the donor or donor relatives can be extremely daunting and puts the DCP in a vulnerable position, as they don't know what kind of response they will receive from the other party. They may need to initially contact the donor's extended family to enable them to work out the identity of the donor. The extended family member may be helpful or obstructive. They may be overenthusiastic or actively block the DCP. Contact with the donor's extended family, also, has implications for the donor, as family members may then become aware that their relative has donated and have contact with the donor offspring before the donor does, thus breaching their privacy. It is also possible the DCP may need to contact several possible people before they correctly identify the correct identity of the donor. DCPs may not tell their parents they are seeking donor information out of perceived loyalty to the nonbiological parent.

Implications for Donors Contacted by Their Offspring

Whilst the DCP may have been contemplating trying to find out more information for some time, the donor may not have been expecting any outreach and may feel quite shocked and unprepared for the contact. It might come at a time when they may be experiencing other life stresses. They may question whether the DCP is, in fact, related to them and may fear they are being scammed. They may be concerned that the person's motives are deceitful and may mistakenly believe they could be entitled to make a claim on their estate. They may also be concerned that the DCP wants them to assume a parental role, when this is not the case, or be emotionally needy or unstable.

Even if the donor doesn't doubt the genetic connection or is not concerned about the motivation of the DCP, the unexpected contact is likely to lead to a complex emotional response. Kenneth Leetz, a donor and retired psychiatrist, contacted by a donor-conceived offspring via his daughter, Michelle, who had taken a DNA test, writes eloquently about the flux of emotions and thoughts he experienced,

> Swirling around in my head were questions of responsibility – and to whom and what? ... How would this affect Michelle, and did I need to protect her? From what, though? My view of the world and my genetic place in it, which had focused on the dyad of Michelle and me, was now potentially a triad. The shift was disconcerting initially, but there were twinges of other unanticipated emotions, such as pride in reproductive success, concern for my newly discovered offspring, and a growing cognitive-emotional inconsistency, which felt vaguely discomfiting. It was all indefinable and cognitively dissonant for me [11].

This quote demonstrates that it is a myth that donors are not curious about their offspring [12]. Many donors express an interest to know whether their offspring are happy, healthy and have been loved. Donors may well be open to sharing information and having contact. Some may find their offspring is remarkably similar in personality or appearance and may find they share common interests. Some may enjoy long-term contact with them with strong relationships forming.

Implications for the Donor's Partner and Children

An outreach from a donor's offspring also has significant implications for the donor's partner, who may or may not be aware that their partner donated previously. This may be due to the donor's shame or embarrassment about donating, or because it was thought that there would never be any need to share this information as there would never be any contact with their donor offspring. Some donors may even be unaware their donation resulted in any births.

The donor's partner has no genetic connection to the donor offspring and so may feel like an outsider to this stranger who is the biological son or daughter of their partner. They may experience feelings of jealousy if their partner is spending a lot of time communicating with them. For some partners, it can feel like their partner has had an "affair," as a child has been born outside their relationship, even though of course there has been no sexual infidelity. Contact can also be particularly emotionally challenging if the couple doesn't have children, especially if they experienced infertility. If the donor's partner isn't in favor of the donor having contact, yet the donor would like to, this can lead to conflict. The donor is likely to feel torn between the wishes of their offspring and partner, trying to please each, and the partner can feel guilty about trying to prevent contact when they know their partner would like to.

Conversely, in other situations, the donor's partner may empathize with the DCP and try to actively persuade their partner to share information. Initial concerns may subside in time, when each partner has had time to adjust. As the wife of a donor writes:

> My initial reaction was to feel as though suddenly the window blind had snapped up while I was in the bath – shocked, exposed and even fearful. And then, after discussion and reflection with my husband, we shared a sense of anticipation and just plain curiosity [13].

The donor's children may not be aware their parent donated. They may welcome the contact as Michelle (above) did and become actively involved and may also assist to persuade their parent to have contact, or they may perceive this as an unwelcome intrusion into their family. They may fear that they may be displaced by the DCP or feel some jealousy if they perceive the DCP to be more "successful" than they are.

Whilst the donor, his partner and children may be prepared to provide information to the DCP who contacted them, they may well be concerned about future repeated requests and the pressure this could pose for them and their family. This is naturally exacerbated if there is concern that the donation has resulted in a high number of donor offspring having been born.

Donor Siblings Connecting

Donor conceived people are often extremely interested to connect with offspring from the same donor, to find people like themselves [14]. Research reports many positive connections with strong friendships forming [15]. Single children in a family may express an even greater curiosity. As donors can often be used to produce large numbers of offspring, many donor siblings may potentially find each other. This can be uniquely challenging and complex as they adapt to a continually expanding number of potential connections.

As mentioned previously, donor siblings may not be aware of their conception status. The sibling who is aware they are donor-conceived is in the invidious position of trying to sensitively and tactfully explain how they could be related to the sibling who is unaware. This then results in a DCP discovering they are donor-conceived or that they are the child of a donor from their donor-conceived sibling. This poses unique challenges when potentially navigating a future relationship together. Donor siblings may form close attachments or may not find very much in common. They may have had very different upbringings and may live far from each other, making it challenging to get to know one another.

Recipient parents, more commonly solo mothers or lesbian mums, are also increasingly contacting each other and their children, even when their children are young. This can also potentially result in large numbers of recipient families connecting with each other. Whilst contact between families can be positive, it can depend on whether the parents and their children like each other and have similar values and expectations of contact. There are also implications relating to whether they reside in geographic proximity to each other. As donor

banks export nationally and internationally [16,17], they may be separated by distance, language and cultural differences.

Donor Linking: Broader Implications and Bigger Questions

Terminology: What Do We Call Each Other?

People may have difficulty knowing how to refer to each other and coming up with appropriate terminology is important. What do DCPs call their donor? Donor, biological father/mother, genetic father/mother, father/mother, real father/mother, donor Dad/mum, progenitor, Dad/Mum? What do they call the other people conceived from the same donor? Donor siblings, diblings, genetic half-siblings, same-donor peers, half-brothers/sisters, sort of siblings, kind of cousins? How does a donor refer to the people they helped to create? Biological son/daughter, donor son/daughter, donor offspring, son/daughter [18]? Terminology continues to evolve over time and each person involved in donor conception must find the words that feel right to them.

Connections: Who Are We to Each Other?

It can take years to feel and to establish a comfortable pattern of interaction, and of course some connections may peter out if the connection isn't serving them. The DCP may have received all the information they sought and not be interested in an ongoing relationship, or the donor may not be prepared to have continued contact. Conversely, the relationship may grow and blossom over time. People often describe feeling like they are "walking on eggshells" in the early years of contact, not wanting to behave inappropriately. As there is no etiquette for donor linking, they are likely to continue to feel their way and try not to offend the other person.

Consequently, people joined by donor conception treatment may question what their connection really means. Are we friends, family or something in-between [19]? They may perceive these relationships as a new form of family, for example, donor clans or donor kin or perhaps merely strangers connected by genes. How do they describe these new relationships to others? How do they introduce the new person/people? Again, these complex issues and implications are likely to change overtime as relationships develop (or not).

Navigating Donor Linking

There is no etiquette book for donor linking. Unlike adoption reunion, this is still a relatively new and emerging form of connection, with different outcomes emerging. All parties, whether they are a DCP, a parent or a donor, can feel bewildered and lost as to how best to maximize their chance of having a positive outcome. They may question what is appropriate/inappropriate and lack confidence and experience as to how to contact other genetic relatives sensitively and respectfully.

Service users of the donor registers at VARTA were asked how they would advise others who were embarking on this process [19]? They suggested the following:

- *Timing* – Take it slowly; let the process pace itself as needed and as you need it to; this will be a marathon and not a sprint.
- *Openness* – Have no expectations; what you learn about the other party may be different from what you have been told or expected; be honest with your children/family; avoid judging your parents or your donor.
- *Practical* – The initial letter is critically important so get support to draft it; think about your social media accounts – what impression may the other person have about you if they see this; consider changing your privacy settings; think about next steps and discuss this with the other person.

They advise that, ultimately, it is going to be an emotional and nerve-wracking process.

Donor Linking Counseling

Ideally the fertility counselor works with all parties who are considering making connections with donor relatives. If this is not possible, then the counsellor can support their client to explore possible outcomes and implications for themselves and people close to them, highlight the possible emotional responses of the other party/ies and assist them to navigate their situation as sensitively as possibly, whilst supporting them throughout the process.

Initially it can be helpful to explore what the client hopes to achieve from contact. Do they want information only or are they hoping for a relationship? How would they initially like to contact the donor relative? What would their fantasy and nightmare scenarios of contact look like? Fertility counselors can have a crucial role to help to prepare clients for outreach and possible contact, assist to manage their expectations, and to give advice as to what they may wish to include in the first outreach message. Clients need to be provided with clear information as to

their possible options, have agency over what they decide to do, and the pace at which they wish to proceed. If a DCP client has only recently discovered their conception status, they may need time to process what this means for them before they are emotionally ready to proceed to try to find out more about their donor relative/s.

Fertility counselors can also support clients who have been contacted by donor relatives and explore how they might respond, what the implications are for them and those close to them. Unfortunately, many are left to manage these new connections without professional support. Peer support groups and information/advice are available for DCPs on Facebook or websites. Little support is available for donors and their families. Donor sites tend to be for the recruitment of donors, either for donor banks or for informal recruitment matching donors with potential recipients.

If working with both a DCP and a donor (and potentially more parties), the fertility counselor should remain neutral. It is essential that they don't become an advocate for one party or the other and don't have a particular agenda or outcome in mind. They may act as a mediator/intermediary facilitator if they have contact with both/all parties and each/all are happy for the counselor to do this. The counselor obviously needs to maintain confidentiality. They must only share any information to the other party with the specific consent of the party concerned.

Donor-linking counseling is thus *implications* counseling rather than intensive *therapeutic* counseling. It is important to remember that the client is usually psychologically healthy and that it is normal and expected to have an interest to connect with donor relatives. It takes courage and ego strength for clients to embark on this quest. However, seeking donor relative information may occur with only recent awareness that the person is donor-conceived or for the donor, that there may be the potential for contact. There may be little support from partners, family, the clinic or bank which provided the treatment/donation, or any other organization to guide them. In addition, few societal norms exist about what these relationships should look like. The primary focus of the fertility counselor when donor linking is to prepare and to assist the client to navigate these new and potentially complex relationships.

Donor Linking Process

The Australian and New Zealand Infertility Counsellors Association (ANZICA) has developed donor linking counseling practice guidelines which provide a framework for fertility counselors working at ART units which offer donor linking services to follow. These guidelines can be found in Addendum 13.1.

Please see Figure 13.1 for a suggested process that supports donor-linkage when a fertility counselor is working in an ART unit.

Conclusion

The dramatic increase in the use of DTC DNA testing has had a significant impact on all aspects of donor conception. It has rendered the practice of donor anonymity as unworkable, impractical, ineffectual, unfeasible and ultimately untenable. It has unearthed past secrets which may have previously been taken to the grave. It has vindicated the counseling advice of encouraging parents to tell their children about the truth of their conception. It has provided a unique mechanism for DCPs to find and connect with donor relatives when previously they may not have been assisted by the clinic or bank from which their parents sourced their treatment or donation.

The genie is fully out of the bottle. Fertility counselors and health professionals need to be aware of the implications that DTC DNA testing has for their past, present and future clients. They need to adapt their current clinic practice accordingly to ensure the use of identity-release donors who are fully informed of the potential information needs and interest of their potential donor offspring, only. Current

Figure 13.1 Donor linkage process.

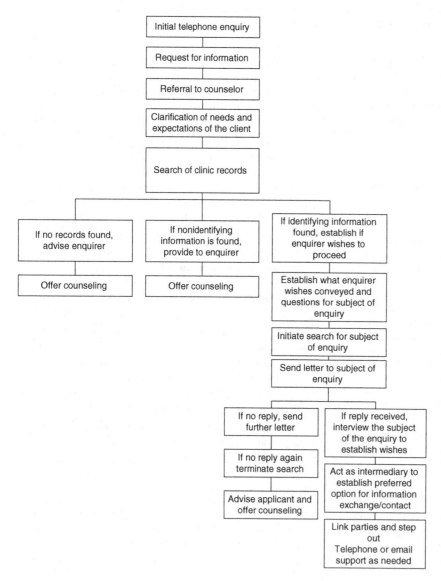

clients, whether they be patients undergoing donor treatment or potential donors, need to be advised of these potential implications for themselves but more importantly for their children.

Counseling may also be needed for past patients and donors who, with the benefit of hindsight, can now be seen to have been poorly advised by their treating clinic or bank, and who may now be experiencing the impacts of past practice with the implications this new technology brings. Most importantly, DCPs need to be provided with support, as they are the unintended victims of what can now be seen as, perhaps, a well-intentioned social experiment which has had unintended, powerful and complex negative implications. Fertility counselors can offer unique support in this emerging and potentially complex web of inter-relationships, to mitigate the impact of any negative experiences and hopefully to help their clients to experience potentially positive outcomes and rich connections with their donor relatives.

References

1. Harper JC, Kennett D, Reisel D. The end of donor anonymity: how genetic testing is likely to drive anonymous gamete donation out of business. *Hum Reprod* 2016;**31**:1135–1140.

2. Regalado A. More than 26 million people have taken an at-home ancestry test, MIT Technology Review. Available from: www.technologyreview.com/2019/02/11/103446/more-than-26-million-people-have-taken-an-at-home-ancestry-test/ [last accessed June 16, 2022].

3. Ancestry.com. Privacy statement. Available from: www.ancestry.com/cs/legal/privacystatement [last accessed June 16, 2022].

4. Vanish Voice. Autumn 2019, pp. 5–7. Available from: https://vanish.org.au/media/95986/vanish-autumn-voice-newsletter-2019.pdf [last accessed June 16, 2022].

5. Shapiro D. *Inheritance, Memoir of Genealogy, Paternity, and Love*. New York, NY: Alfred A. Knopf, 2019.

6. Sarles P. Assisted reproduction: books for parents to help explain assisted reproduction to their children. Available from: https://donorgroupsnyc.blogspot.com/2011/07/patricia-sarles-blogspot-about-books.html [last accessed June 16, 2022].

7. Donor Conception Network. Available from: www.dcnetwork.org/ [last accessed June 16, 2022].

8. Victorian Assisted Reproductive Treatment Authority. Available from: www.varta.org.au/after-donor-conception/telling-children-family-and-others [last accessed June 16, 2022].

9. Golombok S. *We Are Family*. London: Scribe publications, 2020, p. 261.

10. DNA Detectives Facebook group, hosted by CeCe Moore – Genetic Genealogist. Available from: www.facebook.com/groups/DNADetectives/ [last accessed June 16, 2022].

11. Leetz K. An unanticipated outcome of a DNA test. *Am J Psychiatry* 2018;**175**(12):1167–1168.

12. Jadva V. Sperm and egg donors' experiences of anonymous donation subsequent contact with their donor offspring. *Hum Reprod* 2011;**26**:638–645.

13. Victorian Assisted Reproductive Treatment Authority. March 2017. Available from: www.varta.org.au/resources/personal-stories/we-were-sperm-donors [last accessed June 16, 2022].

14. Dempsey D, Kelly F, Horsfall B, Hammarberg K, Bourne K, Johnson L. Applications to statutory donor registers in Victoria, Australia: information sought and expectations of contact. *Reprod Biomed Soc Online* 2019;**9**:28–36.

15. Scheib J, McCormick E, Benward J. Finding people like me: contact among young adults who share an open-identity sperm donor, *Hum Reprod Open* 2020;**4**:hoaa057.

16. Jadva V, Freeman T, Kramer W, Golombok S. Experiences of offspring searching for and contacting their donor siblings and donor. *Reprod BioMed Online* 2010;**20**(4):523–532.

17. Hertz R, Nelson M. *Random Families, Genetic Strangers, Sperm Donor Siblings, and the Creation of New Kin*. Oxford: Oxford University Press, 2018.

18. Kelly F, Dempsey D, Power J, Bourne K, Hammarberg K, Johnson L. From stranger to family or something in between: donor linking in an era of retrospective access to anonymous sperm donor records in Victoria, Australia. *Int J Law Policy Family* 2019;**33**:277–297.

19. Victorian Assisted Reproductive Treatment Authority. Available from: www.varta.org.au/resources/information-sheets/navigating-donor-linking [last accessed June 16, 2022].

Family Life after Donor Conception

Marilyn Crawshaw, Astrid Indekeu and Jane Ellis

Where counseling is delivered in relation to donor conception fertility treatment, incorporating knowledge of the unfolding lifespan experiences of those affected and their networks has the potential to lower risks of later adverse consequences and strengthen parenting potential. In similar vein, later interventions with families, couples or individuals can usefully draw on knowledge about experiences of fertility treatment and involuntary childlessness.

This chapter focuses on the contribution that research, professional practice and personal experiences bring to understanding donor conception (DC) family life. Although there are different family forms according to the type of donation used, we've concentrated primarily on what are shared experiences rather than what is unique. We have not included material specific to donors and their families but invite readers to consider where there may be transferable messages.

Background

For many years, DC was seen as "a solution" to a problem. Embedded in a culture of nondisclosure, pregnancy was considered the end to the need to think about involuntary childlessness. Gradually, awareness-raising by mental health professionals/social workers and especially donor-conceived people themselves challenged this presumption. Today it is more often seen as a family-building process, an ongoing story that unfolds as new questions and challenges arise during family life and beyond. As the evidence base continues to grow, we can slowly understand more about what changes for families and individuals, and what endures, both positive and negative.

Donor conception is also "a story with various storytellers" including grandparents, parents, children and many others, each with their different voices. For a long time, research relied mainly on parents' (mainly mothers) accounts of family life, and observations of DC children.

The addenda referred to in this chapter are available for download at www.cambridge.org/covington-clinical-guide

More recently, the voices of DC people themselves have been gathered, especially those of DC adults, whose parents used an anonymous sperm donor, looking back at their family experiences. The advent of internet forums has facilitated the growth of peer support and evidence-gathering outside of academic research. Nevertheless, the need to fill the continuing gaps is clear, not least as the "family story" is told and co-created by multifamily members with different perspectives and different feelings. This makes it both a creative and a challenging process, including in relation to terminology.

Terminology

Terminology is complex and contested in relation to DC. Terms used can change over time and across contexts, including within families or by individual family members, sometimes creating tensions. One such example is the term "donor." It has been in common usage by professionals and parents (regardless of whether the donor was paid), and although DC people might adopt the term as children, some later prefer a term that they feel better reflects what this person means to them, for example "biological parent."

For the purposes of this chapter, we have elected to use the following:

Donor-conceived (DC) people – to describe those conceived through DC, except when we refer specifically to DC children or DC adults.

Donor – we've used three categories, as each can carry differences, as well as similarities, in implications for family life:

- *Anonymous/unknown donor* – whose identity was not known at the time of treatment and about whom there is no formal mechanism for it to be released at any stage.
- *Known donor* – whose identity was known to the prospective parents at the time of treatment (relative, friend or someone recruited specifically) but about whom there is no formal mechanism for it to be

released at any stage unless they were also recorded as "identity-release."

- *Identity-release donor* – whose identity can be released formally at a later stage to the person conceived with their donated gametes. The age and mechanism for identity-release is usually laid down in either legislation or the policy and procedures of the fertility treatment clinic or gametes donor bank.

We do not cover "informal" sperm donors in this chapter, that is those who donate outside of a clinic or sperm bank setting and who often "advertise" their availability through the Internet.

"Donor-related siblings" or "donor relatives" – we use these terms to describe people genetically/biologically related to each other through the donor.

Finally, we use the term **"biological/genetic" relationships** rather than only "biological" or "genetic." We note the increasing use of "genetic" in professional and policy circles, yet suggest this fails to capture the potentially differing use of, and reactions to, each.

From "Building a Family" to "Being a Family"

We were on a canoe trip with my husband's brother and his family. We were in a canoe with our sons, and his brother and his family (wife and kids) were in a canoe. Paddling alongside each other all of sudden it hit me that my husband shares more genes with his brother's children in the other boat than with our children in our boat ... that's just one of those moments you wonder about genetics, family and all that kind of stuff (Mother through sperm donation)

Prior to treatment, the focus for prospective parents (and counselors) is typically focused on *becoming* a family (or achieving a pregnancy) rather than on *being* a family. The shift happens later. However, the term "family" can itself carry different meanings, including culturally. The use of DC treatment prompts these to be reviewed and managed, including by DC people themselves.

When I found donor-related siblings through online DNA-testing, I also found out that my brother, who I grew up with, and I do not share the same donor as previously told. So he is actually a half-brother. In the same genetic way to me as my donor-related siblings. That was startling at first. 'Cause he is family, and I see him as 'a full brother'. It makes you re-think genetic connections, family. (DC person)

Despite the growth in numbers of same-sex, single and step-parent families, everyday normative understandings of what constitutes a family have been slow to change in most cultures. Mainstream narratives continue to reflect assumptions that "first choice" families comprise a mother, father and their biological/genetic children onto which kinship networks map, and against which other family structures are defined and measured. Our identity and sense of where we fit in "our" world is also constructed through social and collective processes. Thus, a child within a family is situated in relation to key others and wider social networks, commonly underpinned by assumptions of biological/genetic connection.

Using DC interrupts and challenges such assumptions. Although some countries allow open advertising for gametes donors, associated media storylines and diverse family forms, this is not universally so. It is still banned by some religions and countries, and families in some rural or close-knit communities remain conservatively configured. Parents can fear that social disapproval means openness will lead to ostracism for them and their child within their wider family or community.

The new family system, thus, has to seek equilibrium either through getting as close to prevailing norms as possible or by developing or finding new ones, if it is to avoid being in the shadows. A key question it has to address is, "What makes us family, if it is not genetic connections?". Although such social and emotional "work" can appear prominent in the early days, it is increasingly clear that it continues to be needed throughout the family life-cycle with engagement, conscious or unconscious, of all family members, often including extended family. Ongoing family and social conversations, for example, remain influenced by socialized "nature–nurture" messages. Think how often such conversations draw on assumptions about biological/genetic transmission, as well as learned behaviors, of who "takes after" whom or the presumed (or asserted) primacy of "blood ties." They take on different impact and meaning for members of a DC family.

Given that the formative social and emotional work typically falls to the parents, it follows that where a parent(s) is uncomfortable about DC or lacks confidence in discussing it, it will be harder for their children to feel loved and celebrated in their full identity and confident in sharing their DC story as and when they wish. So how does the family manage the sharing of their story?

Different Story-tellers in the Family

I prefer to call him my biological father. He hasn't donated to me and he is my biological father. Donor sounds really clinical, as if I was made in a factory.
(DC person)

My wife and I always used the word donor. But now our daughter (13) talks about her 'biological father'. It makes me feel insecure. What is my role now when she calls him father?
(Father through sperm donation)

Although it is the family unit that has to manage social and cultural assumptions, each member is increasingly likely to do this in their own way and at their own pace. Views and feelings – which might anyway not be static – can collide or diverge between grandparents and parents, parents and children, and siblings. Finding the balance between allowing space for individual differences and staying connected in a shared story can be challenging. It can be especially important to keep in mind that differences are not necessarily a sign of family dysfunction, though they can become so. For example, we referred earlier to potentially different views about the description "donor." Its common use among parents and professionals may reflect that the "donor" is seen to "donate" to the recipient parent(s) or clinic. Donors themselves may also prefer a "gift" narrative to one that emphasizes their contribution to a new life. However, DC people may come to see the "donor" as having provided part of their genes and biography, and therefore warranting the description "biological/genetic parent." Given that terms such as parent and sibling are commonly associated with kinship and hold social and emotional meaning, their use potentially generates relationship tensions or conflicts where any of the parties find it difficult to accommodate terms favored by others (see https://oliviasview.wordpress.com/2020/10/12/that-difficult-word-donor/; and https://isogg.org/wiki/Donor_conceived_or_pre-conception_adopted).

The Family Life-cycle and Challenges with Openness

In discussing this area, we include a note of caution in relation to research findings. Currently, study sizes remain fairly small, as do the numbers and range of studies undertaken. Divergent findings may therefore yet emerge.

In general, developmental psychology research with DC families across all donation types – conducted primarily via mothers through interviews, child/parent–child observations and/or standardized tests until the child(ren) reaches mid-adolescence – shows that the children do well. Although mainly involving sperm-DC children, data on those born following egg and embryo donation are largely complementary. Findings show physical, psychological and social development to be within normal parameters, including on gender development, peer relationships and intellectual development, regardless of awareness of origins. Parents may be more protective towards their children but not significantly so. However, a more variable picture between disclosing and nondisclosing families emerges by mid-adolescence stages (for an overview see [1]). Research with nondisclosing families necessarily has to stop at this stage because it is considered unethical to conduct such studies unless young people are aware of the focus.

Both parents and DC people have reported early openness to have a neutral or positive impact on parent–child relationships. Open parents seem to have less severe disputes with their children and more relational satisfaction than do nondisclosing parents. They appear not to regret disclosing to their children, with some expressing relief at having done so and/or wishing that they had done so earlier. Within disclosing families, more positive family relationships and higher levels of adolescent well-being have been found for those told about their origins before age 7. DC people themselves have reported feeling neutral or curious rather than disturbed about being donor-conceived (at least when told at a young age). Contrary to professionals' fears in the early days, openness does not appear to burden the children and no evidence of associated bullying has been reported. This is not to say that managing the openness process is devoid of challenges.

I thought it was about telling them about the donor conception. And that was it. But now when they are growing up, I realise we still need to tell them they have a different donor . . . so they are not full-siblings . . . and probably have quite a lot half-siblings . . . and that they can request information about the donor . . . still so many steps to go.
(Parent through sperm donation)
I call him "donor-daddy" 'cause I feel guilty and sad my daughter has no real dad like her friends at the playground. But now she starts asking when will her daddy come home . . . so maybe that was not such a good idea . . .
(Solo Mother)

Differences as well as similarities across family-types in relation to patterns of openness have been found. Broadly speaking, lesbian couples and solo mothers using sperm donation appear more open with their children than are heterosexual couples, perhaps because the absence of a father prompts questions. However, this does not necessarily mean that talking about DC is an easier process for one family type over another. For example, same-sex couples using surrogacy seem more open about the surrogate than about the egg donor (where one was used). Indeed, there is growing evidence of the complexity of the task of integrating the DC "story" into family and community life. Despite greater acceptance generally of different family forms, re-constituted families are the largest group and the use of DC can still prompt unique social disapproval, contributing to enduring feelings of shame, stigma or grief in some individuals or couples. It is of note that one research overview concluded that couples across all types were more likely to be open if they felt strong and secure in their relationship [2].

Some parents struggle to get started, even if they believe openness to be important. Given that storytelling is often the vehicle through which information or (healthy) change is managed within and by families – and especially parents – the absence of mainstream DC-related social scripts or codes of conduct can be an inhibitor [3]. This may contribute to at best delaying disclosure and at worst turning to stories that better fit dominant hetero-normative narratives. However, exposure to stories from *outside* the family about the importance of openness about DC can also prompt parents to revisit earlier decisions and/or act as a trigger, even many years later, and peer and professional support can help.

Disclosure is frequently seen as a dichotomous concept: that parents will either disclose or not, a "once-and-for-all" decision. Disclosure is anyway not synonymous with openness, which goes beyond solely "informing" a child about their origins to being able to discuss it throughout the family life-span. Some DC people report that their parents told them once during childhood but never revisited the subject; others remember instructions to either keep it wholly secret or only tell certain people. The resulting parental emotional unavailability for a child needing to keep making meaning of this information over the years ahead can, unsurprisingly, result in adverse repercussions, including internalizing that DC is somehow shameful and hence tainting of their sense of self [4].

In contrast, openness is a process, a story that unfolds in age-appropriate and situation-appropriate ways, with parents responding to questions but also prompting discussion from time to time (see DC Network's guide at bit.ly/3wA30GP). Conversations need to be interactive, with the child(ren) taking an increasingly active role through asking questions, choosing their own descriptions, and gradually taking the lead in deciding who else to tell, when, and how. As their understanding of genetics develops, so too can parents (and others) usefully help DC people incorporate its emerging and potentially fluid meaning to them and their relationship to the donor and donor relatives.

For parents, thinking about their donor's role in their family-*building* is one thing, but being able to incorporate them "as a person" into their family-*being* and respond in nonthreatened ways to their child's interest in him/her draws on different thoughts, feelings and skills. Current research shows no evidence that such interest is driven primarily by poor experiences of family life or parenting, distress or lowered well-being [5]. Nevertheless, talking about the donor together can still feel daunting at times, for all concerned. Children, especially older children, might fear hurting their parents by expressing interest. Parents might find it triggers their insecurities about their parental position or brings to the fore any unresolved feelings about their involuntary childlessness. Being swamped by "here-and-now" adult reactions can reduce their emotional availability as a parent. For those with little information about the donor or donor relatives or opportunity to find more, the adverse impact on this unfolding process is clear. Frustrations can mount, parents can feel guilty about (or regret) their earlier choices of donor type, children can criticize those choices, and the emotional space for fantasy can grow.

Finally, families do not live in a vacuum right from the start. Outside events enter family life through news and media, and children go to school. In classes, questions may be posed about genetic inheritance or ethical values regarding assisted conception, and assignments set to "introduce your family." Parents and children alike can find themselves unexpectedly confronted with such personal issues across different contexts. The rise in popularity of direct-to-consumer DNA testing (which is discussed more fully in Chapter 13) can be one such context. Its use by nuclear and extended family members for other reasons is resulting in increasing numbers learning unexpectedly of their DC origins, or that a relative has been a gamete donor and so on. This highlights as never before the importance of learning how to handle the actual or anticipated reactions of others and maximizing feelings of control through being in the driving seat of openness.

Effects of Continuing Nondisclosure

In the UK, and with a growing consensus internationally, there is now agreement across legal and regulatory frameworks and professional bodies that parents should start the openness process from infancy. This sits well with understandings of child development and these can usefully be shared and discussed with parents, who might otherwise assume a child needs to have reached a level of verbal or conceptual development before openness can commence (see DC Network's guide at bit.ly/2Vt5wBD). Although many will be able to engage nondefensively, this will falter unless any fears about bonding with their child, feelings of shame, stigma or grief, or concerns about the fragility of their family system or wider networks are acknowledged and processed. There is also evidence that parents need concrete help and advice about what disclosure and openness strategies to use, both with the child and others.

Early openness avoids a child being exposed to the risks that might accompany having to later adapt their identity to incorporate a different origins story and understanding of relationships to that which they had previously believed. Accounts from DC adults indicate that disclosure during childhood or adulthood, rather than infancy, can be harmful, including through an identity crisis. For some, it can be difficult to separate out which feelings attach to disclosure and which to desire for information/contact, and this can in turn complicate the processing of feelings about each. Getting the pace right is further complicated, especially in adulthood, by the growth in the size of their networks [6].

Disclosure beyond infancy is less likely to be planned. Outside of DNA testing, here are a few examples of accidental disclosure from our research and practice experiences:

- A father letting slip in a family conversation that childhood mumps had left him sterile;
- Overhearing a parent telling someone else;
- Having medical tests for potential genetic transmission of disease from her father until eventually her mother told her and the doctor that she had been conceived using sperm donation;
- A parent developing dementia and starting to talk openly about DC in her care home; and
- Coming across relevant documents following the death of a parent.

Accidental or later disclosure can lead to loss of trust in parents and others who have held the secret, prompt deep confusion over identity, and be disruptive of a range of relationships, not all of which will be repaired. Some DC people experience anger or distress because they perceive their mother to have prioritized her "wifely" over her parental duties in agreeing to secrecy to "protect" her husband:

> When I probed my mum as to why she didn't tell me as a child, she has always been hazy. She claims that if I had known as a child, I may have been mean to my father about it and not respected him. The most painful thing is this ... to think that she wanted to protect him more than me. Had I been in her position I would have put my child first. (DC adult conceived through sperm donation, quoted in ([4], p. 9))

Others can redefine any prior relationship problems with their father postdisclosure as being caused by biological/genetic difference:

> My father and I never had a bond really, he wasn't terribly interested in me, which affected me very badly as a child. I couldn't understand it. He was unfaithful to my mother continuously throughout their marriage and was almost quite blatant about this. This has affected my relationships as an adult. In some ways I got some closure from learning the truth because I could finally see that we didn't have a bond for a reason and not because of something I had done wrong. (DC adult conceived through sperm donation, quoted in ([6], p. 180))

Conversely, some DC people seem to cope with later planned or accidental disclosure. One study concluded that the experience might be eased where they had a strong relationship with at least one parent whom they felt to be mentally strong and could understand their parents' reasons for seeking treatment and keeping it secret, even if they did not agree with them [7]. Some report relief at disclosure if they had previously felt something amiss in their family relationships and prefer the truth to their fantasies or uncertainties. Nondisclosure has also been a source of sadness where, for example, the truth only emerged after the death of a much-loved nongenetic parent and hence left no opportunity to discuss it with them or affirm their relationship.

There can be additional complexity in secrecy patterns that cause repercussions. Some parents tell friends or family members, perhaps finding it difficult to keep the secret to themselves. As well as creating the potential for these others to later disclose, regardless of parents' wishes, some DC people are distressed at realizing that more people than their parents have withheld the information. Some are told by mothers without fathers knowing, some do not know who else in their family knows including siblings with whom they have been raised, some have relatives who know but act as if they don't, leaving them unsure if this is deliberate or not [6].

The Impact of Family Boundaries: Tight or Permeable?

For me, the donor didn't exist. We needed sperm to build our family. And sperm donation was like blood donation. That's anonymous. I liked it. No need to know anything about the donor. But then our boy was born and started to grow up. And through some characteristics ... the donor became a little bit more visible. Even more, now, I feel confident as a parent and I feel unhappy about donor anonymity as I would like to be able to answer my son's questions about the donor.
(Father through sperm donation)

Despite parents owing the existence of their family to the donor and the emphasis on openness, consideration of the donor as a stakeholder in the ongoing life of the DC family has been relatively neglected, including in research. Whether they are discussed openly, whether they are anonymous/unknown, "known," or identity-release, they play a part in the family system. Parents manage their "presence" in different ways. Some prefer to de-personalize the donor ("We needed cells"; "I just want medical information") and not know anything personal about them, perhaps to protect themselves from the emotional impact of needing a donor, feelings of threat and uncertainty about their position as partner and/or nongenetic parent. Some may acknowledge them as a person but within a closely defined persona ("A kind lady gave us her eggs"). Some set tight boundaries with the donor firmly positioned outside the family system. Others from the outset "invite them in." Others shift their position, albeit sometimes with trepidation, as their perceptions of their child's actual or potential needs alter, or their needs to "kin" and "de-kin" shift following schisms in the family system, such as divorce [8,9].

Birth can be a transformative experience; taking up the parental role can enhance parental confidence, as can the emerging attachment between the nongenetic parent and child. Where this happens, prior uncertainties and anxieties can fade, allowing parents to feel more relaxed about the donor's contribution and their ability to weave it into their family narrative. On the other hand, the donor can slowly invade daily family life uninvited

through resemblance remarks ("How strange that she doesn't look like either of you") and through elements of their child's everyday life such as inquiries about medical family history. Fielding observations from others can be especially challenging for parents who have opted for secrecy, have sore wounds from struggling themselves to see their child as part of their wider family, feel enduring uneasiness at having used DC, or who feel otherwise threatened by lack of physical or trait resemblance to themselves [10].

As children are growing up, parents can therefore be engaged in ongoing careful negotiation between acknowledging the significance of the donor for their family/their child and safe-guarding their parental authority (especially that of a nongenetic parent) and the family boundaries. Learning to separate their own feelings as "here-and-now" adults from those as parents can be crucial for recognizing how best to cope with such reactions in order to remain emotionally available to their children.

What Do Donor Conceived People Tell Us?

There is growing research understanding of the experiences of DC people as reported by them, albeit still in relatively small numbers and with most conceived through sperm donation (for a review, see [11]).

There are consistent reports that some DC people view the donor as someone who holds information that might be valuable to them, including (but not only) for their identity. There is also a widely held belief in their right to donor information so that they can decide its significance for themselves. It follows that any blocks to such information, especially where it is held in state or clinic records, generate strong negative feelings. This carries implications for those whose parents used an anonymous or known non-identity-release donor, even where they can understand parental reasons for doing so.

Donor conceived people also talk about the meaning to them of genetic "stranger" relationships, and hence of genes. Not surprisingly, meanings evolve rather than remaining static and are informed, not only by their level of conceptual and emotional development but, also, by a social context in which reference to genetics is increasingly commonplace [12].

Others react as if I am over-emphasising genes, but genes are just all over! In the news, in biology class, at the GP ... so yes it makes me wonder [if] they came from a person, not a vial ... who is he? What did I get from him? It has

149

nothing to do with my parents. It's all about me (DC adult conceived through sperm donation)

We have always been open about the donor conception . . . but our daughter (12) never asked anything about it. So we were wondering 'does she still remember?'. And then all of a sudden, after reading a little ad in the newspaper about a man who suddenly had died and it appeared he had a genetic heart condition, she asked "Can I have that as well"? . . . so we had to say, we don't know . . . (Mother through sperm donation)

Interest in the donor can vary greatly from person to person and over time, from little or no interest to intense desire for information and/or contact. Different children in the same family – even if they share a donor – can react in different ways, suggesting that personality as well as age, parenting, family life, and gender can play a part. Interest typically extends to wanting information about the donor as a person, rather than only their physical attributes or medical information: what sort of person they are, what they liked at school, what they do for a living and so on. While some have no interest in contact, others are keen to meet and some (but not all) would welcome an ongoing relationship and maybe want to meet the donor's family [13].

Besides being genetically related to the donor, DC people can share genes with others conceived using the same donor. Many express an interest in learning more about them and perhaps having contact as what have been called "relationship pioneers" [14]. While the donor provides half their genes and hence is a unique source of genetic information from which to reflect on what has been transmitted to them, information about donor-related siblings offers a different sort of information. This can include resemblances, shared traits, and characteristics that appear to have come through (or not) the genes they share through the donor, regardless of having a different second biological/genetic parent. Here again, some are interested in forming relationships and extending their [kinship] network; others may be more motivated by seeking medical information and/or avoiding consanguineous relationships.

There is growing awareness of the challenges as well as the rewards of contact, including the needs of some for peer or professional support. As well as having to manage feelings about meeting close genetic relatives who are "strangers," the numbers involved are not always static. Sometimes it can be a first meeting on both sides; sometimes it involves meeting people who have already been in contact with each other for some time; sometimes first contacts are followed by a regular flow of "newcomers." For those conceived by sperm donation, the numbers can be very large indeed. All have their own life stories and experiences and networks. For younger people, the contact can be negotiated and mediated by parents who may set the "rules" for such relationships, at least in the early days. For example, some parents see their child's donor-related siblings as brothers and sisters, but do not necessarily see the other family members as kin. For DC adults, the contact may be carried out independently but decisions have to be made as to who else to tell and whether this "new" network can or should extend to encompass members of their own network. "How do I see these new relationships, as family, kin, friends, acquaintances?" "How can I get to know them all and/or stay in contact?" "Do my own children belong to this network as well?" "My donor-related siblings raise questions I wasn't ready for." These are complex situations to navigate [15].

In other words, DC people can differ in whether they see the donor and/or donor relatives as "family" or "kin" (and vice versa); not only can this change but it does not necessarily apply equally. For example, some report kinship feelings towards donor-related siblings but not the donor; some feel a strong pull towards some donor-related siblings but not others; and so on. What does emerge is that existing family systems/boundaries themselves either adapt or become tighter as members try to determine where they consider new boundaries should be drawn, not always with the agreement of others.

Implications for Counseling

Direct work with families, individuals or couples requires an awareness of the relationship dynamics of their family system(s) and of the social and cultural context within which it operates. This includes understanding of the family life-cycle and the stage at which any power-sharing changes are occurring, (usually) from parents as primary power holders to children as shared power holders and eventually to children as more autonomous beings outside the nuclear family system on a day-to-day basis. It is of particular importance to look for social, as well as internal, influences on parents' actions and reactions in what we have called their "here-and-now adult" feelings as well as those as parents (or "parents-to-be" if pretreatment). It is additionally important to be alert to the potential for one to be masked by the other, for example, whether reference to epigenetics is driven by parental interest about its health significance or adult longing to emasculate the donor's genes. Recognizing whether the balance has tipped, say, towards unaddressed "here-and-now adult" feelings or "parents-as-parents" needs for help in developing disclosure and openness strategies enables counseling responses to be tailored accordingly.

Throughout the chapter we have referred to the potential for unresolved or mixed feelings to return at any stage posttreatment and impact parents' confidence. Parents can usefully be advised that such feelings are not unusual. If unattended or otherwise pushed away, however, they can become toxic. Given that DC and involuntary childlessness can also still attract social disapproval and hence felt and ascribed stigma, the impact on the whole family cannot be underestimated. It can be therapeutic for parents and children (where appropriate) to understand where the source of their reactions can be identified as external rather than only internal.

In such sensitive areas of work, well attuned professionals need to not only be well informed about DC-related research and personal experiences, child development and family life-cycles, but also be able to respond to complex and often entangled feelings that can affect the whole family system. That said, professionals also need to be alert to the dangers of parents (or themselves) attributing difficulties to DC without allowing other influences to be considered that might lead to re-imagining and normalizing their experiences.

Counselors may at times usefully raise issues proactively while remaining attuned to and responding to the triggering of strong feelings, rather than only discussing what the client raises. Using a blend of being proactive as well as reactive, while always seeking attunement, can improve engagement through lowering defences and reducing stigma, especially where people have heightened anxieties, fears and ambivalences (for fuller discussion, see [16]).

As said at the start, DC families come in different forms. No "one-size fits all" support exists and a range of different and complementary sources, both professional and peer, can prove useful across time and context. For many, access to peers who are parents, DC people or whole families can be enough. Collective experience through organizations such as Donor Conception Network (some of whose parent members are also therapists) or internet forums, is an invaluable resource for building/rebuilding confidence, increasing emotional literacy, prompting insights, offering reality checking, and suggesting strategies. Professionals can

also benefit from such contacts, especially if they have limited opportunity to otherwise learn about posttreatment family life.

Finally, we acknowledge that knowledge regarding professional support for DC families is still very limited, whether through research, peer support experiences, professional exchanges and personal accounts. We look forward to seeing this grow.

References

1. Golombok S. *Modern Families: Parents and Children in New Family Forms.* Cambridge: Cambridge University Press, 2015.

2. Wyverkens E, Van Parys H, Buysse A. Experiences of family relationships among donor conceived families: a meta-ethnography. *Qual Health Res* 2014 (online). https://doi.org/10.1177/1049732314554096

3. Nordqvist P. Telling reproductive stories: social scripts, relationality and donor conception *Sociol* 2021 (online). https://doi.org/10.1177/0038038520981860

4. Frith L, Blyth E, Crawshaw M, van den Akker O. Secrets and disclosure in donor conception *Sociol Health Illn* 2018;**40**:188–203. https://doi.org/10.1111/1467-9566 .12633

5. Indekeu A, Maas A, McCormick E, Benward J, Scheib J. Factors associated with searching for people related through donor conception among donor-conceived people, parents and donors: a systematic review. *F&S Rev* 2021a;**2**:93–119.

6. Frith L, Blyth E, Crawshaw M, van den Akker O. Searching for 'relations' using a DNA linking register by adults conceived following sperm donation. *BioSocieties* 2017;**13**:170–189.

7. Mahlstedt PP, LaBounty K, Kennedy WT. The views of adult offspring of sperm donation: essential feedback for the development of ethical guidelines within the practice of assisted reproductive technology in the United States. *Fertil Steril* 2010;**93**:2236–2246.

8. Jociles MI, Rivas AM, Alvarez C. Strategies to personalise and to depersonalise donors in parental narratives of children's genetic/gestational origins (Spain). *Suomen Antropologi* 2017;**24**:25–50.

9. Indekeu A, D'Hooghe T, Daniels K, Dierickx K, Rober P. When "sperm" becomes "donor": transitions in parents' views of the sperm donor. *Hum Fertil* 2014;**17**:269–277. https://doi.org/10.3109/14647273 .2014.910872

10. Isaksson S, Sydsjo G, Svanberg AS, Lampic C. Managing absence and presence of child-parent resemblance: a challenge for heterosexual couples following sperm donation *Reprod Biomed Soc*

Online 2019 (online). https://doi
.org/10.org/j.rbms.2019.07.001

11. Blyth E, Crawshaw M, Frith L, Jones C. Donor-conceived people's views and experiences of their genetic origins: a critical analysis of the research evidence. *J Law Med* 2012;**19**(4):769–789.

12. Indekeu A, Hens K. Part of my story: the meaning and experiences of genes and genetics for sperm donor-conceived offspring *New Genet Soc* 2019;**38** (1):18–37.

13. Canzi E, Accordini M, Facchin F. 'Is blood thicker than water?' Donor-conceived offsprings' subjective experiences of the donor: a systematic narrative review. *Reprod BioMed Online* 2019;**38**(5):797–807.

14. Hertz R, Nelson M. *Random Families*. New York, NY: Oxford University Press, 2019.

15. Indekeu A, Bolt S, Maas A. Meeting multiple same-donor offspring: psychosocial challenges. *Hum Fertil* 2021b (online). https://doi.org/10.1080/14647273.2021.1872804

16. Crawshaw M, Daniels K. Revisiting the use of 'counselling' as a means of preparing prospective parents to meet the emerging psychosocial needs of families that have used gamete donation. *Fam Relatsh Soc* 2018 (online). https://doi.org/10.1332/204674318X15313158773308

Chapter

15

The Male Experience with Fertility and Counseling

Brennan Peterson and William Petok

Introduction

Historically, there are few situations where men's experiences have been marginalized. The experience of infertility, however, may be one of those rare occurrences. Because pregnancy and the majority of infertility treatments occur within a woman's body, it is frequently believed that female factors are the primary cause of a couple's infertility. This fallacy has contributed to cultural myths and misconceptions about fertility that have lasted for centuries. Fortunately, this is changing, as the World Health Organization, and the International Glossary on Infertility and Fertility Care, provide more inclusive definitions of infertility, noting it can also be caused by an impairment in a partner's reproductive capacity [1].

The worldwide prevalence of male infertility is difficult to calculate, due to wide variations in fertility rates by country and geographic location. In addition, limitations in research methodologies and underreporting of male infertility due to cultural norms and values contribute to this challenge. For example, the prevalence of male infertility in the United States (US) is based only on men utilizing Assisted Reproductive Treatments (ARTs) which underrepresents the general population [2]. Nevertheless, the best global estimates are that 50% of all infertility cases include some form of male-factor infertility [2,3], and around 30 million men are infertile throughout the world, with the highest rates occurring in Africa and Eastern Europe [3].

A male-factor diagnosis is caused by medical, behavioral and environmental factors including low sperm count, poor sperm motility and abnormal sperm morphology. In addition, disruption of testicular function, treatments for testicular cancer, and lifestyle factors such as alcohol use, smoking or anabolic steroids can also play a role. The risk factors for male infertility also increase with male age, although the rate is not as dramatic compared to women.

The past several decades have seen a rapid rise in research examining the psychological impact of infertility. However, due to men's omission from research designs, as well as their overall reluctance to participate in studies, the majority of these studies focus on women, causing men's infertility journeys to be underrepresented and often misunderstood. Many people incorrectly believe that men are not emotionally impacted by infertility. However, recent studies show a different reality. Men actually experience a variety of complex emotional reactions to an infertility diagnosis, including feelings of failure, helplessness, and threats to their masculinity. Men also experience grief when confronting unfulfilled expectations of not having a biological child to mentor, teach and pass on generational traditions. When engaged in medical treatments, men commonly report feeling they have little to contribute and feel pushed to the margins – even when it is a male-factor diagnosis.

The purpose of this chapter is to provide fertility counselors and healthcare professionals with a nuanced understanding of the male experience of infertility. The chapter will highlight how men's experience of infertility is embedded in cultural discourses of masculinity. It will also highlight empirical studies that illuminate new perspectives on the psychological impact of infertility on men. Finally, the chapter will provide suggestions for fertility counselors and healthcare professionals to involve men in the treatment process. This increased involvement can improve men's journey through the infertility experience, by helping them obtain support and giving them tools and strategies to cope with this significant life stressor.

Culture and Masculinity

It is well understood that historical and cultural messages about masculinity strongly influence men's attitudes, beliefs and behaviors. Hegemonic masculinity, which emphasizes

The authors would like to thank Bella Bendix for her invaluable contributions in preparing and editing the manuscript.

dominant or hierarchical narratives of male behavior and power, is common in traditional and patriarchal societies [4]. Research guided by this framework provides a context for understanding men's emotional reactions to infertility, as well as men's reluctance to access healthcare services both pretreatment and postdiagnosis [5].

Other perspectives contrast with hegemonic masculinity to provide a greater understanding of men's relationship to infertility. Ethnographic research emphasizing "emergent masculinities" underscores men's ability to act in novel and transformative ways that defy the hegemonic discourse [4]. Anthropologic research using this framework enabled researchers to study new forms of masculinities in the Middle East and Mexico, two regions with long-standing cultural traditions of male dominance and strength [4]. While these traditions have led to widespread stereotyping of men's roles and reactions to stress, men in these cultures are finding new ways of acting that provide greater flexibility to historically rigid scripts of male behavior.

Broader cultural beliefs about childbearing also impact men's experience with infertility. Studies find that men in more child-oriented cultures report greater depression when compared with men in less child-oriented cultures [6]. In pronatalist societies, adjustment to infertility is challenging. In Chinese culture, where the family lineage comes through the male line, male infertility can be a source of shame and emotional distress. In many African countries, men face stigma and intense pressure from family members and relatives, increasing psychological stress. The patriarchal traditions of Ghana, for example, link masculinity with a man's ability to father a child. Furthermore, men are culturally considered blameless for infertility, putting the responsibility solely on women – even when it is male-factor, often leading to intense guilt for men [7].

Stigma, Help Seeking and Openness about Fertility

Social stigma occurs when individuals have characteristics or experiences that leave them open to unfavorable judgments and opinions of others. In the case of infertility, men are more likely experience stigma from peers when compared to women, who may be shown more sympathy [8]. Male fertility is also frequently associated with virility, and male-factor infertility is incorrectly linked with sexual dysfunction. Because of this, male infertility is frequently experienced as shameful and is hidden from others.

One of the negative consequences of hiding an infertility diagnosis is the barrier it creates to receiving social support – an important protective factor in reducing psychological distress when faced with stressful life events. Men reporting discomfort with emotional sharing limit the amount of support received, which increases the likelihood of psychological distress. Cultural norms about masculinity and strength are one of the key reason's men report limited openness about infertility. A 2017 qualitative study identified three potential insights into why men may be reluctant to discuss their infertility diagnosis: (1) they did not want to be the focus of attention or have others feel sorry for them; (2) they did not want to risk being the subject of ridicule from other men (i.e., "shooting blanks"); and (3) they believed that infertility was linked with virility and feared if people knew about their diagnosis, others might view them as weak or incapable [5].

Recent studies shed important light on men's willingness to share their infertility struggles with others and its relationship to male depression. In a study of 170 Italian men, those with a male-factor infertility diagnosis did not report higher depression scores when compared with men in couples with female or combined factor infertility. However, men who had a male-factor diagnosis and who also were less open with others about their infertility were at greater risk for depression. This novel finding highlights an important aspect of the relationship between male-factor infertility and depression, as male-factor infertility alone might not be a predictor of male depression, but rather, a vital variable when interacting with levels of openness with others about the diagnosis [9].

Researching the Psychological Impact of Infertility

Research over the past several decades has increased our understanding of the psychological impact of infertility, particularly for women. However, men's experiences have been far less studied. A key reason for this is the methodological challenges of including men in research [10]. Men's lack of involvement has been due to the high frequency of studies conducted during clinical appointments – which men are less likely to attend. In addition, men are less likely to participate in research overall, and fewer designs have been aimed at understanding the male experience. In studies that include male participants, the reliance on quantitative instruments to measure psychological distress may underreport men's inner experiences. Collectively, these factors have unintentionally underrepresented men's voices in the infertility literature.

Male-factor Diagnosis

One area that has received the most attention is the relationship between a male-factor infertility diagnosis and psychological stress. Although studies have produced varied results, men with a male-factor diagnosis commonly report increased psychological distress. One reason for this is that a male-factor infertility diagnosis is often a threat to a man's perceptions of his masculinity, which leads to feelings of helplessness, inadequacy and role failure [8,11].

Men as Protector of Partner

Evidence suggests that men experience infertility indirectly through the effect it has on their partner, and that men's relationship satisfaction is most strongly related to their partner's reports of satisfaction [12]. Men report suppressing emotional expression to be strong for their partner and to protect their partner from the pain of the infertility experience. A study of 22 men found that every participant reported hiding their feelings as a means of supporting their partner, because dealing with their partner's emotional reactions was challenging [5]. Ironically, this lack of openness can result in a partner feeling isolated and unsupported.

Sexual Stress

There is evidence that a male-factor infertility diagnosis can negatively impact a man's sexual satisfaction, while increasing sexual dysfunction and stress [13]. However, the results of studies are mixed, with some finding decreased sexual quality and increased feelings of sexual failure and sexual stress in men, while others have found no relationship [8]. It is not uncommon for men to report increased pressure when having "sex on demand" (the peak of ovulation) which decreases spontaneity and passion, increases anxiety and decreases overall sexual satisfaction.

Discovering Men's Voices through Qualitative Methods

Men's lack of participation in research, coupled with methodological limitations in studies where they are included, have limited our ability to fully understand the emotional impact of infertility on men. Qualitative research methods, however, have provided illuminating discoveries into the male experience of infertility. In a review of 19 qualitative studies about men and infertility, Hanna and Gough found that infertility led men to experience stigma and shame (which threatened their masculine identity), and that men possessed similar levels of desired parenthood when compared to women [14]. Men also experience employment and financial stress. A 2019 qualitative study found that men felt significant financial burdens related to infertility and treatment, in addition to workplace difficulties that resulted in decreased productivity and performance [15].

Qualitative designs also allow men a way to express their experiences with infertility in a way not captured by quantitative measures. One man reported:

> It's really tough, I'd walk past a children's playground and get tears, I get quite depressed . . . Even when you're watching TV and someone gets pregnant you get upset and you have to turn it off [16, p. 246]

This rare male disclosure illustrates the value of qualitative research methods, as they can capture previously unspoken aspects of men's inner experience during infertility. An increase of studies using these research designs and methodologies will allow for further discoveries of men's experiences with infertility.

Discussion Boards and Online Forums

While qualitative studies provide vital perspectives into the male experience, they can also be limited by interviews that occur in a couple's context, where men may be reluctant to share specific details about their experience. Thus, there is a call for additional designs which offer men an opportunity to share private reactions independent of their partner's participation [14]. A ground-breaking method in obtaining this independent experience can be found by analyzing men's participation in online forums and discussion boards.

Men's participation in online discussion boards offer a unique forum for researchers to understand men's experiences, while also providing a vehicle for men to receive support and cope with the demands of the infertility experience. Because men are less likely to attend in-person support groups or seek fertility counseling, it has been incorrectly assumed that they do not want or need to share their infertility stories. However, an examination of men's participation in online discussion boards finds otherwise. Online discussion boards provide a dedicated space for men to share their collective experiences, and provide a window into hidden experiences of men through the infertility journey. The anonymity of the Internet provides an antidote to the stigma, shame and possible judgments men may encounter during in-person meetings. This forum also provides men the autonomy and privacy to post what they want, when they want and where they want. Men can also choose to opt out of formal participation, but still be involved by reading other's experiences.

Findings from analyzing online forums show that many men are adopting new definitions of masculinity, which allows for greater emotional intimacy and support seeking between themselves and other men [17]. Studies have also found that men value the opportunity to have a space for emotional sharing with other men, a result that calls into question traditional views of male stoicism and emotional restraint. For some men, infertility was an all-consuming force over which they had little control – a finding that does not support previous notions that men feel minimal psychological distress when confronted with infertility [17].

> [Infertility] has taken my pride, my dignity, my privacy, my time, my self-esteem, my money and changed my goals and life's plan. It's caused my parents to judge me, my wife to have doubts about me and it's caused me to doubt myself. [17, p. 371]

An overlooked advantage of online discussion boards is the possibility they provide for men to give support to other men. Because support seeking is well known as a protective factor against stressful life events, examining the impact support seeking has on men's adjustment to infertility is imperative. A study of 199 men posting to online discussion boards found that men experienced multiple paths of support, including requesting support, providing support and receiving support [18]. However, while nearly half of the support requested was for information support (defined as direct requests for information or advice), men were more likely to offer appraisal support in response (communicating a shared understanding of the stressor being faced). This unique combination of advice and understanding resulted in the normalization of men's experiences, reduced stigma and increased feelings of support and well-being among those seeking support [18]. Some men provide support by creating personal blogs to educate and connect with others, while others use online posts to facilitate artistic expression as a means to sharing unique aspects of the male experience (see http://saltwaterand honey.org/blog/zero).

Future Research Methodologies

While the use of online discussion boards and forums captures important elements of the male experience, it is not a perfect research design. These studies can be limited by selection bias, as more distressed and more emotionally open men may seek out and use such resources. Thus, these findings may not be generalizable to all men. There are also other considerations when using qualitative research, such as in-depth interviews, where men may be more reluctant to engage in face-to-face interactions with researchers. For example, in a 2017 study of men's experiences of infertility, over 50 men recruited for the study gave their contact information to the researcher. However, when contacted about participation, over half decided not to participate [5]. Of the 22 who agreed to participate, only one (5%) agreed to be interviewed in-person while the remaining 95% chose to be interviewed via the telephone, with many citing the ability to remain relatively anonymous as a deciding factor. Researchers, thus, are faced with a challenge of involving men in ways that allow them to participate fully in research studies, while also capturing the experiences of those who may be reluctant to engage in studies using traditional methods.

One possible solution may be the use of mixed methods approaches such as qualitative questionnaires. In a 2020 study, this method was used for the first time to examine men's experiences with infertility [19]. Using a survey with 15 open-ended questions, findings from 41 men revealed three key themes: failing at masculinity, feelings of invisibility and the trauma of infertility. Men reported significant challenges to their identity because of their infertility diagnosis and guilt for not being able to provide a child for their partners. They also reported a high degree of stigma about their infertility, resulting in hiding the diagnosis and failing to seek support.

Fertility Awareness

Fertility awareness is defined as having an understanding of reproduction and individual risk factors related to infertility, as well as awareness of societal and cultural factors that affect family planning and family building [1]. A systematic review of 43 studies examining men's knowledge, attitudes and fertility-related behavior found almost all men value parenthood, greatly desire to become fathers and planned to have at least two children on average [20]. In ideal circumstances, they also wanted to ensure they were in a stable relationship, had completed their education, and had obtained a job with a dependable income prior to beginning a family.

However, the review also found men had low levels of fertility awareness, even when they believed it was high.

While much of the focus on fertility awareness and age-related fertility decline has been related to the decreased quality and quantity of a woman's oocytes, few studies have examined men's awareness of male fertility. Daumler and colleagues conducted one of the first large-scale studies on the issue by examining the knowledge of male fertility of 701 men ages 18–50 [21]. While nearly 90% of the men considered themselves knowledgeable about men's fertility issues, only about half were aware of modifiable risk factors for infertility and were even less knowledgeable about fixed risk factors and other health issues associated with male fertility. The study also found that while most men would prefer to receive fertility information from health professionals, men are less likely to ask questions and get information from professionals when compared to women. This apparent discrepancy has led researchers and clinicians to propose changes to the healthcare delivery system for men and improve the quality of information delivered, as well as the services received.

Men's Relationships with Healthcare Professionals

In the US, men aged 15–44 are 2 to 2.5 times less likely to visit a physician compared to women of the same age [2]. Men are also less likely to seek fertility care and be involved in treatment. While many speculate that a primary cause of men's lack of help-seeking is related to cultural beliefs about male socialization and masculinity, the entrenched belief that fertility is a "woman's issue" continues to emerge in studies as a factor of men's lack of engagement in reproductive health discussions, even when the belief is viewed favorably [22].

Because of the complicated history of men's lack of involvement in the fertility treatment process, healthcare professionals commonly lack a workable map or script to interact with male patients. Men's experiences of being side-lined in the treatment process, particularly in cases of male-factor infertility, lead to feelings of decreased self-esteem and powerlessness [19]. When healthcare professionals unintentionally exclude men's participation in treatment, especially in the case of male infertility, men can feel the same type of marginalization and stigma they experience in their other social networks.

The Four "I's": Guidelines for Healthcare Professionals

Because models for healthcare professionals are lacking, they are often faced with the question, what can "I" do to help engage men more fully in treatment. The following section details four key "I's" to include men in the treatment process and, thus, move them from the periphery to the center of the treatment.

Invite

Studies have found that men are less likely to participate fully in treatment without a direct invitation that acknowledges their contributions are needed and wanted [22]. In fact, most conversations between healthcare professionals and patients are aimed at women, primarily because they attend more appointments and seem more open and engaged in healthcare discussions. When men do attempt to be more involved, it can often be met with awkwardness or indifference. Studies have found that men want to be involved in fertility discussions but defer to women because women's bodies are commonly the focus of treatment – even in cases of male-factor infertility [22]. Men also reported feeling they had less of a voice in treatment discussions and decisions. Because men report that invitations to participate more fully in treatment rarely occur, professionals who extend a basic invitation for men's increased involvement during the initial treatment consultation increase the possibility of improved male patient engagement. Table 15.1 provides sample scripts which healthcare professionals can use for each of the four "I's."

Inform

Men prefer to receive information about the psychological impact of infertility from their healthcare professionals [23], putting physicians and fertility staff in a unique and influential position to help male patients. While healthcare professionals may find it easier to direct treatment towards the female partner, men's experience can be improved if they are provided detailed and easily accessible educational material about common reactions to fertility treatment [11]. Healthcare professionals can prepare written and online pretreatment documentation that summarizes how men are likely to respond to treatment (even in cases of female-factor infertility) and provide men access to these resources.

Providing men information at the start of treatment increases patient compliance, reduces stress and is highly valued by patients. According to the European Society of

Human Reproduction and Embryology (ESHRE) evidence-based guidelines, healthcare professionals can effectively inform patients about treatment by: (1) providing patients written information that is treatment-relevant and understandable; (2) informing patients about diagnostic procedures, treatment options, and potential treatment results; and (3) providing customized information that is relevant to the patient's diagnosis and treatment plan [24]. Some men have suggested having the opportunity to meet physicians alone to discuss the emotional rollercoaster they face may provide an environment of increased openness [16]. Healthcare professionals can also provide men links to online resources that inform men about treatment issues, such as the use of at-home tests to evaluate sperm motility, which may further reduce men's reluctance to engage with healthcare professionals.

Involve

A 2016 systematic review of men's psychological adaption to treatment recommended that healthcare professionals involve men more directly in all diagnostic cases [11]. This intentional inclusion of men in the treatment process could significantly reduce the heightened feelings of marginalization men frequently report. Men often convey they have little knowledge in how to be involved – especially when the treatment was directed towards their partner. A simple and overlooked way to increase men's involvement is by giving them permission to do so. Because men can feel ambivalence about their involvement in treatment, this simple act can give men increased confidence that their actions will be helpful, since they are following the directives of professionals. An unexpected benefit of increased involvement may be men's increased well-being. In one study, a man reported: "What I try to do is just participate in [the treatment] as much as I can with her . . . I found that once I started trying to be more involved it really helped me cope and heal myself" [18, p. 669].

Intervene

For many men, infertility can be a life-changing experience associated with heightened psychological distress. Fortunately, healthcare professionals can help men adapt to this stressor by intervening directly with patients. Healthcare professionals and clinic staff can have male patients complete the SCREENIVF (www.res earchgate.net/publication/309479209_SCREENIVF_Eng lish_version_20) and FertiQoL (http://sites.cardiff.ac.uk/fertiqol/) assessment tools at the outset of treatment to

assess for emotional risk factors that make patients vulnerable to the emotional stresses of fertility treatment. Screen IVF is a 33-item measure assessing risk in five key areas: state anxiety, trait anxiety, depression, cognitions and social support [25]. FertiQoL consists of 36 items that assesses how patient quality of life is impacted by negative emotions, changes in physical health, challenges to a couple's relationship and the positive or negative impact of social support or stigma [26]. When healthcare professionals find scores above the cut-off on one or more risk factors for SCREENIVF, and FertiQol scores indicating low quality of life, they can intervene by providing a referral to a fertility counselor – an empirically supported treatment option [24]. Healthcare professionals who are reluctant to refer patients for counseling due to cultural stigma may find it useful to use supportive and neutral language to normalize a fertility counseling referral (see Table 15.1).

Table 15.1 Men on the periphery: strategies to increase the participation of men in the fertility treatment process

Strategy	Sample script
Invite	*"Because treatment focuses so much on a woman's body, it's easy to think that infertility is simply a 'woman's issue.' But we know that men's views, engagement, and participation are just as important in the process. Attending appointments, asking questions and letting us know your perspective can be extremely helpful in providing you and your partner the best treatment possible."*
Inform	*"Approximately 40–50% of all infertility cases are due to male factors. This can often cause men to experience a lot of unexpected reactions, which some refer to as a roller coaster. Even in cases of female infertility, it is common for men to experience stress. Here is some information about your treatment and some answers to frequently asked questions that other men have found helpful."*
Involve	*"Sometimes men feel on the sidelines because treatments focus so much on the woman's body. We want you to feel involved in the process and know that your contribution is essential. You can be involved by participating in all areas of the treatment, letting us know your concerns, and by sharing your thoughts and perceptions with us as treatment goes forward."*
Intervene	*"For many men, the experience of infertility can be stressful and unexpected. A lot of men don't talk about it with anyone other than their partner. Fertility counselors are in a unique position to help, particularly in situations where men haven't talked about it with other people. Meeting just a few times can be really helpful. Here are a few names of counselors we trust who have helped other men in the past."*

Fertility Counseling

A key role of fertility counselors is to help men cope with the stigma of infertility, reduce the shame associated with a male-factor diagnosis, find ways to seek and receive social support and provide guidance about disclosing infertility to others in instances of donor insemination (DI). Fertility counselors must also be aware of the impact of culture and gender socialization when working with men. For instance, Petok noted that men may prefer to talk with a male counselor, but female fertility counselors outnumber male counselors by about 10 to 1 on average [8]. Fertility counselors can coordinate care with medical teams to provide patient-centered treatment, most notably in instances where men experience infertility as hopeless, are considering using donor sperm, and have not disclosed their infertility to anyone other than their partner [6,23].

Fertility counselors can engage men in the counseling process by normalizing behaviors stemming from socialized norms of masculinity. Because these cultural scripts often function outside of awareness, they can be perceived as unchangeable truths. Fertility counselors can help men examine these ideas by discussing them with curiosity and openness. When cultural norms negatively intersect with a partner's need, some men may find themselves in what feels like an unwinnable situation (trying to fill the masculine script of being strong for their partner while simultaneously suppressing more vulnerable emotions that may lead to interpersonal connection).

Studies have found that psychological interventions aimed at reducing infertility stress, depression and anxiety are effective for men and women. However, research has found that when faced with challenges, men are less likely to seek mental health services and are more likely to cope on their own [27]. In addition, men are more likely to attribute more shame and blame to mental illness than women.

Due to socialized scripts of masculinity, men may equate help-seeking and counseling with weakness, and as such, are more likely to be passive observers rather than active participants in counseling. This can manifest itself when men mask their discomfort by assuming a supportive role of their partner and assure the counselor they do not need help themselves. Because cultural portrayals of counseling invoke images of emotional expression and vulnerable disclosures, these perceptions may conflict with masculine identities that link emotional stoicism with strength [27].

Similar to healthcare professionals, fertility counselors can help involve men in counseling by inviting them to participate in counseling by attending appointments and sharing their experiences. Fertility counselors can help men view counseling as a team effort, no matter who has been diagnosed with infertility. Counselors can also emphasize that men's participation provides an opportunity for themselves and their partner to discuss vital relational issues such as communication, coping, decision-making and decreasing sexual stress (see also Chapter 4 of this volume).

It is also important to note that not all male clients experience discomfort with vulnerability, and many men will be open to participating without hesitancy. However, in instances where men are reluctant to engage, fertility counselors can frame counseling as a strength-based solution that takes determination and strength for one's partner, as opposed to weakness and resignation.

Donor Insemination

Donor insemination (DI) is the process where the sperm from a donor (commonly anonymous/unknown) is used to fertilize the female partner's oocyte. In heterosexual couples, DI can be used as a family-building option for men and their partners in cases where other treatments fail (such as intrauterine insemination (IUI), or intracytoplasmic sperm injection (ICSI) – where a single sperm is injected into an oocyte). Fertility counselors must be aware that men considering DI are not only coping with the original stresses and difficulties of the initial infertility experience, they also must consider the complexities of how DI challenges their beliefs about themselves, their future parenting, and the importance they may place on maintaining a genetic link to their children, which can result in feelings of grief and loss [6].

Because of these factors, the use of DI is considered by many to be one of the most challenging aspects of the infertility treatment process [19]. Some men worry using DI will make them less important in their child's life than the biological donor. They also express concern about protecting their child from possible rejection related to DI, as well as feelings of uncertainty in how to discuss the issue with children [6].

Secrecy and Disclosure

Fertility counselors play a critical role in helping men normalize the stress associated with DI and contemplate its meaning and implications. They can also help men develop awareness of personal boundaries and strategies for disclosing DI to their children and others [6]. Historically, secrecy and shame about DI have been common in heterosexual couples because of the stigma linked with male virility and masculinity. Because of this, men may find it difficult to discuss DI with others outside of trusted family members, and also with their children as they get older. Fortunately, fertility counselors have created guidelines for disclosing DI to children that promote adjustment and healthy development. It is generally agreed upon that disclosing DI to children is best at an early age (typically between 3–6 years) in order to avoid family secrets which can challenge children's future identity [6]. Fertility counselors can also help men understand that disclosure is not a one-time event, but an unfolding process. The use of DI for lesbian couples and single women is a specialized area of fertility counseling, and more information about these topics can be found in the Section III of this book.

Adjustment over Time and Life after Fertility Treatment

Few studies have examined men's adjustment to life following infertility treatment. However, the limited evidence available shows that men's psychological adjustment over time is healthy – regardless of whether they have a child or not. Martins and colleagues conducted a systematic review examining men's psychological response to unsuccessful treatment [11]. While men had poorer adjustment in infertility stress, depression, social support and sexual functioning in the year following an infertility diagnosis, men's adjustment often returned to pretreatment levels in the years afterward. Men's use of protective factors such as support-seeking, emotional expression and meaning creation shielded them against depression and declines in relationship satisfaction [11].

For men who have a child following treatment, a study of 172 first-time Israeli fathers examined if the stress of infertility would continue to impact men's life after parenthood. The study compared the anxiety and relationship quality of 76 men who became fathers after using ART (such as IVF), and 96 men who became fathers after their partner had a spontaneous pregnancy. No significant differences in marital quality and life satisfaction were found between the two groups, providing hope to men that the stresses of infertility and treatment likely return to normal levels in early fatherhood and do not impact future life satisfaction [28]. These findings are in line with a five-year longitudinal study of men undergoing fertility treatments that showed no differences in the quality of life between men who became fathers compared to men who did not [29].

Conclusion

The male experience of infertility has been widely misunderstood, largely due to cultural scripts and methodologic limitations that limit men's expression. While it was once believed men were only mildly impacted by infertility, men actually experience a variety of complex emotional reactions, including depression, helplessness and threats to their masculine identity. Even in cases of male-factor infertility, men commonly feel that they have little to contribute to treatment and feel pushed to the margins when engaging with healthcare professionals. Qualitative research has provided insight into the complex inner landscape men frequently experience when navigating infertility. Fertility counselors and healthcare professionals are in a unique position to help men cope with the stresses of infertility and increase men's involvement by inviting, informing, involving and intervening. The four "I's," coupled with appropriate referrals to fertility counselors, can help men navigate the infertility journey by giving them tools and strategies they need to cope with this unexpected life stressor, increase social support and enhance their overall quality of life and well-being.

References

1. Zegers-Hochschild F, Adamson GD, Dyer S, et al. The international glossary on infertility and fertility care. *Fertil Steril* 2017;**108**(3):393–406.

2. Mehta A, Nangia AK, Dupree JM, Smith JF. Limitations and barriers in access to care for male factor infertility. *Fertil Steril* 2016;**105**(5):1128–1137.

3. Agarwal A, Mulgund A, Hamada A, Chyatte MR. A unique view on male infertility around the globe. *Reprod Biol Endocrinol* 2015;**13**(1):1–9.

4. Inhorn MC, Wentzell EA. Embodying emergent masculinities: men engaging with reproductive and sexual health technologies in the Middle East and Mexico. *Am Ethnol* 2011;**38**(4):801–815.

5. Dolan A, Lomas T, Ghobara T, Hartshorne G. 'It's like taking a bit of masculinity away from you': towards a theoretical understanding of men's experiences of infertility. *Sociol Health Illness* 2017;**39** (6):878–892.

6. Wischmann T, Thorn P. (Male) infertility: what does it mean to men? New evidence from quantitative and qualitative studies. *Reprod BioMed Online* 2013;**27** (3):236–243.

7. Naab F, Kwashie AA. 'I don't experience any insults, but my wife does': the concerns of men with infertility in Ghana. *S Afr J Obstet Gynaecol* 2018;**24**(2):45–48.

8. Petok WD. Infertility counseling (or the lack thereof) of the forgotten male partner. *Fertil Steril* 2015;**104**(2):260–266.

9. Babore A, Stuppia L, Trumello C, Candelori C, Antonucci I. Male factor infertility and lack of openness about infertility as risk factors for depressive symptoms in males undergoing assisted reproductive technology treatment in Italy. *Fertil Steril* 2017;**107**(4):1041–1047.

10. Culley L, Hudson N, Lohan M. Where are all the men? The marginalization of men in social scientific research on infertility. *Reprod BioMed Online* 2013;**27**(3):225–235.

11. Martins MV, Basto-Pereira M, Pedro J, et al. Male psychological adaptation to unsuccessful medically assisted reproduction treatments: a systematic review. *Hum Reprod Update* 2016;**22**(4):466–478.

12. Greil AL, Slauson-Blevins K, McQuillan J, Lowry MH, Burch AR, Shreffler KM. Relationship satisfaction among infertile couples: implications of gender and self-identification. *J Family Issues* 2018;**39**(5):1304–1325.

13. Wischmann T. 'Your count is zero' – Counselling the infertile man. *Hum Fertil* 2013;**16**(1):35–39.

14. Hanna E, Gough B. Experiencing male infertility: a review of the qualitative research literature. *SAGE Open* 2015;**5**(4):1–9.

15. Hanna E, Gough B. The impact of infertility on men's work and finances: findings from a qualitative questionnaire study. *Gender Work Organization* 2020;**27**(4):581–591.

16. Arya ST, Dibb B. The experience of infertility treatment: the male perspective. *Hum Fertil* 2016;**19**(4):242–248.

17. Hanna E, Gough B. Emoting infertility online: a qualitative analysis of men's forum posts. *Health (London)* 2016;**20**(4):363–382.

18. Richard J, Badillo-Amberg I, Zelkowitz P. "So much of this story could be me": men's use of support in online infertility discussion boards. *Am J Mens Health* 2017;**11**(3):663–673.

19. Hanna E, Gough B. The social construction of male infertility: a qualitative questionnaire study of men with a male factor infertility diagnosis. *Sociol Health Illness* 2020;**42**(3):465–480.

20. Hammarberg K, Collins V, Holden C, Young K, McLachlan R. Men's knowledge, attitudes and behaviours relating to fertility. *Hum Reprod Update* 2017;**23**(4):458–480.

21. Daumler D, Chan P, Lo KC, Takefman J, Zelkowitz P. Men's knowledge of their own fertility: a population-based survey examining the awareness of factors that are associated with male infertility. *Hum Reprod* 2016;**31**(12):2781–2790.

22. Grace B, Shawe J, Johnson S, Stephenson J. You did not turn up . . . I did not realise I was invited . . . : understanding male attitudes towards engagement in fertility and reproductive health discussions. *Hum Reprod Open* 2019;**2019**(3):1–7.

23. Fisher J, Hammarberg K. Psychological aspects of infertility among men. In: Simoni M, Huhtaniemi I, Eds. *Endocrinology of the Testis and Male Reproduction.* Switzerland: Springer, 2017, 1–31.

24. European Society of Human Reproduction and Embryology. Routine Psychosocial Care in Infertility and Medically Assisted Reproduction – A Guide for Fertility Staff [Internet]. 2015 [cited June 26, 2021]. Available from: www.eshre.eu/Guidelines-and-Legal/Guidelines/Psychosocial-care-guideline [last accessed June 16, 2022].

25. Ockhuijsen HDL, van Smeden M, van den Hoogen A, Boivin J. Validation study of the SCREENIVF: an instrument to screen women or men on risk for emotional maladjustment before the start of a fertility treatment. *Fertil Steril* 2017;**107**(6):1370–1379.e5.

26. Boivin J, Takefman J, Braverman A. The fertility quality of life (FertiQoL) tool: development and general psychometric properties. *Hum Reprod* 2011;**26**(8):2084–2091.

27. Pattyn E, Verhaeghe M, Bracke P. The gender gap in mental health service use. *Social Psychiatry Psychiatr Epidemiol* 2015;**50**(7):1089–1095.

28. Taubman-Ben-Ari O, Skvirsky V, Bar Shua E, Horowitz E. Satisfaction in life among fathers following fertility treatment. *J Reprod Infant Psychol* 2017;**35**(4):334–341.

29. Schanz S, Häfner HM, Ulmer A, Fierlbeck G. Quality of life in men with involuntary childlessness: long-term follow-up. *Andrologia* 2014;**46**(7):731–737.

Chapter 16

Counseling Lesbian, Gay, Bisexual and Queer Fertility Patients

Sarah Holley and Lauri Pasch

Introduction

This chapter provides information related to counseling lesbian, gay, bisexual and queer (LGBQ)[1] women and men as they engage in the family-building process. The path to parenthood often presents same-sex couples with a number of challenges, including making complex childbearing decisions, navigating a fertility treatment system designed for infertile heterosexual couples, and confronting barriers such as accessing insurance coverage and uncertain legal rights. This chapter highlights the primary issues that many LGBQ patients and partners confront, and provides guidance for fertility counselors on specific considerations to factor in when working with this growing population of prospective parents. Many aspects of fertility treatment are no different for same-sex couples as for heterosexual couples and thus are covered elsewhere in this book. This chapter examines aspects of family building that are particular to same-sex couples. And while this chapter focuses on couples, many of the issues covered here also pertain to LGBQ individuals who may seek treatment as a single parent by choice.

The composition and experiences of LGBQ families are highly diverse. A dyad with two women is often termed a lesbian couple, though members of a same-sex female couple may identify their sexual orientation as bisexual, queer, pansexual, demisexual, and so on. The same goes for a dyad with two males, which is often termed a gay couple. For the purposes of this chapter, we will focus on family building for same-sex couples, with full recognition that within each dyad, any number of sexual orientation identities may be represented. Further, as a convenience and with appreciation of all the identities these terms encompass, we will use "female couple" as a term to represent all same-sex female

couples, and "male couple" as a term to represent all same-sex male couples. It should also be noted these couples may include one (or more) transgender individuals. See Chapter 17 for family-building counseling specific to transgender patients.

Clinical Issues: Decisions, Decisions, Decisions

For same-sex couples on the path to parenthood, there are no "oops babies" or opportunities to just try "naturally." Rather, the process is an inherently intentional one that requires considerable planning and coordination. A series of choices must be evaluated and decisions made: What reproductive options to pursue? Whose eggs will be used? Whose sperm will be used? Who will carry the child? Will adoption be considered? Where can LGBQ-friendly services be found? What are each partner's legal rights? Will any of this be covered by insurance? A primary function of the fertility counselor is to help couples understand their options and the implications of their choices, as well as to support them through the process of treatment. The counselor must additionally take into account complex interrelationships between social, legal, political and economic factors that may uniquely impact family-building options for LGBQ patients [1].

Routes to Parenthood

One of the first major decisions is what route to take to parenthood. For female couples, there may be many possible options, while for male couples, options are typically limited to surrogacy with egg donation or adoption. Specific family-building options and considerations for same-sex couples are highlighted below.

Home Insemination

Female couples may use home insemination. This route involves vaginal insemination performed at home, either with the help of a known donor or with sperm from

---

The addenda referred to in this chapter are available for download at www.cambridge.org/covington-clinical-guide

[1] In this chapter, we are using "lesbian, gay, bisexual, and queer" and the acronym "LGBQ" as umbrella terms for all sexual minority individuals. We recognize the diversity of sexual identities, and that identity can change over time.

a sperm bank. Couples can use what has been called "turkey-baster technology" (e.g., a needleless syringe, eye dropper, cervical cap). Home insemination does not need to involve any medical staff, and couples may therefore feel a greater sense of intimacy or autonomy [2]. Further, it often represents the least expensive route.

There are, however, important considerations to keep in mind with home insemination. Some couples carrying out self-insemination may not feel supported or have access to medical assistance should they need it [2]. If using fresh sperm from a known donor, the donor may not have been screened for sexually transmitted diseases, so there may be a higher level of health risk. Finally, and perhaps most crucially, in some jurisdictions, known donor sperm must pass through the hands of a licensed medical professional and/or a legal contract must be in place, otherwise the donor may be granted legal rights and responsibilities for any resulting offspring.

Clinic-based Treatments

Clinic-based treatments may involve an initial meeting with a gynecologist or reproductive endocrinologist, a fertility evaluation, and genetic testing. Some clinics require a meeting with a fertility counselor. A common starting point for female couples is intrauterine insemination (IUI), but couples can make use of the full range of fertility treatment options depending on their needs. Often multiple medical interventions (e.g., blood work, ultrasounds, medications) are also part of the treatment. Some couples may be uncomfortable with the degree of medicalization, while others will welcome the interventions as helpful tools for conception [1].

Clinic-based treatments can offer certain benefits as compared to home insemination. If working with a known donor, the donor will have to undergo screening and infectious disease testing. Working with a clinic offers greater protections of parental rights, as the treatment process requires legal documentation defining parental status [1]. If pregnancy does not occur, fertility interventions can be added to the treatment protocol as needed. Conversely, some clinic policies may seem involved and cumbersome. Furthermore, these procedures can add a great deal of time and cost to the process.

Surrogacy

For male couples, a possible route to parenthood is gestational surrogacy with egg donation. Surrogacy allows one of the partners to have a genetic link to the offspring, which is often valued by couples. In most parts of the world, however, surrogacy is either illegal or highly restricted. In some jurisdictions, surrogacy is legal but must be purely altruistic, meaning the carrier cannot be financially compensated other than for direct expenses; this, in turn, tends to make finding an appropriate surrogate very difficult. In most of the United States (US) and in some other countries, financial compensation is permitted, making surrogacy much more available but often very expensive. In the US, surrogacy laws vary from state to state, with some states considered surrogacy-friendly and others not. Some states further have additional restrictions that may prevent same-sex couples from accessing these services. For example, in Louisiana, surrogacy is legal *only* when the intended parents are a married heterosexual couple who are both genetically related to the child.

Generally speaking, couples need to be aware of the laws in their home state/country, the laws of the gestational carrier's home state/country, and the state/country in which the child is to be born. Surrogacy is a relatively complicated process because it means involving several outsiders, usually including an egg donor, a gestational carrier, as well as a fertility doctor, legal counsel, and often an agency to help find the donor and carrier. As highlighted in Chapter 12, intended parents will need to work closely with a family law attorney to get the necessary legal contracts in place defining the rights and responsibilities of all parties involved throughout the family-building process.

Adoption or Foster Care

While adoption or foster care is an option for prospective LGBQ parents, they may face certain barriers. Couples must first determine the policies of the state from which they are attempting to adopt or foster. According to the Movement Advancement Project, as of 2021, 19 states have no protections against discrimination based on sexual orientation, and 11 states allow state-licensed child welfare agencies to refuse to provide services to same-sex couples if doing so conflicts with their religious beliefs. Policies for international adoptions can also vary dramatically. Due to the extreme variability of the laws, couples should find out about laws in their jurisdiction and seek consultation at the outset of the adoption or foster process from either a family lawyer, state equality organization, or a national organization like the Human Rights Campaign [3].

Adoption agencies themselves can either function as supports or barriers. While many agencies work with LGBQ families and are very helpful, others may not accept them as clients or may be less likely to place a child with same-sex parents. Some agencies may operate on a "don't ask, don't tell" policy, which can be upsetting and confusing for clients [4,5]. Prospective parents should ask the agency about its track record in placing children with LGBQ families [3].

Complex Arrangements

Until recently, same-sex couples were frozen out of the institution of marriage and more "traditional" family structures. As a result, some couples have chosen to fully redefine what the notion of family entails and created extended parental or kinship structures. For example, a female couple and a male couple may decide to conceive children together and rear them together [6]. Other researchers have found that some female couples may seek out gay donors, in part to give the donors an opportunity to take part in a parenting role that they might not otherwise have had [4]. Given the diverse paths LGBQ prospective parents may take to family formation, fertility counselors need to be open-minded in supporting patients who may be creating relatively unique family structures. In these cases, the primary role of the counselor may be to help all parties involved consider the roles, rights and responsibilities of all of the individuals involved in family-building and the family system.

Which Partner Will Provide Gametes?

Another major decision stems from whose gametes (i.e., sperm and egg) will be used. For same-sex couples, presuming intact fertility in both partners, decisions will be based on a number of factors such as age, health history, family relationships and intensity of the desire to be a genetic parent. In some cases, infertility actually is an issue, which may then dictate which partner is able to provide gametes. Many times, some combination of any or all of these factors will be weighed in deciding which partner will provide half of the needed genetic material [7].

Some couples know in advance that they want to try to have more than one child, so then it becomes a question of whose gametes to use first. Male couples planning surrogacy sometimes choose to fertilize half the eggs with each of their sperm, respectively, so that both partners can have the possibility of having a genetically related child. Sometimes men will ask that two embryos, one fertilized by each partner, be transferred at the same time, but that is less common in recent years because of the move toward single embryo blastocyst transfer in surrogacy to avoid the risks associated with multiples. Although some couples ideally would like to have more than one child so that both can have a genetically related child, age and financial barriers may make this unlikely or difficult. For example, if the first pregnancy produces twins, a couple may be less likely to have more children. Further, family building with surrogacy is often limited by legal barriers, financial constraints, or low availability of appropriate candidates, thus only one surrogacy arrangement may be feasible.

Same-sex couples are typically accepting of the fact that the child will only have a genetic link to one of the partners [4], though one job of the fertility counselor will be to work with the couple to process any perceived loss around this issue. Occasionally, same-sex couples will plan to have a child with a genetic connection to both partners by using the gametes of one partner and the gametes of a genetic relative of the other partner (this is usually either a sister or brother of the non-gamete providing partner). This can be a special family-building option but often is not possible or practical given age and sibling relationships, and it must be comfortable for all involved parties.

Which Partner Will Carry?

For female couples, the choice to use one partner's eggs and which partner will carry often go hand in hand, though that is not always the case. Some couples are interested in *reciprocal IVF* (also called *co-IVF, shared conception*, or *shared maternity*), wherein the eggs from one woman are retrieved and fertilized then transferred to the partner's uterus. One of the most significant determining factors for female couples in selecting which partner will carry tends to be related to who has the greatest desire to experience pregnancy and childbirth. Other factors that can impact the decision of who carries include: the age of each partner, medical history, insurance benefits, attitudes of extended family and the presence of existing children [7]. Additional considerations stem from practical implications, such as who has the most job flexibility or can most easily take time off.

Who Will Be the Donor?

For same-sex couples, a third-party donor will inevitably be a part of the picture, but the decisions around the donor can vary greatly. For some, having a known donor (e.g., friend or family member) is viewed an important part of the family-building process [1]. Prospective parents may want to give the child the opportunity to have a relationship with the donor as they grow up [4]. Others prefer a known donor because they feel it gives them more control over the insemination process, or because they want more direct access to the donor's health or genetic history. Regardless of the motivation, an important consideration for couples using known donors is to openly discuss, in advance, what role that individual will play in the family unit, as well as to have a legal agreement in place wherein the known donor relinquishes all legal rights and responsibilities to the child. There are also couples who might prefer a known donor in theory, but do not know anyone they feel comfortable asking or who is willing to be a donor.

Conversely, some couples have a strong preference for an unknown donor. Two major motivations stem from legal reasons (i.e., nobody else can lay claim to the child) and from the desire to raise the child without outside interference from a third party [4]. Many sperm banks have "identity-release" (or "willing-to-be-known") options, wherein the donors allow the sperm bank to pass along requests for contact information from the offspring after they turn 18 [7]. This can often be an appealing option for couples as it enables them to engage in family building without the involvement of an outside party, but still provides the offspring the later possibility of obtaining information about their genetic origins.

Specific Challenges for LGBQ Patients

It is important to have a sense of the various social and political forces that may influence LGBQ patients' feelings about pursing fertility treatment, their access to services, or the attitude of healthcare professionals. Historically, LGBQ parents typically had children within a heterosexual relationship then came out after the relationship dissolved [4]. Now, many LGBQ individuals choose to become parents within the context of a same-sex relationship. The trend will likely continue now that same-sex couples have gained access to marital rights and as social attitudes shift toward greater acceptance.

Fertility treatments, however, have not always been accessible to same-sex couples. In the past, discrimination against LGBQ patients was overt, with healthcare professionals citing legal, ethical or moral arguments against same-sex parenting [1,2]. While this remains the case in some countries, fortunately the situation in many places has improved. In the US, in 2006, the Ethics Committee of the American Society for Reproductive Medicine (ASRM) declared, "The ethical arguments supporting

denial of access to fertility services on the basis of marital status or sexual orientation cannot be justified" [8, p. 1333]. ASRM went on to conclude that there is no basis for denying LGBQ patients access to treatment, highlighting the absence of scientific evidence that parenting effectiveness is affected by parental sexual orientation. In the US, the ethical directive garnered some legal enforcement in 2008 when the California Supreme Court ruled that refusal to treat a lesbian based on the physician's religious views violated state law.

In Europe, a European Society of Human Reproduction and Embryology (ESHRE) task force released a statement in 2014 to address "assisted reproduction for people in what may be called 'non-standard' situations and relationships" (i.e., lesbian and gay couples, along with "singles" and "transsexual people") [9]. While they concluded that "categorically denying access to any of these groups cannot be reconciled with a human rights perspective," the statement also reflected the tenuous nature of access to treatment, as it noted individual doctors with "conscientious objections" can refuse service provision and called for more research into "the welfare of children growing up in nonstandard situations" [9, p. 1864]. More recently, a consortium within ESHRE found that Europe remains a patchwork of local legislations, with notable differences in access to treatment from country to country (only 18 out of 43 countries reportedly offer treatment to female couples, and only five offer treatment to male couples) [10]. But there are some countries that have firm protections in place (e.g., Canada), with laws unequivocally protecting those seeking reproductive services from discrimination on the basis of sexual orientation [11].

Even in countries that provide ethical and legal protections, however, potential barriers and stressors unique to same-sex couples are still present. These types of stressors and their effect on LGBQ prospective parents may best be understood through the sexual minority stress model (Figure 16.1). Sexual minority stress is defined as psychosocial stress resulting from stigmatization and marginalization in a heterosexist society [12]. Sexual minority stress can take many forms, including actual experiences of discrimination and bias (distal stressors), as well as expectations of rejection, efforts to conceal sexual identity, and internalized homophobia (proximal stressors). Sexual minority stress is considered chronic and socially based (i.e., it stems from processes and structures beyond the individual), and it necessitates sexual minority individuals to engage in adaptation efforts above and beyond that required by nonminority

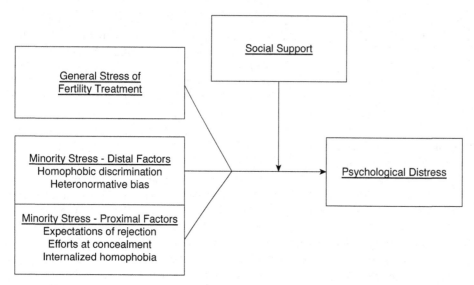

Figure 16.1 Fertility treatment and sexual minority stress.

Note: Adapted from Meyer's Sexual Minority Stress Model [12]. In the context of fertility treatment, LGBQ patients experience the general stress associated with treatment and must additionally contend with stressors specifically associated with their sexual minority status.

individuals in similar circumstances [12]. As applied to fertility treatment, this means the already stressful process of using fertility treatment often has extra layers of stress stemming from the couple's sexual minority status. Social support and other supportive resources may serve as protective factors, or a lack thereof may constitute an additional set of stressors. Cumulatively, these stressors may contribute to experiences of psychological distress for same-sex couples during their family-building process.

The following section will explore challenges related to sexual minority stress, as well as highlight specific considerations related to cost and legal issues. While each area is addressed individually, it should be recognized that these social, institutional, economic and legal forces are often inextricably interwoven in ways that may significantly affect fertility treatment for LGBQ prospective parents.

Minority Stress: Distal Factors

Confronting Homophobic Discrimination

With firm support from organizations like ASRM and some degree of legal protection in various places, overt discrimination against treating LGBQ fertility patients appears to be waning. Unfortunately, that does not mean it has disappeared. At the most severe, discriminatory policies against LGBQ parents may prevent access to services altogether. This is certainly true in countries that prohibit same-sex couples from receiving treatment, but

it may also be the case where services are theoretically available. And while the ASRM issued a clear ethical directive, the guidelines are not legally binding, and different clinics may have widely discrepant access policies [11].

For example, a survey of assisted reproductive technology (ART) programs in the US in 2005 found that (of those with data on sexual orientation), 17% reported they were likely or very likely to turn away a lesbian couple wanting donor insemination, and 48% reported they would turn away a gay couple wanting to use surrogacy [13]. A subsequent study in 2010 found that 14% of practicing obstetrician-gynecologists would discourage a woman in a lesbian relationship from using ART, and 13% would not help the woman obtain services [14]. And while the number of clinics offering services to same-sex couples appears to be steadily rising, data from as recently as 2014 indicated that only 235 (60.2%) of the 386 Society for Assisted Reproductive Technology (SART) clinics reported treating female couples, and only 178 (46.1%) of the clinics reported treating male couples [15]. Further, providing a window into patient care attitudes, a study in 2017 found that only 53% of SART clinics had LGBT content on their websites [16]. Other forms of homophobic discrimination that couples may experience within the treatment setting include healthcare professionals' difficulty with eye contact, inappropriate questioning, or overt homophobic slurs and comments [17]. Thus, while overt discriminatory acts (such as refusal of service) may be less common today than in the past, they do still occur and can leave same-sex couples feeling isolated, unsupported, and serve as barriers to accessing care.

Navigating a Heteronormative System

Bias against LGBQ patients may also be manifest in more subtle ways, even by clinics with inclusive practices and policies. The majority of fertility treatment services are targeted toward heterosexual women, and partners are presumed to be husbands. This heteronormative approach is reflected in the very term "infertility counseling" or "infertility treatment" that is commonly used by ART providers. That is, these services were designed for people who met the criteria for infertility (defined as 12 months of regular, unprotected heterosexual intercourse without a successful conception). This construct does not create space for the experiences of same-sex couples. Take the example of a perfectly healthy female couple in the US, with no known risk factors for infertility, using anonymous donor sperm, who go to a fertility clinic for IUI treatment. Based on clinic policy (and in accordance with ASRM guidelines), this patient may be required to receive a medical workup, genetic testing and psychological counseling. These requirements can feel unfairly burdensome to couples who are not actually experiencing infertility, and can medicalize or pathologize a relatively straightforward path to parenthood [11].

The heteronormative framework has far-reaching implications for same-sex couples attempting to access services. On a practical level, it may create a mismatch between clinic practices and patients' needs. A common example of this is clinic forms, which often are not designed appropriately for same-sex couples (e.g., they may specify "husband" and "wife," or "mother" and "father") [17,18]. This can be very off-putting for LGBQ patients, sending the implicit signal that the clinic's services are not really intended for them. Further, the literature or orientation seminars provided by clinics may presume infertility and focus on coping with loss, and clinics may fail to provide psychoeducational materials tailored to same-sex couples [18,19]. In addition, particularly for female couples, the nonbirth mother may experience a sense of invisibility during the entire treatment process, with healthcare professionals failing to acknowledge the partner on office visits [4,19]. Of note, in heterosexual couples, male partners may also experience a similar sense of invisibility (see Chapter 15), so this may be a more general "partner inclusion" issue that healthcare professionals should take care to address. However, for female couples, the nonbirth mother may *attribute* the lack of inclusion to bias or discrimination, which can make the experience that much more

deleterious. Finally, aside from adding stress to the family-building process, the heteronormative framework can also have significant implications for legal rights or insurance coverage for same-sex couples, as will be explored in more detail in the following.

Minority Stress: Proximal Factors

At its most insidious level, stigmatizing attitudes about LGBQ parents may be internalized and contribute to feelings of defectiveness or shame, or they might foster a sense of anxious anticipation [12]. Yager and colleagues [20] found that lesbian and bisexual women who were trying to conceive described expectations of encountering biased attitudes when meeting with ART healthcare professionals. LGBQ patients have further described feeling like they were repeatedly "coming out" to healthcare professionals throughout their treatment process [17]. And unlike their heterosexual counterparts, same-sex couples have the added worry of whether disclosing their sexual identity could negatively affect their treatment experience or quality of care. This anticipation of discrimination, even absent actual discrimination, may contribute significant psychological distress to LGBQ patients during the fertility treatment process [12,20].

Such proximal minority stress factors can make it feel like a major struggle to access supportive and appropriate care [18]. As an example, for same-sex couples, the process of selecting a treatment clinic will not just involve finding a qualified professional, but will also entail assessing the level of homophobia or bias expected from a healthcare professional or healthcare system. Extra steps may involve reviewing websites for representative material, calls to assess how the clinic feels about having same-sex couples as patients, or seeking referrals from others for healthcare professionals known to provide inclusive care [17]. At best, these proximal stressors will create extra anxiety and effort for LGBQ patients, and at worst, they may keep them from seeking treatment at all.

Minority Stress: Social Support Considerations

Social support from friends, family or support groups is important for anyone going through the fertility treatment or adoptive process. Novel issues may arise, however, for same-sex couples. It may be difficult to find support groups oriented toward LGBQ family building. In addition, some individuals may not have disclosed their sexual orientation to family members – the transition to parenthood may end up "outing" them [19]. Families, in turn, may or may not be supportive.

Research further indicates that some couples encounter a lack of support, or in some cases, overtly negative attitudes from the LGBQ community when they become parents [20]. In such cases, it may be that their entry into parenthood goes against the norms that have been established within that group. Conversely, some couples find that their desire to parent is more understood and accepted by heterosexual friends, for whom parenthood tends to be an expected stage of the lifecycle [4]. For many, they may not know how people will react until it happens.

The LGBQ transition to parenthood may be associated with significant social network shifts. These changes may stem both from the aforementioned issues with family/friend attitudes, as well as from a general realignment of priorities. In a study examining gay men adopting children, Goldberg [21] found that many fathers reported a sense of alienation from gay nonparent friends and increasing closeness to heterosexual parent friends. The shift from nonparent to parent friends is common for new heterosexual parents as well, but as Goldberg notes, the shift for gay couples is qualified by the fact that their friendships with gay nonparents are not easily replaced by friendships with gay parents. This may be particularly true for couples living outside of major urban areas, where there are simply fewer LGBQ parents in the vicinity [5]. Some LGBQ parents may therefore feel they lack a community of parent friends who really "get" their full experience.

Cost Issues

Fertility treatments are expensive, and these costs can be prohibitive for any couple, regardless of sexual orientation. As such, many treatment options remain the exclusive province of those with access to resources or insurance coverage [22]. For same-sex couples, however, the cost burden may be even higher as compared to their heterosexual counterparts, due to second-parent adoption costs, the need for legal counsel, and so forth.

Even for those couples who have insurance, barriers may still exist in accessing the coverage. The insurance policy may require a diagnosis of infertility (which, defined in medical terms, presumes heterosexual sex) or have other criteria written with the presumption that the patient is in a heterosexual relationship (e.g., specify that the patient's eggs be fertilized with her spouse's sperm) [22]. Insurance will rarely cover sperm or egg donation, which are necessary components of family building for same-sex couples. Thus, even for straightforward treatment plans (e.g., a female

couple who want to use IUI), the costs can add up quickly and become a limiting factor for prospective LGBQ parents.

Legal Issues

The legal considerations for LGBQ prospective parents can be complicated and may vary dramatically based on geography. As noted above, different states within the US and different countries have differing policies regarding LGBQ adoption and surrogacy, and these policies are subject to change. In the US, there currently is no federal policy regulating access to ART. As a result, the law has limited ability to respond to LGBQ barriers, and the question of who legally qualifies as a child's parents may be up for significant debate [6]. Therefore, consultation with attorneys who specialize in family law may have to be an integral part of LGBQ family creation. Such legal issues can add cost, time and stress to an already long and arduous process.

A major issue for same-sex couples pertains to getting legal recognition in place for both parents. For example, when a female couple conceives a child, sometimes only the birth parent is recognized on the birth certificate. However, even when both parents are able to include their names on the birth certificate, and even when they are married, same-sex couples still have to go through a "second-parent" or "step-parent" adoption. These two forms of "confirmatory" adoption allow the nonbiological parent to adopt the child without termination of the first parent's rights, thereby providing all parties with legally recognized relationships with one another [7]. LGBQ stepparent adoption is now legal in all states, and second-parent adoption is available in 18 states. However, the process can be expensive, time-intensive and invasive (e.g., it may involve an evaluation and home visit by a social worker). Further, this process entails a period of ambiguity after the birth of the child wherein the nonbiological parent has to wait for her or his rights to be instated. It can also feel discriminatory to same-sex couples, particularly since married heterosexual couples who use donor gametes typically do not have to take these extra steps to secure parental rights.

Guidelines for General Best Practice

Fertility counselors are in an excellent position to identify areas where treatment services can better support LGBQ family building. To do so, fertility counselors need to develop the necessary *cultural competency* for working with LGBQ patients. In this context, cultural competency involves recognition of the types of challenges highlighted throughout this chapter that same-sex couples may encounter during treatment [18,20].

As a starting point for delivering culturally competent care, a primary task is for the fertility counselor to be aware of contemporary conventions for appropriate LGBQ-related terminology, and to be cognizant of the fact that these conventions evolve over time. In current practice in the US, the words "lesbian," "gay," and "bisexual" are used as adjectives, not nouns (e.g., "Sam is a gay individual," rather than "Sam is a gay.") The term "homosexual" has largely fallen out of favor and should generally be avoided. Conversely, the term "queer" is coming back into use as a self-affirming umbrella term encompassing all nonheterosexual identities; fertility counselors, however, should only use this term if there is a compelling reason for doing so (e.g., quoting someone who self-identifies as queer). Helpful resources can be found online (see Addendum 16.1). In general, the best rule of thumb is to determine what terms the patient prefers, and to honor those preferences.

Below are additional suggestions to help to establish a set of best practices in serving LGBQ patients, based on our experience and a review of the literature. This list is not comprehensive but at minimum provides a basic set of guidelines for fertility counselors (and fertility treatment clinics) to provide supportive services to the LGBQ patient population.

- Check printed and online materials for heteronormative biases. In particular, forms should reflect possible variability in family structure. Either make forms gender neutral or have alternative versions available for different family-building configurations. In addition, websites and clinic literature should include language and images that are inclusive of LGBQ families.
- Be aware of the messages that are communicated verbally. Use neutral terms (e.g., partners instead of husband/wife). Frame treatment in terms of family building, rather than solving the medical problem of infertility.
- Be sure to involve the partner. The partner who is not providing gametes (and/or serving as the gestational carrier, in the case of female couples) may be overlooked throughout treatment. They will be equal parents to any offspring and should therefore not be marginalized during the treatment process.
- Be able to direct patients to appropriate literature sources. This minimally includes resources that do not just focus on infertility or refer to "husband and wife," and ideally includes psychoeducational resources that are developed specifically for LGBQ patients.
- Be knowledgeable about supportive services that address the social and emotional support needs of LGBQ prospective parents, such as local or internet-based LGBQ-specific support groups.
- Be aware of the laws for marriage, adoption and surrogacy in your state or country as they pertain to same-sex parents, or where to direct patients to look for finding out this information (see Addendum 16.1 for resources). Have referral information available to LGBQ-friendly adoption agencies and family planning lawyers in your area.
- Fertility treatment clinics may want to consider adapting policies so that certain service components (such as a full pretreatment fertility workup, or fertility counseling) are recommended but optional, after discussing with the patient the type of information they may miss by opting out.
- If fertility counseling is mandatory for same-sex couples, fertility treatment clinics should take care to articulate the rationale for this meeting (i.e., to provide guidance and support to *all* couples using third-party donors) so the requirement is not perceived as an assessment of parenting fitness or a gatekeeping barrier targeting LGBQ families.
- To provide the highest level of transparency, fertility treatment clinics should provide clear, written, defensible treatment policies for all patients. Clinics can additionally provide a detailed description of patient demographics, thus enabling prospective patients to know the extent to which the clinic is welcoming of LGBQ patients.
- Be aware of healthcare professionals who may be creating an uncomfortable environment, and make efforts to provide psychoeducation. Or proactively provide education to all clinic staff, addressing any discomfort or concerns they have about treating LGBQ patients, and encourage all to adopt the types of inclusive practices outlined here.

Summary

Fertility care for LGBQ patients has changed dramatically in the past few decades. A "debate" article published in 1994 in the journal *Human Reproduction* on the use of insemination services for lesbian women stated, "The sexual minorities now have an increased confidence which has led them to assert their rights for social recognition, encouraged by a new talk of tolerance towards minorities (even if it does not always fit in with reality)" [23, p. 1969]. The author's clinic had decided to welcome these "special requests" for donor insemination using a stringent psychological screening protocol. He noted the decision to treat lesbian women was not for everyone, and that "every practitioner must have the right of nonparticipation should their moral conscience tell them so." That this was the prevailing dialogue of the day (and one that represented an "inclusive" attitude at the time) reflects the extent to which the decision to deny fertility treatment services to LGBQ patients was both socially and medically sanctioned. Since that time, research has resoundingly debunked questions about LGBQ parental fitness, and prominent medical and ethical governing bodies have made clear statements supporting equal rights to fertility treatment services. As a result, the debate regarding fertility treatment has made a profoundly important shift from *if* LGBQ patients should be treated to *how to best* deliver treatment to this steadily growing patient population.

Fertility counselors working with same-sex couples have the important task of helping to facilitate family building within a societal framework that is often not fully supportive. A major challenge fertility counselors face is that patients may view our role through a lens colored by previous experiences of discrimination – as a result, developing a positive working alliance can be hard. Overcoming this challenge requires creating an inclusive environment, openness to diverse family-building scenarios, staying up to date with new developments, and seeking consultation from colleagues when faced with unfamiliar concerns. The fertility counselor can play a critical role in providing LGBQ patients guidance, psychoeducation and support as they work to build their families and navigate a treatment system that was not necessarily designed with their needs in mind.

References

1. Mamo L. *Queering Reproduction*. Durham, NC: Duke University Press, 2007.

2. Wykes KA. Fertility services for same-sex couples: policy and practice. *Br J Nurs* 2012;**21**(14):871–875.

3. Child Welfare Information Gateway. Frequently asked questions from LGBTQ+ prospective foster and adoptive parents. Washington, DC: U.S. Department of Health and Human Services, Children's Bureau, 2021.

4. Goldberg AE. Lesbian and gay parents and their children: *research* on the family life cycle. Washington, D.C.: American Psychological Association, 2010.

5. Kinkler LA, Goldberg AE. Working with what we've got: perceptions of barriers and supports among small-metropolitan same-sex adopting couples. *Fam Relat* 2011;**60**(4):387–403.

6. Patterson CJ. Children of lesbian and gay parents: psychology, law, and policy. *Am Psychol* 2009;**64**(8):727–736.

7. Amato PR, Jacob MC. Providing fertility services to lesbian couples: the lesbian baby boom. *Sex Reprod Menopause* 2004;**2**(2):83–88.

8. Ethics Committee of the American Society for Reproductive Medicine. Access to fertility treatment by gays, lesbians, and unmarried persons. *Fertil Steril* 2006;**86**(5):1333–1335.

9. De Wert G, Dondorp W, Shenfield F, et al. ESHRE Task Force on Ethics and Law 23: medically assisted reproduction in singles, lesbian and gay couples, and transsexual people. *Hum Reprod* 2014;**29**(9):1859–1865.

10. Calhaz-Jorge C, De Geyter CH, Kupka MS, et al. Survey on ART and IUI: legislation, regulation, funding and registries in European countries: the European IVF-monitoring Consortium (EIM) for the European Society of Human Reproduction and Embryology (ESHRE). *Hum Reprod Open* 2020;**2020**(1):hoz044.

11. Corbett SL, Frecker HM, Shapiro HM, Yudin MH. Access to fertility services for lesbian women in Canada. *Fertil Steril* 2013;**100**(4):1077–1080.

12. Meyer IH. Prejudice, social stress, and mental health in lesbian, gay, and bisexual populations: conceptual issues and research evidence. *Psychol Bull* 2003;**129**(5):674–697.

13. Gurmankin AD, Caplan AL, Braverman AM. Screening practices and beliefs of assisted reproductive technology programs. *Fertil Steril* 2005;**83**(1):61–67.

14. Lawrence RE, Rasinski KA, Yoon JD, Curlin FA. Obstetrician-gynecologists' beliefs about assisted reproductive technologies. *Obstet Gynecol* 2010;**116**(1):127–135.

15. Carpinello OJ, Jacob MC, Nulsen J, Benadiva C. Utilization of fertility treatment and reproductive choices by lesbian couples. *Fertil Steril* 2016;**106**(7):1709–1713 e4.

16. Wu HY, Yin O, Monseur B, et al. Lesbian, gay, bisexual, transgender content on reproductive endocrinology and infertility clinic websites. *Fertil Steril* 2017;**108**(1):183–191.

17. Gregg I. The health care experiences of lesbian women becoming mothers. *Nurs Womens Health* 2018;**22**(1):40–50.

18. Kirubarajan A, Patel P, Leung S, Park B, Sierra S. Cultural competence in fertility care for lesbian, gay, bisexual, transgender, and queer people: a systematic review of

patient and provider perspectives. *Fertil Steril* 2021;**115** (5):1294–1301.

19. Chabot JM, Ames BD. "It wasn't 'Let's get pregnant and go do it'": decision making in lesbian couples planning motherhood via donor insemination. *Fam Relat* 2004;**53** (4):348–356.

20. Yager C, Brennan D, Steele LS, Epstein R, Ross LE. Challenges and mental health experiences of lesbian and bisexual women who are trying to conceive. *Health Soc Work* 2010;**35**(3):191–200.

21. Goldberg AE. *Gay Dads: Transitions to Adoptive Fatherhood.* New York, NY: New York University Press, 2012.

22. Kawwass JF, Penzias AS, Adashi EY. Fertility – a human right worthy of mandated insurance coverage: the evolution, limitations, and future of access to care. *Fertil Steril* 2021;**115**(1):29–42.

23. Englert Y. Artificial insemination of single women and lesbian women with donor semen. Artificial insemination with donor semen: particular requests. *Hum Reprod* 1994;**9** (11):1969–1971.

Transgender Assisted Reproductive Technology

Jamie Joseph, Trystan Reese and Molly Moravek

Introduction

Transgender Literacy 101

This chapter introduces information needed for fertility counselors working with transgender people who require assisted reproductive technology (ART) to attempt to preserve their future fertility or grow their families. Throughout this chapter, when using the word "transgender," it is the intent of the authors that it is used as an inclusive term to describe any individual whose gender identity does not align with the sex assigned to them at birth. This is consistent with current nomenclature to designate full inclusivity of the multiplicity of transgender identities. Understanding common terminology used to describe transgender peoples' experiences, concerns and expansiveness is necessary for fertility counselors to provide inclusive care and support for community members who require ART to grow their families. While this may seem a simple task, it is not. As is the case with most marginalized communities, there are many different terms used across generations, geographic regions and identities.

When communicating with ART patients who are transgender, fertility counselors should work to understand language generally used to describe trans experiences, while also working to be active listeners and hear and identify how each transgender ART patient personally describes themselves, how they communicate about and explain their bodies, and what their unique situation and needs are. If unclear about what a specific term may mean for a patient personally, a respectful request for clarification can convey acceptance and validation of their unique experiences.

Here, we cover basic terminology relating to transgender people; all fertility counselors should know these terms at a minimum when working with transgender

patients. This is not a comprehensive list and should be considered an introduction for fertility counselors seeking to provide inclusive support for transgender people who are considering ART for their family planning needs.

Sex assigned at birth refers to one's original designation as either male or female on a birth certificate. Sex assigned at birth is often associated with the physical attributes of chromosomes, hormone prevalence and external and internal anatomy. A person's ***gender identity*** is their internal knowledge and conceptualization of themselves as male or female, both, neither or other. Gender identity is how a person sees themselves; it is self-defined.

In a ***gender binary*** system, gender is constructed to fit into two exclusive categories of male and female. Conversely, ***gender nonbinary*** is an adjective describing people who do not identify exclusively as male or female. They may identify as being both male and female, somewhere in between or as falling completely outside of those two categories. ***Gender expression*** is the external way a person wears, displays or shows their gender, through dress, hairstyles, speech patterns (voice), mannerisms and overall appearance. When a person's sex assigned at birth aligns with their gender identity, the term ***cisgender*** is used. When a person's self-identified gender differs from their sex assigned at birth, the term ***transgender*** is used.

Gender dysphoria is a psychological state characterized by feelings of distress and negative emotionality and can occur when sex assigned at birth is different from the gender an individual identifies as. As a clinical term, gender dysphoria is accompanied by impairment in social, occupational or other important areas of functioning. Importantly, the *discrepancy* and resultant *distress* between assigned gender and self-identified gender is the area of concern for any treatment [1]. Gender dysphoria, when severe, can lead to significant depression, impairment and even death by suicide. However, it may not be present for all transgender people and for others, it may not be persistent when appropriately addressed [2].

The addenda referred to in this chapter are available for download at www.cambridge.org/covington-clinical-guide

If a transgender person goes through a gender-affirming *transition*, this refers to the period when they begin to live in ways that match their gender identity, rather than the sex they were assigned at birth. The duration and nature of any one person's gender transition is completely individualized and no two are exactly alike. There are no specific orchestrated steps necessary for a person to go through a gender transition; rather, each person makes changes that work for them based on what is available to them, what they can access and what they need to feel comfortable in their body. Some people may go through a *social transition*, whereby they express themselves and live in the gender that is authentic to them outwardly to society. Some people may also go through a *medical transition*, which involves modification of the body to align it with their gender identity, utilizing hormone treatment and/or surgery. Importantly, not all transgender people want to, can or will medically transition. *Legal transition* involves changing one's legal name and/or gender marker on legal documents. For some, transition can be a shorter process while for others, it can be lifelong, evolving over time. Fertility counselors working with transgender ART patients may interface with people in any area of their transition process.

Depth versus Breadth of Training for Fertility Counselors

Fertility counselors working with transgender patients need to provide compassionate, respectful, culturally competent fertility and family planning counseling to transgender individuals and couples who may need ART to build their families. When providing care, it is important to keep in mind the idea of "depth vs. breadth of training" [3]. This means the fertility counselor is aware there are many different reasons why a transgender person would seek mental health consultation. When seeing mental health consultation for a social or medical gender transition, the depth of knowledge required by the mental health professional for accurate assessment, differential diagnosis and treatment or recommendations is expansive. This level of expertise is beyond the level of competency needed by mental health professionals working in the capacity solely as "fertility counselors." For exclusively fertility concerns, counselors need at least a "breadth" of competency that allows them to be culturally responsive and skillful when interacting with transgender clients who seek their services purely in relation to fertility and family building. Chang and colleagues highlight this difference in level of training that can be applicable to fertility and family-building counselors, which is different from the level of training for professionals who provide transition-related clinical care in an ever-evolving complex field [3].

Desire for Family Creation

The drive to create a family is nearly ubiquitous, transcending history, geography, culture, religion, race, socio-economic status, biological sex and gender identity. Case histories, anecdotal reports and research indicate that transgender people want to build families for many of the same reasons cisgender people do. These include, but are not limited to, closeness, nurturance and intimacy [4]. Therefore, family formation and parenting can be a natural and important part of a transgender person's life trajectory just as it may be for many cisgender people [4,5,6]. A growing body of research data shows that children are not harmed by having a transgender parent and The American Academy of Child and Adolescent Psychiatry maintains there is no evidence that connects a parent's sexual orientation or gender identity as an adverse indicator of children's development [7].

Brief Background and History

Over recent decades, modern science, progressive thinking, cultural advances and intense advocacy efforts have brought attention to the health and healthcare experiences of the transgender population. As a result, many major medical and health organizations have established guidelines and initiated training on how to provide inclusive care for the transgender community. Among those involving fertility concerns are the World Professional Association for Transgender Health (WPATH), American Society for Reproductive Medicine (ASRM), The Endocrine Society and the American College of Obstetrics and Gynecologists (ACOG). Additionally, recent research on infertility and childlessness in the transgender population indicates that many people have a desire to access fertility preservation and reproductive services in relation to family building [8,9]. However, "Despite the burgeoning scholarship on transgender health and healthcare, the literature on transgender reproduction and reproductive medicine remains limited" [10, p. 517].

The reasons for this dearth of research, information and knowledge of transgender people's desire for family formation, reproduction and ART is multifactorial. First, transgender people continue to experience substantial marginalization, disempowerment and discrimination in all areas of life around the globe. Until recently, and in many areas around the world it is still the case, transitioning to one's affirmed gender meant unintentional and/or coerced sterilization [11]. For example, in the 1960s in the United States (US), those seeking gender transition were advised to sever contact with their established life, including relationships with their own children if they had transitioned after becoming a parent. Transitioning parents were advised to tell young children that their parents were divorcing or that the parent had died, which, at the time, was considered a better alternative for a child than having a parent who was transgender [12]. As of 2018, 23 European states (13 of which are in the European Union) required medical sterilization to issue a legal affirmation of gender status [13]. Laws such as these around the world have meant that in many cases, to transition to one's identified gender, a person had to give up their reproductive potential; they must surrender their ability to become a parent to their own progeny in the future, any possibility for becoming a parent in other ways, and, at times, the option to continue parenting children that they already had prior to their gender transition.

Medical Gender Transition and Fertility

Institutional Support and Informed Consent

Since 1979, the WPATH has established and published internationally accepted Standards of Care (SOC) for the medical and mental health treatment for transgender individuals with gender dysphoria who want to medically transition, and they are updated with new scientific information periodically [14]. These guidelines are designed to promote the health and welfare of transgender people around the globe. In 2001, the WPATH introduced a single paragraph to the SOC to address fertility concerns for transgender people prior to initiating hormone therapy. Later, in 2011, the seventh edition of the SOC devoted an entire chapter on the topic. The chapter specified that many transgender people would want to have children and acknowledged that hormone therapy may limit fertility. Specific recommendation was made for healthcare professionals (including mental health professionals) to discuss reproductive options with all transgender patients prior to the initiation of any medical treatment that may impact fertility (including hormone therapy and surgeries).

The SOC-7 also emphasizes the expectation that healthcare professionals should discuss reproductive options even if patients are not interested in fertility and reproductive issues at the time of gender-related medical treatment. They acknowledge many younger patients may express lack of interest in future reproduction but stress the importance of fertility counseling anyway. This is especially true for adolescents who initiate gender transition via medical treatment which can impact their future fertility potential or, in some cases, may render them infertile completely. The SOC eighth edition, which is currently under review at the time of writing of this chapter, will likely expand on those concerns, offering further guidance for fertility and reproduction.

Like WPATH, The Endocrine Society has published guidelines that recommend all medically transitioning individuals be counseled about the effect of treatment on their fertility and be educated on and offered options for fertility preservation before they transition [15]. The ASRM published Ethics Committee Opinions in 2015 and updated them in 2021, stating that transgender and nonbinary people seeking reproductive technologies should not be restricted, but rather they should be informed about the limited but reassuring data on long-term outcomes for patients and their offspring [5]. Furthermore, the ASRM states that ART programs should treat all requests for treatment without regard to gender identity; encourages the collection of outcome data that explores the emotional well-being of transgender and nonbinary persons and their offspring and recommends fertility programs become educated on providing culturally competent care [5].

Regarding fertility counseling, the ASRM's 2021 Ethics Committee Opinion specifically recommends transgender people undergoing ART should be offered psychological counseling by a qualified mental health professional to assist them with questions about disclosure to offspring and others, the use of donor gametes, disclosure of the parents' transgender status, as well as to provide support for the biopsychosocial impacts of treatment. Furthermore, the ASRM suggests "additional areas of counseling exploration might include the impact of discontinuing hormone therapy to achieve pregnancy, the impact of fertility treatments on gender dysphoria, and the need for emotional support and resources. Further research is needed on the psychosocial counseling needs of transgender patients receiving reproductive care [5, p. 876].

Despite WPATH, The Endocrine Society and ASRM's support for reproductive and fertility counseling and ART for transgender people, many healthcare professionals, from all medical and behavioral backgrounds, have not been formally trained, nor are they familiar with the unique concerns, specifics and history regarding transgender people. Moreover, no practice guidelines for providing this fertility-specific care have been offered by ASRM, WPATH or The Endocrine Society. In lieu of this absence of guidance, it is imperative that mental health-care professionals in the ART field seek multiple sources of continuing education and ongoing cultural competency for providing fertility services to transgender individuals and couples about reproduction and family formation.

Decisions about Medical Transition and Future Fertility

Though more data would certainly be welcome, some transition steps may reduce or even eliminate reproductive possibilities. Regarding planning medical transition, some transgender prospective parents may have to decide between transitioning now with a plan to cease gender-affirming hormone treatment at some point (in the hopes of regaining fertility later), or postponing part or all of their medical transition in order to undergo a fertility preservation or reproductive process. These decisions can be distressing, as either option can feel equally challenging. One requires taking the risk that reproductive capacity may not fully return down the road, while the other requires the delay of medical treatment that may increase happiness and well-being for the later goal of having genetically related offspring or ability to carry a pregnancy. Tables 17.1 and 17.2 outline the reproductive and fertility preservation options for people with sperm or oocytes.

Gender-affirming Hormone Therapy

Several guidelines on providing gender-affirming hormone therapy already exist in the literature and are outside the scope of this chapter. Briefly, the overarching goal of postpubertal hormone therapy is to induce secondary sex characteristics congruent with one's gender identity and, eventually, cause some regression of already established incongruent secondary sex characteristics. In transmasculine individuals, hormone therapy is principally with testosterone, administered either by injection (intramuscular or subcutaneous) or transdermally, titrated to serum testosterone and estradiol levels typical of cisgender men [16]. Amenorrhea is typically achieved by 3 months of hormone therapy initiation [17], but testosterone cannot be considered an effective contraceptive as unpredictable ovulations have been shown to occur while on testosterone therapy [18]. For transfeminine individuals, the principal hormone is estradiol (injectable, oral or transdermal), usually in combination with androgen blockers such as spironolactone or finasteride, similarly titrated to serum testosterone and estradiol levels typical of cisgender women [19]. For transgender and nonbinary youth presenting at an early stage of puberty, puberty blockade is possible with gonadotropin-releasing hormone (GnRH) agonists to halt puberty and prevent further development of incongruent secondary sex characteristics [15].

Gender-affirming Surgery

Gender-affirming surgery ranges from cosmetic changes, such as facial feminization surgery or tracheal shaving, to major genital reconstruction. Surgeries that remove reproductive organs (ovaries or testes) are sterilizing, so fertility goals should always be discussed prior to these surgeries. Additionally, even when the ovaries are left in place, vaginectomy (removal of the vagina) and other masculinizing surgeries in the genital region make oocyte retrieval technically challenging and, in some cases, impossible.

Table 17.1 Fertility options for people with sperm who desire genetic children

Fertility preservation only	Partner with oocytes	No partner with oocytes
Postpubertal: - Semen cryopreservation - Testicular aspiration **Prepubertal:** - Testicular tissue cryopreservation (experimental)	**Partner willing/able to carry pregnancy:** - Intercourse - Intrauterine inseminations - In vitro fertilization **Partner not willing/able to carry pregnancy:** - In vitro fertilization with embryo transfer into gestational carrier	In vitro fertilization using donor oocytes and a gestational carrier

Table 17.2 Fertility options for people with oocytes who desire genetic children

Fertility preservation only	Partner with sperm	No partner with sperm
Postpubertal: - Oocyte cryopreservation - Ovarian tissue cryopreservation **Prepubertal:** - Ovarian tissue cryopreservation	**Patient willing/able to carry pregnancy:** - Intercourse - Intrauterine inseminations - In vitro fertilization **Patient not willing/able to carry pregnancy:** - In vitro fertilization with embryo transfer into gestational carrier	**Patient willing/able to carry pregnancy:** - Intrauterine inseminations with donor sperm - In vitro fertilization with donor sperm **Patient not willing/able to carry pregnancy:** - In vitro fertilization with donor sperm with embryo transfer into gestational carrier or partner with uterus

Assisted Reproductive Technology Clinic-based Treatments

Transgender individuals should have all the same options available to them in the fertility clinic as cisgender individuals do, and those options rely upon the same factors: whether the individual is partnered, what gametes and organs the patient has (and those of their partner, if applicable), and whether the patient (and/or their partner) is willing and able to carry a pregnancy. Various options based on these factors are presented in Tables 17.1 and 17.2. If third-party reproduction (donor oocytes or sperm, or gestational carrier) needs to be utilized, costs increase substantially.

Gametes

Use of donor gametes is an option for transgender people just as it is for cisgender counterparts, if viable oocytes or sperm are not available. For individuals who cryopreserved gametes prior to starting hormone therapy and are not able to attempt conception without medical assistance, it is probably best to use those stored gametes, given the limited data on effects of hormone therapy on reproductive capacity, or whether there may be effects in offspring created from hormone-exposed gametes. Without cryopreserved gametes, transfeminine patients can try to produce a semen sample while remaining on hormones or may be able to regain spermatogenesis after several months off hormone therapy. A retrospective study evaluating 69 semen analyses at the time of cryopreservation in 29 transgender women found that patients who had never been exposed to hormone therapy had significantly higher sperm concentration and motility compared to transgender women previously (but not currently) on hormone therapy, but only patients who

were currently on hormone therapy had abnormal semen parameters according to the WHO criteria [20]. Of note, of the seven current hormone users, three were azoospermic. Other studies reporting pathology findings at the time of gender-affirming orchiectomy have reported histological abnormalities in the structure of the testes and varying degrees of impaired spermatogenesis in transgender women on hormone therapy [21,22]. Interestingly, studies evaluating semen analyses at the time of cryopreservation in transgender women who have never been exposed to hormone therapy have found an increased incidence of abnormal semen parameters compared to cisgender men [23,24].

Similarly, the effects of masculinizing hormone therapy on reproductive capacity have not been fully elucidated. There have been widely publicized pregnancies in transgender men previously on testosterone, as well as survey studies of transgender men who have had a live birth, so we certainly know that pregnancy is feasible after testosterone exposure, but it is unclear whether overall fecundity or pregnancy outcomes differ, as there are currently no studies following transmasculine individuals actively attempting conception without medical assistance [25]. There have been several histological studies performed on ovaries attained at the time of gender-affirming surgery for transgender men on testosterone, but the results of these studies vary, and many were from transgender men who had only been on testosterone for 1–2 years [26]. In the largest of these studies, 40% of ovaries had completely normal histopathology and 6% had pathology consistent with polycystic ovary syndrome [27]. The only parameter associated with duration of testosterone therapy was ovarian volume. Another one of these studies isolated oocytes from the tissue and found that the oocytes were able to be matured in vitro into mature oocytes with mostly normal spindle structure [28]. Clinically, case series of transgender men seeking assisted reproductive technology for fertility preservation or current fertility have been reassuring, with successful oocyte cryopreservation and live births reported, even in those who had previously been on testosterone [29,30]. Of note, case series to date have discontinued testosterone therapy prior to ovarian stimulation, so the question of whether equivalent outcomes can be obtained without discontinuing hormone therapy, and thereby decreasing risk of increasing gender dysphoria during treatment, remains. For transmasculine patients who wish to carry a pregnancy, hormone therapy should be discontinued prior to attempts at conception.

For individuals that had puberty halted with GnRH agonist, there is concern that the reproductive organs and respective gametes may not have matured enough to enable future reproduction. There are currently only two case reports of oocyte cryopreservation in transmasculine youth who started peripubertal GnRH agonists [31,32]. Though stimulation protocols differed between the two reports, mature oocytes were able to be cryopreserved in both cases (4 and 22 oocytes), providing proof of concept that it is theoretically possible to preserve fertility in this population. To the authors' knowledge, there are not any cases of sperm cryopreservation from transfeminine youth who had puberty halted with GnRH agonist, nor are there any reports of oocytes or sperm obtained from individuals who had puberty halted with GnRH agonist, then went directly into treatment with gender-affirming testosterone or estradiol before attempting to obtain gametes.

Gestational Carriers

If an individual is not able/willing to carry a pregnancy and they do not have a partner who is able/willing to carry a pregnancy, then the individual/couple will need to undergo in vitro fertilization (IVF) with implantation into a gestational carrier. Gestational carriers may be known or unknown to the individual/couple, and unknown carriers may be found through agencies that specialize in third-party reproduction or through less formal channels, such as social media platforms. Depending on the route chosen, it can be quite costly to use a gestational carrier, with potential charges including agency fees, payments to the carrier, covering travel/childcare, etc. for the carrier, legal fees to create a contract, paying for the IVF itself (and potentially for donor eggs or sperm) and other associated medical expenses. Additionally, laws regarding gestational carriers and the rights of intended parents vary widely from state to state and may affect the availability of a desired carrier.

Alternative Parenting/Family Structures

While there isn't clear data on the relationship arrangements of the transgender community, anecdotally it seems as though LGBTQ people, and transgender people specifically, are more likely to have less common relationship and/or family structures that include multiparent households, intentional solo parents, co-parenting with platonic friends, people who are parenting in community with other families and/or people who practice gender-creative parenting (which may include not assigning a gender to their child in utero or during early childhood). Intake paperwork and forms should include space for transgender patients undergoing ART to share information on who they're in a relationship with, whether they're going through the process with or without a romantic partner, and how they plan to raise their future child/ren within those relationship arrangements. Fertility counselors should ask open-ended, nonjudgmental questions that don't have embedded assumptions in them. For example, when seeing a new client, asking "Who is with you today?" or "Tell me your story." Phrasing of questions in this manner conveys inclusivity and acceptance.

As with any decision made by a prospective parent, it is important to apply a harm reduction lens to these types of conversations. Ask open-ended questions to discern why they are making the choices they are, and work to find options that can mitigate some of the risks while honoring the very real values or fears they may hold. Utilizing an informed consent model can help people to understand the possible risks and benefits of their family formation choices.

Financial and Psychological Concerns About Assisted Reproductive Technologies

As with anyone going through a fertility process, ART-related expenses for the transgender community add up quickly and are rarely covered by insurance. Given that transgender people are four times as likely to live at or below the poverty line compared to the national average, these expenses are even more likely to be unaffordable for the transgender community [33]. Additionally, transgender people are more likely to have experienced insurance problems in the past (55% have been denied surgery coverage and 25% have been denied hormone coverage) so they may be hesitant to even try to secure coverage for fertility processes [33].

These variables, or some version of them, may be at play for any transgender prospective parent. Fertility counselors should not assume an individual would want to become pregnant (or that they wouldn't want to become pregnant), that they could afford a surrogate, that they would feel comfortable giving a sperm sample, or any of the fertility processes that may seem simple and straightforward as may be for cisgender people.

Family Building Outside of Clinic-based Approaches

Because of the high prevalence of medical trauma in the transgender community (see "Trauma-informed Care" later in this chapter), many transgender people actively avoid seeing a healthcare professional, even when they need medical care [33]. As a result, some transgender people may prefer to work with a known donor, for example, attempting conception at home rather than in a medical clinic. Aside from any possible medical concerns (such as sexually transmitted infections) or future legal concerns (if the donor later decides they would like to play a role in the child's life), there is the consideration of sperm quality. Given that many transgender people would like to expedite the conception process (especially if they have transition concerns), it can be devastating to realize that their known donor does not have high enough quality sperm (either in morphology, concentration or motility) to easily achieve a pregnancy.

Affirmative Fertility Counseling for Transgender People

The Affirmative Movement, Model and Approach

Roots for affirmative practice date to the 1970s and early 1980s and assume that "sexuality and gender identity different from heterosexual and cisgender experience were normal and, moreover, that acknowledging and affirming identity and experience was a critical component of helping clients integrate their identity with the rest of their lived experience" [33, p. 31]. Affirmative care in behavioral, emotional and healthcare delivery is when organizations, programs and healthcare professionals

recognize, validate and support the identity of the individual served and is considered inclusive, validating and best practice for working with the LGBTQ+ community [34,35,36]. Therefore, the "Gender Affirmative Model" is a multifaceted approach to working with and supporting transgender people and is valuable with family planning, fertility care and ART. Because medical and behavioral health training programs have not historically included curriculum on transgender health and concerns, continuing education and humility training in transgender issues is imperative for understanding the unique aspects of transgender people who present for assisted reproductive fertility services.

Eight Ways Fertility Counselors Can Affirm Transgender People Seeking Assisted Reproductive Technology

1. *Be gender literate.* Knowing and understanding basic terms and concepts within the transgender vernacular and population is imperative for providing culturally responsive care. Half of transgender patients have reported they needed to educate their healthcare professionals about their health needs, the language they use to describe themselves, their experiences and the world [33]. This can be very frustrating to transgender people seeking fertility counseling support, given that infertility is in and of itself a stressful process to navigate. Familiarity with the terms and concepts discussed at the outset of this chapter can serve as a link to validation of a transgender person's experiences and be affirming and rapport building.

2. *Use names and pronouns the person specifies to be known by.* In showing respect to a transgender person(s), it is imperative to use the pronouns and names they designate when addressing and referring to them. At times, legal names on insurance documents, identity documents, etc. may be different from what the person uses to refer to themselves. Fertility counselors should always inquire on written intake forms and in conversation if the person wants to be called by something other than what is on their legal documents. This may be due to the fact they have not been able to or chose not to change their legal name, but do not want to be called by it. Likewise, pronoun usage is personal and fertility counselors are advised to ask for the correct pronouns a person wants to be referred to with. Pronouns

should never be assumed based on presentation, sex, gender or anything else. Inquiring about what name and pronouns a person uses is a way of showing respect for their identity.

3. *Keep in mind that sex and gender are different.* Often the words "sex" and "gender" are used interchangeably, such as during the so-called gender reveal parties sometimes thrown during pregnancy. However, sex and gender refer to two different aspects of identity. Given this, we really cannot genuinely know a person's gender until they are able to tell us what their self-defined concept and understanding of themselves is. Therefore, the popular fad of revealing an unborn fetus's gender by showing pink or blue smoke, cakes or other creative manifestations is inaccurate. The correct terminology would be a "Sex Reveal Party" since the fetus or newborn child cannot vocalize their self-perceived gender. Even then, newborn infants are not able to understand or express their gender identity, which is thought to be formed around the age of three developmentally, and some parents may choose to rear their younger children with "**gender neutral parenting**." This approach emphasizes raising children without assumption of their gender identity and not assigning a gender to them as male or female based on their sex at birth, but waiting for children to be able to voice their authentic, self-defined gender.

4. *Gender identity and sexual orientation are related but different.* The concepts of gender identity and sexual orientation are often conflated, but they are not the same. The fertility counselor should understand that gender identity is a person's self-defined sense of who they are, while sexual orientation is who they are sexually and emotionally attracted to. Moreover, any person's gender identity and sexual orientation is dictated and defined by them, and fertility counselors need to respect these facets of their human experience with dignity, sensitivity and inclusivity.

5. *Gender dysphoria "may or may not" be a concern in relation to fertility and reproduction.* Gender dysphoria, the intense negative psychological state, distress and persistent discomfort with primary and secondary sex characteristics a transgender person may experience, varies in intensity between people. Some people experience extreme discomfort with the incongruence of their bodies in relation to their gender identity, while others may suffer mildly or not at all. It is important for the fertility counselor to inquire about how the person has experienced gender dysphoria historically and presently. Additionally, where the person is in their transition at the time of the ART is relevant, especially if that person's gametes will be harvested and/or if they intend to use their uterus to carry the pregnancy. The extent to which the individual's gender dysphoria has or has not been resolved is of importance. The fertility counselor is advised to ask transgender persons seeking ART whether they have experienced gender dysphoria in the past, how they dealt with it, and to think about changes that will come about in their body when harvesting gametes or carrying a pregnancy.

People who had difficulty and even trauma during their gender transition may be at higher risk than others whose dysphoria may have been mild. Previous experiences with gender dysphoria are important to discuss in fertility counseling sessions to provide psychoeducation about what individuals may anticipate during treatments they may need to undergo to create their family. However, caution is given to not assume that prior experiences are a necessary predictor of a difficult time with fertility treatment or pregnancy. Each person is different, and their unique situation should be explored with the fertility counselor.

For example, a recent study of 22 transmasculine individuals who had experienced one or more pregnancies [11] found that the experience of gender dysphoria during pregnancy and birth varied widely between people. Two people indicated that they did not see their bodies as female, but they did feel that pregnancy is a female activity which triggered feelings of gender dysphoria. In relation to bodily focused gender dysphoria, seven participants indicated they had an increase in dysphoria in relation to the chest, hips, voice, hormone changes and imbalance, body fat distribution or combinations of these. Gender dysphoria was at times centered around the pelvic area, pelvic-related medical procedures or the process of giving birth. One participant reported he was surprised by some of the body changes he had experienced and thought that had he been able to predict them in advance of his pregnancy, he may have been able to cope better with them. Some participants were able to implement coping strategies to help them manage the gender dysphoria related to their family building. These strategies included focusing on the temporary nature of pregnancy and the utility of it as a means to an end to form a family.

Regarding dysphoria and procreation, some transgender people decide not to have biological children because they cannot imagine themselves utilizing their gametes in a way that feels, to them, to be gendered. There are not many cultural examples of mothers who have contributed sperm to a pregnancy or fathers whose eggs have resulted in children. Pregnancy, egg harvesting, ejaculation and ovarian stimulation are processes which can feel emotionally difficult or impossible for some transgender individuals, given the complicated nature of their relationships to their bodies or experiences of trauma. At times, the impossibility to use one's own gametes or body to form a family may not be medical but is a psychological barrier that is insurmountable depending on the individual.

6. *Intersectionality is reality.* When working with transgender people, the concept of **intersectionality** is imperative. This means understanding that a person's gender identity is just one part of themselves, and all people are highly multifaceted. People's identities outside of gender include their cultural, racial, religious and spiritual identities to name a few, in addition to other characteristics such as intelligence, education, talents and abilities, social class, etc. [3]. Overfocusing on the person as one dimensional (i.e., transgender) greatly reduces the complexity of the person because all these different facets of a person intersect to form who they are and their experiences.

7. *Cisnormative and heteronormative biases discriminate against transgender patients seeking ART.* In Chapter 16, the authors discuss how a **heteronormative bias** exists in fertility treatment, where services are directed toward women and their husbands. In addition to the heteronormative biases transgender prospective parents experience is a **cisnormative bias**. This is the assumption that cisgender is the norm and that all people's gender identity matches their sex assigned at birth. Fertility counselors and the larger fertility industry need to stop treating all people seeking their services as if they are cisgender. For example, a man may have a uterus and be pregnant, just as a woman may have a penis and not be able to carry a pregnancy.

8. *Use a trauma-informed lens of care.* Many transgender clients have experienced trauma not only in their daily lives, but also while seeking medical and mental health care. For example, in the US alone, in a 2015 study on transgender discrimination [33], pervasive mistreatment and violence in the home, work and community were revealed in addition to severe economic hardship, instability, mental and physical illness and homelessness at substantially higher rates than those of the general population. Practicing through a **trauma-informed care** lens is important [37]. Trauma-informed care recognizes the presence of trauma symptoms and acknowledges the role that trauma may play in a transgender person's daily life and while seeking medical and mental health services. A trauma-informed approach to fertility counseling with transgender individuals seeking ART recognizes the widespread impact of trauma and the signs and symptoms of traumatization in transgender people and responds by seeking to reduce re-traumatization by showing acceptance, inclusivity, validation and careful listening and responding.

Summary

Over recent decades, reproductive justice for transgender people has made strides in recognition to varying degrees around the globe. The extent of equality and inclusivity does vary across different countries and legal systems. Options for transgender people to preserve their fertility and reproductive capacity have been advanced not only by modern scientific advances but also through the ongoing recognition that the psychological well-being and outcomes for children raised by a transgender parent(s) are positive. This chapter has introduced a brief history of this journey and growth. We have outlined some essential concepts for fertility counselors to know about transgender people to provide more inclusive and culturally expansive services to those who require ART to preserve their fertility options prior to medical transition to their affirmed gender and/or grow their families using this technology. Addendum 17.1 provides the fertility counselor with additional resources for transgender intended parents.

It is the hope of the authors that this chapter serves as a springboard for fertility counselors to continue to expand their understanding of working with transgender people and how they build their families. Indeed, use of ART is just one way to form a family. Adoption, fostering, chosen families, blended families, step-parenting extended families, among others are all valid, meaningful and rich ways for transgender people to parent and care for others.

References

1. American Psychiatric Association. *Diagnostic and Statistical Manual of Mental Disorders*, 5th ed. Washington, DC: American Psychiatric Association, 2013.

2. Health Care for Transgender and Gender Diverse Individuals: ACOG Committee Opinion, Number 823. *Obstet Gynecol* 2021;**137**(3):e75–e88.

3. Chang SC, Singh AA, Dickey LM. *A Clinician's Guide to Gender-affirming Care: Working with Transgender and Gender Nonconforming Clients*. Oakland, CA: New Harbinger Publications Inc., 2018.

4. Dickey LM, Ducheny KM, Ehrbar RD. Family creation options for transgender and gender nonconforming people. *Psychol Sex Orientat Gend Divers* 2016;**3**(2):173–179.

5. Ethics Committee of the American Society of Reproductive Medicine. Access to fertility services by transgender and nonbinary persons: an Ethics Committee Opinion. *Fertil Steril* 2021;**115**(4):874–878.

6. American Psychological Association. Guidelines for Psychological Practice with Transgender and Gender Nonconforming People. *Am Psychologist* 2015;**70**(9):832–864.

7. American Academy of Child and Adolescent Psychiatry. Gay, lesbian, bisexual or transgender parents. Published 2013. Available from: www.aacap.org/AACAP/Policy_Sta tements/2008/Gay_Lesbian_Bisexual_or_Transgender_Pa rents.aspx [last accessed June 16, 2022].

8. De Sutter P, Verschoor A, Hotimsky A, Kira K. The desire to have children and the preservation of fertility in transsexual women: a survey. *Int J Transgend* 2002;**6**(3).

9. Wierckx K, Van Caenegem E, Pennings G, et al. Reproductive wish in transsexual men. *Hum Reprod* 2012;**27**(2):483–487.

10. Besse M, Lampe NM, Mann ES. Experiences with achieving pregnancy and giving birth among transgender men: a narrative literature review. *Yale J Biol Med* 2020;**93**:517–528.

11. MacDonald TK, Walks M, Biender M, Kibbe A. Disrupting the norms: reproduction, gender identity, gender dysphoria, and intersectionality. *Int J Transgend* 2021;**22**(1–2):18–29.

12. Green R, Money J. *Transsexualism and Sex Reassignment*. Baltimore, MA: John Hopkins Press, 1969.

13. Transgender Europe – *Trans Rights Europe Index, 2018*. Produced by: The International Lesbian, Gay, Bisexual, Trans & Intersex Association (ILGA) Europe. Brussels, Belgium.

14. World Professional Association for Transgender Health. Standards of care for the health of transsexual, transgender and gender variant people. Version 7. Available from: www .wpath.org. Published 2012.

15. Hembree WC, Cohen-Kettenis P, Gooren IJ, et al. Endocrine treatment of gender-dysphoric/gender incongruent persons: an Endocrine Society clinical practice guideline. *J Clin Endocr Metab* 2017;**102**:3869–3903.

16. Moravek MB. Gender-affirming hormone therapy for transgender men. *Clin Obstet Gynecol* 2018;**61**(4):687–704.

17. Defreyne J, Vanwonterghem Y, Collet S, et al. Vaginal bleeding and spotting in transgender men after initiation of testosterone therapy: a prospective cohort study (ENIGI). *Int J Transgend Health* 2020;**21**(2):163–175.

18. Taub RL, Ellis SA, Neal-Perry G, Magaret AS, Prager SW, Micks EA. The effect of testosterone on ovulatory function in transmasculine individuals. *Am J Obstet Gynecol* 2020;**223**(2):229.e1–229.e8.

19. Randolph JF Jr. Gender-affirming hormone therapy for transgender females. *Clin Obstet Gynecol* 2018;**61**(4):705–721.

20. Adeleye AJ, Reid G, Kao CN, Mok-Lin E, Smith JF. Semen parameters among transgender women with a history of hormonal treatment. *Urology* 2019;**124**:136–141.

21. Kent MA, Winoker JS, Grotas AB. Effects of feminizing hormones on sperm production and malignant changes: microscopic examination of post orchiectomy specimens in transwomen. *Urology* 2018;**121**:93–96.

22. Matoso A, Khandakar B, Yuan S, et al. Spectrum of findings in orchiectomy specimens of persons undergoing gender confirmation surgery. *Hum Pathol* 2018;**76**:91–99.

23. Li K, Rodriguez D, Gabrielsen JS, Centola GM, Tanrikut C. Sperm cryopreservation of transgender individuals: trends and findings in the past decade. *Andrology* 2018;**6**(6):860–864.

24. Marsh C, McCracken M, Gray M, Nangia A, Gay J, Roby KF. Low total motile sperm in transgender women seeking hormone therapy. *J Assist Reprod Genet* 2019;**36**(8):1639–1648.

25. Light AD, Obedin-Maliver J, Sevelius JM, Kerns JL. Transgender men who experienced pregnancy after female-to-male gender transitioning. *Obstet Gynecol* 2014;**124**(6):1120–1127.

26. Moravek MB, Kinnear HM, George J, et al. Impact of exogenous testosterone on reproduction in transgender men. *Endocrinology* 2020;**161**(3):bqaa014. https://doi.org/10.1210/endocr/bqaa014

27. Grimstad FW, Fowler KG, New EP, et al. Ovarian histopathology in transmasculine persons on testosterone: a multicenter case series. *J Sex Med* 2020;**17**(9):1807–1818.

28. De Roo C, Lierman S, Tilleman K, et al. Ovarian tissue cryopreservation in female-to-male transgender people: insights into ovarian histology and physiology after prolonged androgen treatment. *Reprod Biomed Online* 2017;**34**(6):557–566.

29. Leung A, Sakkas D, Pang S, Thornton K, Resetkova N. Assisted reproductive technology outcomes in female-to-male transgender patients compared with cisgender patients: a new frontier in reproductive medicine. *Fertil Steril* 2019;**112**(5):858–865.

30. Adeleye AJ, Cedars MI, Smith J, Mok-Lin E. Ovarian stimulation for fertility preservation or family building in a cohort of transgender men. *J Assist Reprod Genet* 2019;**36** (10):2155–2161.

31. Rothenberg SS, Witchel SF, Menke MN. Oocyte cryopreservation in a transgender male adolescent. *N Engl J Med* 2019;**380**(9):886–887.

32. Martin CE, Lewis C, Omurtag K. Successful oocyte cryopreservation using letrozole as an adjunct to stimulation in a transgender adolescent after GnRH agonist suppression. *Fertil Steril* 2021 (online). https://doi .org/10.1016/j.fertnstert.2021.02.025.

33. "USTS Reports – 2015 U.S. Trans Survey." Available from: www.ustranssurvey.org/reports [last accessed 16 June, 2022].

34. Mendoza NS, Moreno FA, Hishaw GA, et al. Affirmative care across cultures: broadening application. *Focus* 2020;**18**:31–39.

35. Gates TG, BrianK. Affirming Strengths-Based Models of Practice. Social Work Practice with the LBGTQ Community, 2017, pp. 235–248. Retrieved from Loyola eCommons, Social Work: School of Social Work Faculty Publications and Other Works.

36. Hidalgo M, Ehrensaft D, Tishelman A, et al. The gender affirmative model: what we know and what we aim to learn. *Hum Develop* 2013;**56**:285–290.

37. *SAMHSA's Concept of Trauma and Guidance for a Trauma-Informed Approach*. HHS Publication No. (SMA) 14–4884. Rockville, MD: Substance Abuse and Mental Health Services Administration, 2014.

Chapter 18

A Racially and Culturally Sensitive Approach to Fertility Counseling

Kimberly Grocher and Trudie Gerrits

Introduction

Fertility counselors see an array of clients who may be diverse in terms of countries of origin, ethnicity, race and/ or cultural background. These diverse backgrounds may affect their views, emotions, experiences and options regarding their fertility challenges, child-wish, use of assisted reproductive technologies (ARTs), third-party involvement in procreation and resulting forms of family compositions and parenthood. All these features may also affect the issues clients are confronted with and how they want to see them addressed in counseling sessions [1].

This chapter will address the following questions: What do fertility counselors need to know about addressing racial, ethnic and cultural diversity issues of the clients they see? How can fertility counselors approach working with clients from a culturally sensitive and anti-oppressive practice perspective?

These are not easy questions to address. These questions can be highly political and sensitive. The answers to these questions are complex and nuanced. Unfortunately, scientific evidence in this field is limited and what does exist cannot fully address the lived experience of every individual of a particular race, culture or ethnicity. With this in mind, we offer a number of concepts and ideas in this chapter in an effort to "start the conversation" about race and cultural dynamics in fertility counseling, rather than a rulebook of "do's" and "don'ts."

We begin the chapter with several principles to guide this conversation. These principles include understanding how we consider race, ethnicity and culture while emphasizing the importance of not "essentializing," that is not lumping members of given racial and ethnic groups together, irrespective of social context and variations within these groups [2]. The chapter continues with a brief overview of the meaning and consequences of infertility in various places worldwide and among migrant, ethnic and racial minorities,

how this can affect access to, use of and experiences with fertility treatments and ARTs. Finally, we offer considerations for a racially and culturally sensitive clinical approach in fertility counseling.

Considering Race, Ethnicity and Culture

Race, culture and ethnicity are socially constructed terms that help us begin to understand and locate social identities on a spectrum; however, they fail to encapsulate the entirety of a person or their lived experiences. These terms are not finite among themselves and can overlap with one another. Before defining these concepts, it is important to briefly explore critical factors that contribute to these concepts.

There are huge differences between categories used to describe ethnic minority groups in different societies around the globe [3]. The phrase "ethnic communities" tends to conjure up or reinforce the idea that there are compartmentalized moral worlds, located in spaces neatly separated by ancestry, religion, cultural and social positioning [4]. The vast origins and history of ethnic and racial minority groups around the globe can vary drastically. For example, in the United States (US), Australia and New Zealand, current ethnic minority groups include groups who were the original habitants of the land in addition to groups who migrated (recent or over the course of centuries) [1]. This latter group can be further divided into groups who migrated by force (such as in the slave trade), political refugee groups and those who migrated for economic advancement. Ethnicity is produced within particular social and historical contexts, making cross-country comparison and statements problematic [1].

Ethnic identity can also be a source of pride and belonging [1]. It is produced and negotiated within a particular social context, which embodies individual interpretation and preferences in relation to the values of significant others. Ethnic identity emerges as flexible, negotiable and contingent: a resource which could be used creatively to support a person's sense of who he/she is, while simultaneously sustaining disadvantage and discrimination [1].

The addenda referred to in this chapter are available for download at www.cambridge.org/covington-clinical-guide

For the purpose of this chapter, when we refer to *race,* we acknowledge that race is a social construct that is created by, and reinforced by, social and institutional practices as well as individual attitudes, experiences and behaviors [5]. When referring to *ethnicity* we are considering the relationships and communities formed around ethnic similarity [6]. When we refer to *culture,* we are considering ideologies, practices and rituals that are learned or socially transmitted, that can change over time and context [6]. By framing these explanations as considerations instead of definitions, we acknowledge the overlaps that exist between these concepts and their shifting meanings based on the context and geographical location.

It is, also, important to understand the concept of racism with an emphasis on Anti-Black racism when discussing these challenges. Racism can be considered a system of advantage based on race that includes institutional, cultural and interpersonal practices that create advantages for people that are legally defined and socially constructed as "White" [5]. Anti-Black racism includes this schema where white represents dominant culture, standards and beliefs, while black represents anything "other." The primary orienting "category" is racism, but it also accounts for an individual's other social identities that include gender, colorism, nationality, ethnicity, geography, age, sexuality, health, ability, etc. (see Figure 18.1). Anti-Black racism is historically rooted in systems, institutions, policies and practices that perpetuate inequality and favor the dominant culture at the expense of anything or anyone not of the dominant culture, the "other." While it incorporates intersecting identities, Blackness, in its many forms across the globe, is the root and foundation of Anti-Black racism.

Not Essentializing Ethnicity, Race and Culture

It is becoming common practice for health professionals, psychologists, counselors and social workers to consider racial and cultural diversity in health care. Under umbrella terms such as "cultural competence," "cultural sensitivity" or "cultural humility," professionals are encouraged to adapt their practices and address prejudices in care delivery, decrease health disparities and improve quality of care for a diverse patient/client population [7]. While such practices may help medical professionals become more aware of diversity issues in their consultation rooms, these approaches are also critiqued.

A major point of critique refers to the conceptualization and use of the notion of culture. "Culture" is often used in reference to the cultural and exotic "other" or stranger, not to the standard/dominant group within a country. Often

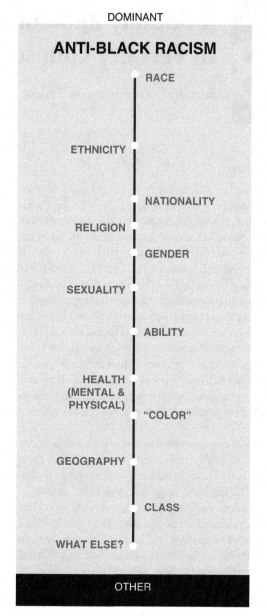

Figure 18.1 Schema of Anti-Black racism.

culture, nationality, race, religion and country of origin are lumped together (as opposed to being considered as distinct aspects of the individual) to refer to people's identity. Subsequently, these broad and fixed categories are used to depict the "other," their ideas and behavior, in rather stereotypical and static ways. Finally, this category is then presented as the direct cause of certain problematic conditions (physical or psychological) or behavior, without explicitly acknowledging intermediate contextual factors (such as uncertainty about residence situation, housing condition, financial problems, norms and values, life style and the social and political context that may impact these factors), which may explain a correlation between a person's condition and background/circumstances, but certainly does not apply equally to all members of a particular ethnic or racial category [1,7].

Views and experiences of migrants are not necessarily the same as those of citizens living in their home country. Migrants, whether recently migrated or years before, may not adhere to the views and values they brought when they moved to the country where they currently reside. Their views may have become more or less similar to the "dominant" views in the country where they currently reside, depending on many factors and circumstances [1]. Contrarily, however, some of them may stick to the values they brought from home, even while these may have changed there. Migrants may be aware of these changes or not, and they may agree with them or not. Thus, care should be taken not to generalize research finding about migrants' home countries to migrants.

To summarize, we are cautioning fertility counselors against broad generalizations and essentializing culture. Clients should not be *essentialized* based on the background category they belong to, which is not equivalent to assuming a color-blind approach (where the fertility counselor operates from a "we are all the same, race, culture, etc. doesn't matter" mindset) in fertility counseling [8]. We consider fertility "not simply as a medically diagnosed reproductive impairment, but a socially constructed reality" where people's (cultural) background and their (marginalized) position may and do matter in how they view fertility problems, the treatment options they seek, have access to and the care they need and receive [1].

Meaning and Consequences of Infertility

As we discuss the meaning and consequences of infertility from various parts of the world, we invite fertility counselors to consider the research and scenarios presented as "signposts" to consider when navigating the fertility journey with clients, as opposed to statically applying these principles to clients that may identify with these cultural groups. Since the 1990s, research studies worldwide have shown the social construction of infertility and its myriad of consequences for women and men impacted by infertility. This is especially true in countries located in the global south where reproducing is often culturally

mandated, and where a substantial number of migrants to western countries originate [9,10]. While huge differences exist between and within different sociocultural, religious and economic environs, these studies depict how infertility may affect different aspects of life.

Emotional Consequences

Infertility can affect people emotionally, often leading to a range of emotions that include sadness, worthlessness, jealousy and/or depression. While this applies to women, who in many societies bear the blame for infertility, even when the male identifying partner is the source of infertility issues, studies that include men increasingly show that they are also deeply emotionally affected by infertility [11,12].

Relational Consequences

Infertility can also influence a couple's relationship. In some cases, a woman may be treated disrespectfully by her partner, enduring physical violation, abandonment or divorce in cultures where infertility is an acceptable reason to take another or additional partner. In many contexts, having children is an extended family affair, adding social pressure on the couple to conceive. In-laws may mistreat childless women and encourage or pressure their male family member to divorce or attempt to conceive with or marry another woman.

Differences can exist in partner and family dynamics, based on how descendance is (traditionally) perceived. Matrilineal societies, where the children born by a woman belong to her lineage, are generally more protective for women who can't conceive than patrilineal societies [13]. To be sure, there can be variances in patrilineal societies with how men and their families treat women facing fertility problems.

Communal Consequences

At the community level, both childless women and men may be isolated, stigmatized and discriminated against. Men may feel emasculated. Male fertility challenges are often equated with sexual impotence. In some cultures, that may impede a male's ability to be considered for leadership roles [12]. In order to "protect" their infertile husband, women may claim that the fertility problem is theirs [12,14].

Economic Consequences

Fertility challenges may also lead to economic hardship, as intended parents often spend a large part of their income on treatments. Their social security might be negatively impacted since they may not have children to take care of them in illness or as they age. Women and men who are experiencing fertility challenges and are childless may also be concerned about what happens to them when they pass away: who will bury them, mourn them and fulfill the cultural, ancestral or religious rituals [13]?

Alternate Experiences

While these consequences are relevant for many across cultures and nationalities, there are alternate views and experiences as well. Women experiencing fertility complications who have a relatively high status in the community, as for example in Ghana, tend to be less stigmatized than other women experiencing fertility challenges [15]. In addition to these women having resources, such as higher education and/or capital, to achieve a respectful societal position beyond motherhood, disparity in experiences also relates to uneven access to quality infertility care. While IVF clinics are rapidly expanding globally, they are generally only accessible to the wealthy who can afford the expensive treatments in their own country or can travel abroad for fertility services [14,16]. Yet, when ARTs are widely accessible and used, even when only affordable for a few, they affect the way infertility is perceived and handled [14].

Migrant and Racial Minorities: Meaning and Consequences of Infertility

Clearly, context, including the availability of ARTs, matters. What does this mean for individual's views and experiences when they leave their home country and become migrants in a country in the global north? There is a dearth of literature to address this question. Compared to the abundance of studies on infertility in the global south, there is a lack of such studies among ethnic and racial minority groups who travel or live north [1,17]. It has been suggested that, at least in the US, infertility is framed as an issue for white, well-educated and wealthy women looking for IVF, while Black women are seen as "hyper-fertile" and who should be encouraged to procreate less rather than more [1]. This false perception that Black women are hyper-fertile can lead to isolation when they experience fertility challenges and reluctance to seek treatment [18].

Several studies among ethnic and racial minorities show that having children is often still considered mandatory, often soon after marriage, as it was in the

country of origin for many of the participants in these studies. This applies, for example, to Turkish couples in the UK and the Netherlands, for Arab American couples and Latinos/as in the US, South Asian communities in the UK, and Hmong women in Australia [1]. See Addendum 18.1 for more information on studies addressing infertility care among ethnic or racial minorities.

However, the extent to which the cultural, religious mandate and/or social pressure to reproduce is experienced differs highly among these groups. The Hmong women, for example, were predominantly stuck to traditional patrilineal and patrilocal notions: women were only respected within their family and clan when they produced children, preferably male children. While among the South Asian communities in the UK, there appears to be more space for change and individual agency: the younger generation feels less obliged to conceive immediately after marriage or to have a boy and aspire to a lower number of children in total compared to the older generation [1]. Overall, in this community, pursuing higher education is considered a good reason to postpone marriage and childbearing; "social class, gender and generation" thus matter [1].

Muslim couples with an Arab background in the US also continue to highly value parenthood as a mandatory "route to adult personhood, as the ingredient for happiness and commitment within a marriage, as the key to social acceptance in the community, and as the only guaranteed path to future immortality" [11]. While in the Middle East women rarely initiate divorce when their husband is the origin of the couple's fertility problem, in the US some of them do take the initiative, pointing to possibilities of social change when moving to a different context [11].

Another theme emerging in the infertility literature about ethnic and racial minorities is the meaning of male fertility and men's fear of emasculation [1,19]. For Latinos in the US, the stigma of infertility is even bigger for men than for women, as they generally conflate infertility with sexual impotence. Latino men feel denigrated by others and subsequently, according to the women in this study, are often unwilling to submit semen for analysis [1]. For Arab American men who had to flee their country (for example due to the war in Iraq) and had lost everything that was important for them, the experience of not being able to reproduce, "in a cultural and social world where children were a confirmation of a man's selfhood and his future immortality," represented "a genuine existential tragedy" [11]. These Arab American men – contrary to the Latinos – were most willing to undergo diagnosis and treatment and even went for testing on their own.

Ethnic and Racial Minorities Fertility Care and Counseling

Seeking Treatment and Experiences with Fertility Care

While ARTs are offered globally, people belonging to racial and ethnic minorities in North America and Europe make less use of these technologies [11,17]. This disparity may be due to economic reasons; yet, a similar tendency is observed in countries where health insurances fully cover ARTs [17]. This disparity reflects "stratified reproduction," the idea that "some people, because of structural and/or cultural factors are more empowered to reproduce than others" [20]. What makes people belonging to racial and ethnic minorities be less empowered and/or inclined to utilize ARTs? And how do they experience the fertility care available? A recent systematic review of qualitative studies by Kirubarajan and colleagues summarized five key "barriers" to fertility care for racial and ethnic minority groups, affecting the use of fertility care: "stigmatizing cultural beliefs, low fertility knowledge, language barriers, discrimination and lack of institutional trust" [17] (see Addendum 18.2 for information on the studies included in the review.) Supporting the position that "current inequities are a stark remnant of the unethical history of obstetrics/gynecology in North America and Europe" [17] we first discuss discrimination and lack of institutional trust. These concepts, related to this history, are fundamental to understand the experiences and needs of racial and minority groups in fertility health care and counseling.

Lack of Institutional Trust and Discrimination

Medicine has evolved tremendously over its long history and includes many advances that benefit humans across the lifespan. However, the field of medicine has a dark past when it comes to the treatment of marginalized and oppressed groups, roots that continue to influence our medical systems today. For example, James Marion Sims, commonly considered the father of modern gynecology, developed tools and procedures that have had a tremendous impact on women's reproductive health; however, he used enslaved women as involuntary test subjects for his new techniques, without anesthesia. In the twentieth century, the infamous Tuskegee experiment, where Black men who agreed to be research participants were unknowingly infected with syphilis, destroyed the lives of many Black families. Jews in concentration camps across Europe during World War II were also made to be subjects of painful and at times, terminal, medical procedures for the purpose of research. Medicine's history of abusing and exploiting marginalized members of society to advance science has for many people of racial and ethnic marginalized groups resulted in distrust of the healthcare system that continues today.

This historically informed distrust in medicine is reflected in some of the studies reviewed by Kirubarajan et al. [17], often in combination with experiences of racial discrimination and ethnic stereotyping. Awareness of the mistreatment of the Black population throughout history was explicitly mentioned to cause distrust in current medical practices among fertility patients in the US and made immigrant women in Canada facing fertility problems reluctant to share information with health staff [17]. In other studies, patients suspected their fertility doctors were not motivated to provide optimal care to women from their own ethnic group, respectively African American women, and Turkish migrants in the Netherlands, as they were assumed to have too many children, or because doctors would rather foreigners didn't have more children. Some study patients described experiencing racial discrimination, perceiving to be "stereotypically" judged on their physical appearance (assumed as not being able to afford ARTs) and therefore felt treated differently, which may have led to people not returning to the clinic. Studies in the UK and US found that fertility providers held ethnocentric, discriminatory and stereotypical assumptions about patients pertaining to ethnic minority migrants, which affected the fertility care they received [4,11].

One study noted the persisting reproductive racism and discrimination in the US geared towards Arab men. These men are often "vilified as dangerous and untrustworthy 'others' in American society" [11]. Arab couples in the study described interactions with American healthcare professionals as dismissive, patronizing and offending, especially when the women were wearing hijab. They were stereotyped as fundamentalist, religious, hyperfertile and suffering from patriarchal suppression by their husband.

A study exploring the risks of stereotyping South Asian (SA) patients in the UK found that health professionals tend to assume that within these "minoritized communities," culture and religion, rather than personal choices, shape decision-making about infertility management, which would be in sharp contrast with white patients who are supposed to respond autonomously, in a culture-free way [4]. Other generalized assumptions are that SA patriarchal families deny autonomy to their adult children, that they are all strongly pro-natalist and, consequently, secretive about fertility problems. This "secretiveness" in SA communities is seen as and referred to as a desire for confidentiality in white communities. However, sharing or not sharing information about anything related to reproduction and reproductive technologies can be done for many reasons in all communities.

These assumptions lead health professionals to think that discussing fertility problems and ARTs is taboo or offensive [4]. As a result, they may withhold information and thus undermine the practice of informed choice regarding medical treatment. Cultural sensitivity doesn't deny differences among and within groups, but at the same time should ensure equality of access to healthcare options [4].

Stigmatizing Cultural Views

While we continue to caution against stereotypical views that may not do justice to personal values and needs of people belonging to ethnic or racial minority groups and may lead to discriminatory practices, studies also show that (internalized) stigmatizing cultural views may impact the suffering from infertility and impede people in seeking fertility treatment [17]. These stigmatizing views in particular refer to the previously discussed cultural mandate to procreate (and to have large families) in various minority groups, and the resulting shame, and for men the fear of emasculation, when they don't succeed. In addition, several patients of different ethnic-religious communities expressed concerns about the acceptability of ARTs according to their religion and may be a reason for not using certain ART options (i.e., gamete donation among some Muslims).

Research reflects the unique nuances of each individual experience by also revealing alternate patterns: the urge to procreate may also lead to frantic help-seeking in an early stage, searching for ways that enable the use of ARTs [11]. An ethnographic study among Arab migrants in the US, for example, shows that in a context where parenthood is mandatory and strongly wished for immediately after marriage, and infertility – especially male fertility challenges in particular – is highly stigmatized,

many men were willing to undergo diagnosis and treatment. To by-pass cultural barriers, these men found Muslim physicians in the US who understood their social plight of infertility, spoke the Arab language and shared the religious sensibilities of their local moral worlds [11]. Sunni Islam men with serious male infertility problems seriously considered ICSI as this was their only option, because their religion does not allow sperm donation or adoption. Unfortunately, as ICSI is even more costly than ordinary IVF, it was not affordable for most of them, which underlines again the stratification of (assisted) reproduction [11].

When exploring the views of South Asian migrants (not fertility patients themselves) in the UK regarding gamete donation, researchers noticed that these views were not set in stone [4]. While gamete donation raised religious concerns (which were different for Muslim, Hindu and Sikh participants), they also could understand it as "a strategy of last resort," and as an altruistic means (for donors) to ease the suffering of childless people. Donor nonanonymity, however, raised gendered concerns, among others related to the strong link between biological paternity and inheritance of property for Muslims; while women were mainly worried about the emotional turmoil of nonanonymity for themselves and their families in the future. This study draws attention to the huge variety of attitudes to reproductive options within and between ethnic and religious groups – some of which may be highly stigmatizing – and those views also change over time.

Limited Fertility Literacy

Limited fertility literacy, that is lack of understanding around the biomedical processes involved in fertility treatment, can be seen as a barrier to care. Kirubarajan [17] and associates explored the effect that fertility literacy can have on seeking care among migrant and minority populations. This includes inaccurate ideas about possible causes of infertility (e.g., a man producing sperm being always considered fertile or that smoking does not impact one's fertility), the functioning of the reproductive system, fertility treatment options or their possible side-effects. Patients may feel embarrassed to acknowledge their limited fertility literacy. Low fertility literacy often was related with language barriers: fertility services and information were often only provided in a country's dominant language, while professional translators were not always available. When fertility patients then used informal translators, often their partners, miscommunication still occurred, partly resulting from their embarrassment about the information to be translated. Not surprisingly, patients in various studies provided suggestions for improvement of communication, education and fertility literacy, which is also relevant for fertility counselors including writing care plans in layman's terms, culturally relevant marketing geared towards minority and immigrant populations, providing translated documents, and having providers from diverse backgrounds on staff.

Fertility Counseling with Racial and Culturally Marginalized Groups

Different groups may have different views of counseling and other types of mental health treatment. There can be stigma and preconceived notions about who seeks such treatment ("crazy," "weak," etc.) resulting in feelings of shame about deciding to or feeling the need to seek treatment. Racial minorities and other marginalized groups may have had negative experiences related to treatment they have sought in the past, especially if the counselor was unable or unwilling to work effectively from a culturally sensitive framework.

While it's important to call attention to the barriers, the informal means that different groups may use to cope with emotional and psychological stressors must be considered. It can't be assumed that resistance to therapy or counseling in a medical context means that a person is not open to receiving support to cope. Other means of obtaining support may come from community members, religious leaders and institutions, and peer support networks. Many ethnic groups across the globe have a collective and community philosophy around support and caregiving, where the community is responsible for caring for the needs of its members. When a member is in need, they turn to the community for support first. It is important for fertility counselors to be prepared to explore community, spiritual and other supports that are amenable to the client.

Fertility Counseling: Racially and Culturally Sensitive Clinical Approaches

Racially and culturally sensitive clinical practice is a complex topic indeed. To guide the discussion, we will be sharing approaches that are informed by an anti-oppressive practice and a social justice lens [21,22]. These approaches are grounded in a reconceptualization of practice that's informed by critical social and cultural theory. Critical social and cultural theories challenge us to consider questions of power, difference and domination. They assert that our daily life experiences are shaped and constrained by structural forces including the social, economic, cultural and political systems in which we live, as we have demonstrated earlier in this chapter. While all of this may still seem far-fetched from what happens in the fertility counselor's virtual or physical office, it does have an impact on how we practice, when we consider and integrate racial and cultural dimensions into our work with fertility clients.

The ideas in this section may not be an entirely new way of working for some fertility counselors; however, it asks us to shift our mindset and be cognizant of racial and cultural factors that exist beyond the treatment room. It also requires us to be aware of how they influence and need to be considered during the fertility counseling process.

The counselor's mindset and internal work around bias are critical to this process. While understanding the definitions and principles around racial and cultural issues is relevant, investigating, acknowledging and working through our own internal biases is at the heart of this work. It is critical as fertility counselors to understand our positionality, identities and social location and how it influences our view of the world, as well as how it may be similar or different from the client(s) in front of us [22]. Acknowledging the inherent power structure that exists in the therapeutic relationship, and its reflection of the unjust social practices and systems that we are living in, is part of our work as clinicians. By asking ourselves questions like "What are my assumptions about the client in front of me? Their needs? Their perspective about this process? What resources do they have access to (or don't have access to)? How might my assumptions be different if their identities were different? Do I know their identities as they view them? What type of work have I done around my own biases?," the fertility counselor is making a commitment to uncertainty in this work. The fertility counseling landscape is inherently complex and unpredictable, and even more so when race and culture are considered in the therapeutic process.

Phases of Racially and Culturally Sensitive Treatment

Racially and culturally sensitive treatment occurs from pre-intake to termination and builds on the key concepts of meaning, context, power, history and possibility that are found in Table 18.1 [21,22]. The accompanying chapter in the *Case Studies* volume illustrates this approach and the five phases of treatment.

Table 18.1 Key concepts in racially and culturally sensitive treatment [21,22]

Key concepts	
Meaning	How do people give meaning to the experiences and conditions that shape their lives? How do people give meaning to the fertility journey? It's important to gain an understanding of what meaning fertility has for the client with whom you are engaging. What does it mean for them personally? What does it mean for them socially?
Context	What are the contexts in which those experiences and conditions occur? How does this larger context impact the context of the fertility journey?
Power	What forms and relations of power shape people and processes? How do power dynamics (whether social, political or interpersonal) impact this client's fertility journey and the fertility counseling process? How do they perceive their power in this process?
History	How does history make people and how do people make history as they engage in struggles over questions of meaning and power? This can include the larger historical context of your client's identities as well as their personal history.
Possibility	How might an appreciation of these struggles help us imagine and claim a sense of possibility in the practice of racially and culturally sensitive fertility counseling?

Pre-engagement/Engagement

Relationship is at the heart of our work with our fertility clients and the engagement phase sets the tone throughout our work with our clients [22]. It sets the context for our relationship and acts as a holding container for the work that is to be done in the fertility counseling process. It is shaped by mutual understanding, empathy, compassion, sincerity, humility, dedication and commitment.

It continues throughout the therapeutic process and in some cases, beyond. A consultation may take place at the beginning of the pre-engagement/engagement phase. The initial consultation is a good time to begin establishing rapport with potential fertility counseling clients. Oftentimes, as fertility counselors, we are taught to view this as a gatekeeping process where we are the experts making decisions and recommendations about what's right for the client, based on the information they provide. However, when we shift our mindset and practice to a culturally sensitive framework, we begin to see this phase as a process of listening, communication, translation and connection that begins to address questions of trust, power, intimacy, difference and conflict, and their potential within the therapeutic relationship

as well as in the larger context of the client's life and fertility journey [21]. In practice, this may look like expressing respect and concern for the client while providing a space for clients to be themselves and express themselves freely, while understanding that this may take time for clients who are accustomed to the rigid, formal, "expert knows best" power dynamic of many medical offices and facilities. It can also look like making decisions by consensus rather than by coercion. For example, inquiring about a client's treatment preferences, where choice is available, making suggestions on treatment options and inquiring about the client's point of view about this suggestion. In situations where the client has little choice about the recommendations made (such as for safety reasons or because limited options are available), delivering those recommendations in a way that fully explains the reason for the recommendation, and creating space for the client to express their thoughts and feelings about the recommendation and what it means for them, is important.

Teaching and Learning

What we typically think of as "assessment" becomes known as the "teaching and learning" phase of treatment from a racially and culturally sensitive framework. Traditionally, fertility counselors are taught that an assessment is a list of questions that need to be asked of the client to formally begin the treatment process. Yes, there is information that needs to be gathered to adequately help the client, but all too often these assessments can turn into interviews and interrogations. Thus, the hierarchy between patient and fertility counselors is not only evident but becomes centered, reinforcing the dynamics that are seen in social and political structures in larger societies and decentering the client from this very personal process.

Shifting our mindset and vernacular to teaching and learning begins to create a reciprocal relationship in this phase of treatment. In this sense, the fertility counselor honors their expertise but allows space for genuine curiosity about the client, whereby they are open to acknowledging that they don't know it all and want to learn about the client. This includes their lived experiences as referenced through the client's social location in their world and the meaning, context, power, historical and possibility factors that form the foundation of that lived experience.

The teaching and learning phase also gives the client agency to be in the teacher role vs. an interviewee or the interrogated. They are sharing knowledge that will be used to co-create the fertility counseling process, allowing their agency to be an inherent part of the process as opposed to other frameworks where the client is granted agency by the fertility counselors.

Action and Accompaniment

The phase traditionally known as "intervention" is reframed as "action and accompaniment" through this culturally and racially sensitive lens. It involves the fertility counselor collaborating with the client to determine the actions that will occur during the counseling process and determining how the fertility counselor can best support or accompany the client with carrying out the agreed upon actions. For example, a client may be having challenges with explaining some of their concerns about a physician's "bedside manner" during IVF procedures to the physician, fearing creating conflict or being turned away from treatment and being deemed a "difficult" patient. In this phase of treatment, the fertility counselor may help the client process their experience, while also helping the client explore possible actions they'd like to take, if any, in this situation. The client may decide that they'd like to voice their concerns. The fertility counselor would then inquire about how best they could help the client with this endeavor, possibly using expressive techniques such as role play, empty chair, writing a letter, etc. However, the key element is inquiring on how best the fertility counselor can support, or accompany, the client with their desired action. The client may decide that being able to bring their concerns to the counselor is what they need, or they may decide that it would be more meaningful and relevant for the fertility counselor to speak to the physician on their behalf. This seemingly simple, but powerful shift in the way we approach accompanying our clients on their journey, as opposed to directing them, leaves room and consideration for their needs, beliefs and values to not only be stated, but allows them to fully engage in the therapeutic process.

Participatory Evaluation

Participatory evaluation is another "phase" that takes place throughout the therapeutic process. It involves working alongside the fertility client to evaluate how the process is unfolding, whether the outcomes of the counseling process have been met or do they need to be shifted. It is, also, an evaluation of how effective the therapeutic relationship is for the client and the fertility counselor, including the understanding of racial and cultural factors as well as the integration of relevant cultural factors for the client into the process.

There is a shift from how we typically think of evaluation where the fertility counselor may be looking at objective data such as measures or scales. There may be some input from the client, but it is more of an interview/interviewee style. There is still a clear hierarchy, and the fertility counselor is driving the process and deciding what gets evaluated.

Objective data, such as data obtained from a psychological test or screening instrument, can also be part of the participatory evaluation process, but the difference is that the tools and means used for evaluation are decided upon by the fertility counselor and client together at the beginning of their work together. Questions such as, "How will we know that our work together is working for you?" or "How often should we check in to see if we are accomplishing your goals/moving toward your outcomes or need to adjust our process in some way?," can help to begin the discussion about how participatory evaluation will work in the context of your therapeutic process with your client.

Termination

The termination process is also an opportunity to honor important cultural factors as they relate to your fertility client. It's important to consider what the circumstances for termination are? Is the termination planned? In many cultures there are rituals of acknowledgement of endings and new beginnings and whatever the terms of termination, it usually signifies the ending of a phase and the beginning of a new one.

Navigating Sensitive Conversations Pertaining to Race and Culture

Having conversations pertaining to race and culture with our fertility clients can be a slippery slope and, as we mentioned throughout the chapter, there isn't a one size fits all approach. It is often said that counseling and therapy are both a science and an art. There is some artistic maneuvering to having these conversations and it requires the fertility counselor to be open to embodying new approaches that are different than the ones we may have been previously taught, as well as exercising self-compassion and being open to acknowledging and learning from our missteps. We'd like to offer a few final suggestions for navigating sensitive conversations pertaining to race and culture.

Guidelines

Aligning with our principles described earlier in the chapter, please use the information from this chapter as well as other sources you've been exposed to, including your own lived experiences, as guidelines and not rules when it comes to understanding your fertility client's identities, social location and the impact it has on the fertility counseling process as well as their entire fertility journey. Guidelines can be amended as needed, whereas rules can be considered hard and fast.

Client-centered

The aforementioned clinical approaches have a singular foundation component in that they are a manifestation of a client-centered approach. The process is navigated, decisions are made, and action is carried out *with* the client, all the while integrating their racial and cultural identities and any associated beliefs, rituals, practices, concerns, etc. that are deemed essential to the process by the client.

Cultural Humility

Cultural competency is replaced with cultural humility. Cultural competency denotes mastery while humility recognizes that engaging with cultural dynamics is an ongoing learning process for the professional.

Checking-in

Understanding that fertility counselors may have knowledge about a certain aspect of the client's background, given their experience working with a particular population or based on shared racial or cultural identities, it is still necessary to check in with clients throughout the therapeutic process and in therapeutic interactions to see if this information is applicable to *this* client. The fertility counselor needs to be asking, "What is the meaning for this client? What is the context that has determined this client's racial and cultural identities as seen and experienced by this client? What power dynamics (intrapersonal, interpersonal, societal, cultural, institutional, etc.) have influence on this client and their fertility journey? How does historical phenomena (either personal or societal) impact this dynamic or other aspects of the fertility journey? Considering all these factors, what is possible for the client on their fertility journey through the fertility counseling process?"

Considering Transference and Countertransference Issues

Race and cultural identities can lead to a host of transference and countertransference issues in the counseling process. This topic could be a chapter by itself, but we'd like to offer possibilities that may emerge for the fertility counselor and their clients as they are engaging in the therapeutic process. Comas-Diaz and Jacobsen [23] suggest that ethnicity and culture can touch deep

unconscious feelings in most individuals and become the target of projection for the client and counselor, thus becoming more accessible during therapeutic interactions. Unacknowledged differences can lead to distrust and suspicion of the therapist by the client. They also point out the importance of the therapist understanding their own ethnicity and culture to truly achieve effective cross-cultural counseling.

There may be a range of transference reactions. These reactions can include: the client's projection of ideas, beliefs and attributes onto the therapist, including overcompliance and friendliness on the part of the client; avoidance of issues related to race or culture by the client; mistrust, suspicion and hostility towards the counselor; and ambivalence where the client may have negative feelings toward the counselor due to racial and cultural factors, but has also developed an attachment to them.

When the fertility counselor and the client share racial and cultural identities, there can also be transference concerns that manifest in different ways. These feelings become increasingly complex if those identities are associated with groups that have been systematically oppressed or marginalized in some way [23]. The client may view the therapist as a "success story" (this is even further complicated if the client sees or has some knowledge of the therapist as overcoming fertility issues) or, at the other end of the spectrum, the client views the therapist as a traitor for somehow managing to succeed despite oppression and marginalization. There is also the possibility that a client may choose not to work with a counselor that shares their identities because they have conflicted feelings about their own identities and may not be ready to address those concerns alongside their fertility challenges.

There can be just as many countertransference challenges: the therapist's projection of ideas, beliefs and attributes onto the client. This may range from complete denial of differences (being "color-blind") to being overly curious about the client's background and seeking a racial and cultural lesson at the expense of the client, as opposed to the benefit of the client's process. Curiosity can be a difficult one to recognize because there may be genuine interest to learn more about the client as suggested in the other counseling phases, but it may be perceived as burdensome and invasive by the client. This is where a checking-in, a seemingly simple concept, accompanied by transparency about the reasons for inquiry, becomes a critical part of the fertility counseling process. Guilt, pity, aggression, ambivalence and survivor's guilt (usually when the therapist is from a racial or cultural identity that has historically struggled economically, politically, etc.) when manifested as countertransference can also impede the therapeutic process. When the therapist shares the same racial and/or cultural identities with the client, there is the risk of overidentification or intentionally distancing themselves from the client to avoid overidentification.

Recognizing possible transference and countertransference issues as they relate to racial and cultural identity and the impact they can have on the counseling process is an important aspect of doing this work effectively, albeit quite challenging. It also highlights the need for ongoing racial and cultural sensitivity training, coupled with quality supervision from a supervisor that has training, experience and is comfortable addressing racial and cultural factors in the fertility counseling process.

Summary

This chapter has discussed the following questions: "What do fertility counselors need to know about addressing racial, ethnic and cultural diversity issues of the clients they see?" and "How can they approach working with clients from a culturally sensitive and anti-oppressive practice perspective?" We have presented several principles to guide this conversation, including emphasizing the importance of not "essentializing" race, ethnicity and culture, in order to avoid easy generalizations and acting on stereotypes. Next, we briefly discussed the meaning and possible consequences of infertility globally and among migrant and racial minorities in particular, and how these may affect access to, use of and experiences with fertility treatments and ARTs. Finally, we offered suggestions for racially and culturally sensitive clinical approaches in fertility counseling. These approaches originate from the idea that people's daily life experiences are shaped and constrained by structural forces including the social, economic, cultural and political systems in which they live and that these systems impact fertility counselors' work with their clients. Acknowledging, investigating and working through the fertility counselor's own social identities and internal biases – regarding ethnic and racial minority groups – is at the heart of this work. Key concepts in this approach are "meaning, context, power, history and possibility," and these should be taken into consideration throughout the counseling process, from pre-engagement to termination. Finally, we have offered suggestions for how to sensitively navigate conversations pertaining to race and culture in the consultation room, highlighting the need for quality

supervision from a supervisor that has training, experience and is comfortable addressing racial and cultural factors in the fertility counseling process. It is our hope that you will continue this journey.

References

1. Culley L, Hudson N, Rooij F van, Eds. *Marginalized Reproduction: Ethnicity, Infertility, and Reproductive Technologies*. London: Earthscan, 2009.

2. Lo MCM, Stacey CL. Beyond cultural competency: Bourdieu, patients and clinical encounters. *Sociology Health Illness* 2008;30(5):741–755.

3. Bradby H, Nazroo J. Health, ethnicity and race. In: Cockerham WC, Ed. *The New Companion to Medical Sociology*. Malden MA: Blackwell, 2010, 113–129.

4. Hampshire K, Simpson B, Eds. *Assisted Reproductive Technologies in the Third Phase: Global Encounters and Emerging Moral Worlds*, Vol. 31. New York and Oxford: Berghahn Books, 2015.

5. Funk M, Varghese R, Zuniga X. Racism. In Adams M, Blumenfeld WJ, Catalano C, et al., Eds. *Readings for Diversity and Social Justice*, 4th ed. New York, NY: Taylor & Francis, 2018.

6. Suyemoto KL, Curley M, Mukkamala S. What do we mean by "Ethnicity" and "Race"? A consensual qualitative research investigation of colloquial understandings. *Genealogy* 2020;4(81):1–24.

7. Zanting A, Meershoek A, Frambach JM, Krumeich A. The "exotic other" in medical curricula: rethinking cultural diversity in course manuals. *Medical Teacher* 2020;42(7):791–798.

8. Phillips A. What's wrong with essentialism? *Distinktion* 2010;11(1):47–60.

9. Inhorn M, Van Balen F, Eds. *Infertility around the Globe: New Thinking on Childlessness, Gender, and Reproductive Technologies*. Los Angeles, CA: University of California Press, 2002.

10. Van Balen F, Bos HM. The social and cultural consequences of being childless in poor-resource areas. *Facts, Views Vision ObGyn* 2009;1(2):106.

11. Inhorn MC. *America's Arab Refugees. Vulnerability and Health on the Margins*. Stanford: Stanford University Press, 2018.

12. Hörbst V. Male perspectives on infertility and assisted reproductive technologies (ART) in sub-Saharan contexts. *Facts, Views Vision ObGyn* 2010;8:22–27.

13. Gerrits T. Infertility and matrilineality. The exceptional case of the Macua. In: Inhorn MC, Van Balen F, Eds. *Infertility around the Globe: New Thinking on Childlessness, Gender and Reproductive Technology*. Los Angeles, CA: University of California Press, 2002.

14. Inhorn MC, Patrizio P. Infertility around the globe: new thinking on gender, reproductive technologies and global movements in the 21st century. *Hum Reprod Update* 2015:**21**(4):411–426.

15. Donkor ES, Sandall J. The impact of perceived stigma and mediating social factors on infertility-related stress among women seeking infertility treatment in Southern Ghana. *Soc Sci Med* 2007;**65**(8):1683–1694.

16. Gerrits T. Reproductive travel to Ghana: testimonies, transnational relationships, and stratified reproduction. *Med Anthropol* 2018;**37**(2):131–144.

17. Kirubarajan A, Patel P, Leung S, Prethipan T, Sierra S. Barriers to fertility care for racial/ethnic minority groups: a qualitative systematic review. *Fertil Steril Rev* 2021;**2** (2):150–159.

18. Jackson-Bey T, Morris J, Jasper E, et al. Systemic review of racial and ethnic disparities in reproductive endocrinology and infertility: where do we stand today. *Fertil Steril* 2021;**116**(1):169–188.

19. Inhorn MC, Fakih MH. Arab Americans, African Americans, and infertility: barriers to reproduction and medical care. *Fertil Steril* 2006;**85** (4):844–852.

20. Gerrits T. Introduction. ARTs in resource-poor areas: practices, experiences, challenges and theoretical debates. In: Hampshire K, Simpson B, Eds. *Assisted Reproductive Technologies in the Third Phase: Global Encounters and Emerging Moral Worlds.* Oxford: Berghahn Books, 2015, 94–104.

21. Finn JL. *Just Practice: A Social Justice Approach to Social Work,* 3rd ed. New York, NY: Oxford University Press.

22. Morgaine K, Capous-Desyllas M. *Anti-Oppressive Social Work Practice: Putting Theory into Practice.* California, CA: Sage Publications.

23. Comas-Diaz L, Jacobsen FM. Ethnocultural transference and countertransference in the therapeutic dyad. *Am J Orthopsychiatry* 1991;**61**(3):392–402.

Resilience in Reproductive Loss

19

Irving Leon

Diverse Meanings, Diverse Outcomes

In common parlance, resilience is the ability to respond adaptively to adversity, indicating bouncing back from a decline in functioning due to adverse stress. Bereavement and trauma experts are more likely to emphasize the ability to resist impaired coping as a response to stress, demonstrating instead an effective adaptation from the start [1]. Others are inclined to focus on the benefits that accrue from weathering the crisis, into the post-traumatic (or post-loss) period [2]. Still others choose to view resilience as having multiple definitions embracing a quick recovery, successful adaptation and positive sequelae [3]. To as broadly as possible tap into the research and clinical work on resilience, I will apply all three understandings.

There are three distinct categories of resilience to consider; that of exploring its impact on infertility, its effects on negotiating pregnancy losses and foundational research on resilience across the spectrum of stressors. Infertility studies on resilience tend to be meager and skewed, often examining impaired rather than improved functioning. One striking exception is the Infertility Resilience Model [4] which evaluates individual, couple and external factors. In that approach resilience is often based on the quality of the couple's communication, their openness with each other, talking out differences, and shared decision-making. Most research supplementing my clinical experience on resilience will be from the reproductive loss literature and broader studies on resilience in general.

A Paradigm Shift

The test of a first-rate intelligence is the ability to hold two opposed ideas in the mind at the same time, and still retain the ability to function.
F. Scott Fitzgerald, The Crack-up, *1936*

Exploring resilience challenges our usual ways of understanding reproductive losses. Instead of our typical clinical goal being the facilitation of grieving, resilience is oriented to minimizing grief. Instead of focusing on maladaptive responses, often labeled as pathologic symptoms, we investigate successful adaptations to loss and how bereavement can instigate gains. This paradigm shift is not intended to replace our earlier more traditional models of identifying disorder, but to expand and integrate our understanding to include more benign and positive responses promoting well-being.

Intense grief, depression and post-traumatic stress disorder (PTSD) are not universal reactions to loss and severe stressors. Resilience, in fact, may be more normative than exceptional. While 50–60% of the US population has experienced traumatic stressors, it has been estimated that only 5–10% demonstrate PTSD [1]. A very large-scale study of over 10,000 women revealed that there is no significantly greater likelihood of mental health symptoms among those who experienced a single pregnancy loss than those who did not [5]. We, as therapists, need to beware of covertly generalizing our clients' distress to the wide, community population, overlooking the likelihood of milder distress among those who do not seek our help.

Resilience is not a capacity that you have or is absent. In evaluating a client for psychotherapy, I always identify that person or couple's strengths and prior psychic triumphs over adversity, not focusing solely on vulnerabilities and sources of distress. It is crucial to remember that those who present with fertility problems or a recent reproductive loss will often demonstrate much distress and impaired functioning in the first meeting, sometimes appearing more "disturbed" than they in fact are [6]. A couple of sessions of empathic listening and responsiveness will often, simultaneously and paradoxically, deepen the discussion on suffering while demonstrating psychological resources to build on, in order to handle that pain. It is not

Table 19.1 The components of resilience

1. Active coping
2. Making meaning of the loss
3. Continuing the bond
4. Secure attachments
5. Positive emotions
6. Post-traumatic growth

uncommon for couples facing multiple issues melding together in the crisis of infertility (e.g., low self-esteem, becoming a parent, separating from one's family of origin and the limits of control) to creatively work out currently viable, if not permanent, adaptations as significant distress goes hand in hand with previously unrealized resilience [7].

Resilience should not be viewed as a singular process. There are multiple, often unexpected, pathways to resilience [1,3], not one road defining the way. Most of this chapter will explore the ingredients of resilience, using brief clinical anecdotes to illustrate the components of resilience in action (see Table 19.1). As with many clinical concepts with multiple aspects, the ingredients amalgamate in unique patterns for different individuals. Certain aspects of resilience will be vital for some and absent for another. Clinical examples will mostly be taken from my own practice, while most of the conceptual underpinning will be drawn from the experts in this field.

Finally, the components of resilience will be operationalized in different ways. Some will be readily learnable; others rooted in disposition and character, much more difficult to alter; and others are transformational, acquired through the post-loss period.

The Components of Resilience

Active Coping

Active coping is the most ubiquitous feature of resilience. In their "dual process model of coping with bereavement" (DPM), Stroebe and Schut [8] conceive of grieving not as the usual discrete sequence of stages to be mastered, but a constant oscillation between two poles: one of actively grieving and the other of coping with daily tasks and changed circumstances oriented to a restoration of new normative functioning. While a stage model envisions an end to grieving and subsequent resumption of regular living, a dual process approach more realistically views grieving alternating with coping from the very start, and gradually diminishing over time without ever coming to a final endpoint. DPM essentially embeds active coping in

all bereavement. One cannot actively grieve without interruption, but instead grief comes and goes, intermittently, as in waves. Between bouts of grief, there are the daily tasks of life to do as well as the new challenges of preparing for a funeral, attending to life changes due to the loss, taking on new roles and relationships, etc.

The dual process model of coping with bereavement appears especially well-suited to illustrate how resilience via active coping usually is embodied in all reproductive losses. Mothers typically grieve such losses with greater intensity and longevity – favoring the task of grieving – than their partners, who concretely problem solve and tend to gravitate to the task of coping. It is usually adaptive to strike a balance between partners, with each having a stake in grieving and coping, despite the different emphases between them. It is more problematic when each partner exclusively inhabits opposite poles, compulsively grieving or coping, resulting in no shared experience of the loss, little communication between the couple and a marked lack of resilience [4].

In such a situation, each may be coaxed out of their corners with the father encouraged to express his loss in whatever way suits him, allowing his wife to feel closer in their shared grief. She in turn, via active coping, can resume doing family tasks, enabling a greater sense of shared family responsibilities. In the process of doing this, his fears of her being overwhelmed by needing to cope, or the family falling apart if he lets down his guard, are confronted and proved inaccurate. This intervention may address not only recent maladaptive patterns emerging in managing marital grieving and coping, but earlier and more chronic versions as well.

Some reproductive losses require mastering complicated issues demanding a rapid oscillation between the tasks of grieving and coping. Assisted reproductive technologies (ART) for infertility demands coping with exacting protocols for IVF, alternating with the intermittent grieving of not being able to create children via intercourse, and the sadness over the possibility of not having biological children should IVF ultimately fail. The option of pregnancy termination for fetal anomaly obligates coping by learning all one can about the abnormality as preparation to decide whether to continue or end the pregnancy – onerous tasks to cope with – oscillating with grieving the loss of the healthy, wished-for baby who is gone.

Active coping can involve engaging with the threat to one's well-being provoked by the loss, through seeking out the help and guidance of family and friends, identifying the particular dangers one fears, and assessing how realistic those threats are. One's self-confidence may be a crucial determinant of whether that threat is viewed as manageable or overwhelming. Importantly it is not the external situation, but the perception and reaction to it, that is decisive to the contribution of resilience and the experienced outcome.

Active coping can paradoxically entail a purposeful and adaptive avoidance or even denial, sometimes called "repressive coping" [1]. When the grief is too much to bear, one can effectively cope by actively suppressing it. A very resourceful mother who was deeply grieving a newborn and then a miscarriage in her second pregnancy sometimes chose to shut down her feelings, putting them in a compartment she could visit at her own chosen time. This avoidant choice enabled her to take joy in effectively coping with parenting a healthy child from her third pregnancy, while reassuring herself that she has not forgotten her losses as there will be time later to return to her grief.

In the beginning, the compartment might be huge, the size of most of the house, with little room to retreat to get away from overwhelming grief. Over time and the diminishing grief, the compartment becomes much smaller. The couple can decide when and for how long it needs to be opened, marking the time period set aside for either partner to talk about the loss. This allows them the freedom of knowing there can be grief-free zones, when they can avoid being sad. This compartment technique can be readily taught as a safe way to get some respite from grieving, allowing the parents more control and self-regulation of their feelings.

Meditation and mindfulness can also be used as effective tools to actively cope by focusing on the immediate present, as a way to distract oneself from becoming absorbed by past painful memories or a dreaded empty future. Adaptive avoidance or denial in the service of resilience should be distinguished from passivity. While the former is an active, strategic choice to temporarily escape from unbearable feelings with the intention of engaging the adversity when one is fortified, passivity is usually a more global, maladaptive retreat without expectation of future confrontation or reconciliation, resulting in unresolved grief.

While defenses are often viewed in psychoanalytic terms as frequently maladaptive ways to pervasively avoid grappling with unconscious conflicts, they can also be understood as tactically effective forms of actively coping temporarily with intolerable situations. Women choosing to terminate a pregnancy due to fetal anomaly can anticipate the procedure with such dread that using

dissociation, mixed with denial to tune out her feelings, can be adaptive. Listening to soothing music or meditatively focusing on calming visual imagery can serve that purpose. Isolation or extreme detachment from one's feelings can be an effective means of coping with the overwhelmingly protracted suffering due to repeated reproductive losses, such as multiple miscarriages. This is evident when, instead of sadness, there is a deadened blandness in describing the losses as one blends into another. Finally, undoing can be understood as a means of reversing the loss through some process, often spiritual sanctification. Of course, for religious clients, this is a declaration of the permanence of the soul and not viewed as a psychological defense mechanism.

Active coping can be engaged often by simply asking about how day-to-day tasks are going, especially self-care behavior. This must not be done in the well-meaning, though insensitive manner, that some family and friends tell the bereaved that after a month or so it is time "to move on." Instead, it is asked, not dictated, with genuine interest and concern, empathically timed to sensing the mother's diminished grief and increased readiness to become involved in new activities and relationships, with the reassurance of returning to the memories of her child as needed. This again illustrates the shifting balance between coping and grieving going hand in hand.

Making Meaning of the Loss

While we are accustomed to calibrating the degree and nature of grieving with the extent of attachment to the deceased, we may neglect giving sufficient weight to the importance of making sense of this loss. Losses often leave a bevy of "shattered assumptions" [9] in their wake. The world can no longer be viewed as the benign, safe, predictable and just place it once was. This is especially so with reproductive losses, which are usually so shockingly unexpected, violating the fundamental belief in the cycle of life, where offspring are expected to bury their parents and not the other way around. Because so much of a couple's life usually becomes intertwined with their children, it is understandable to lose one's purpose and meaning in life when one's baby dies. While the search for meaning can be a solitary journey, more often it is an interpersonal enterprise, embedded in different cultural contexts [10]. This may explain the frequency of accessing support groups as a place not only to express grief, but to offer different reflections and the feedback they elicit. Acquiring a sense of coherence and meaning has been associated with a reduction in intensity of grief [11] and post-traumatic stress symptoms [12] after a perinatal loss. Rituals can have a special value in linking a baby with whom one has few, if any, memories into a symbolic matrix providing meaning to that life in the active participation and timelessness of the ritual [13].

It is difficult to imagine a profound search for meaning which does not address "why," Why did this happen to me? Why did this happen to my baby? Of course, it usually is extremely helpful to have medical questions answered, in order to make sense of what happened physically, as well as to ease the very common attribution by the mother of self-blame. Rarely is the asking of "why" not directed to God and religion as well. There is a wide spectrum of responses to this question, some more reinforcing of resilience and others not. Here are some brief anecdotes to illustrate that variability.

A very devout Catholic woman deeply grieves the death of her son several days after birth due to a rare metabolic disorder. She feels relieved knowing her son is in heaven, healed and whole, which he couldn't be in this world. She never questions the will of God, comforted by knowing there is a reason for his death, even if it's beyond her ken. No search for meaning is taken on or needed as her view of the world and her place in it has not changed.

A moderately religious Protestant woman (more of a believer in God than a church goer) learns that her twentieth week gestation baby dies in utero. She had learned about 8 weeks earlier that this baby had Down's Syndrome. After working through the grief of her expected healthy child, she excitedly threw herself into learning what she could about parenting a child with disabilities. She felt totally betrayed by God upon learning of his demise. After losing a prior child at 2 years old to serious cardiac problems, she can't fathom why she has to suffer so much at the hands of what she experiences as God's punishments. She considers leaving her congregation, but does not, pleased to hear that her pastor warmly supports her having any and all feelings, including rage, at God. She does talk to Him, though they are not on good terms yet.

A 40-year-old woman with a long history of infertility and unsuccessful IVF gives up her plans of trying to have a baby. Within a year, she unexpectedly becomes pregnant. At first, she is furious over being pregnant after so much loss and finally getting to the point of stopping trying. Without explanation, the baby dies in utero at 30 weeks. She is bitter beyond words. She can't fathom how God would let this happen after all she had been through, especially having forsaken plans to become pregnant. She

avows that she will never walk inside a church again or speak to a clergyman. It is extremely difficult for her to discuss her anger, even though it has pervaded her social and family relationships, formerly warm, now marked by irritability and resentment.

These three cases illustrate the range of different religious and spiritual responses in the search for meaning. For the woman who unquestioningly accepts the loss as God's will, her faith remains steadfast, serving as a very powerful source of resilience, which may not diminish grief but buttresses, rather than disrupts her values and order in life. At the other end of the spectrum is a woman who has a total eradication of faith and whatever comfort she might have derived from God, closing the door to any reconciliation and experiencing a pervasive bitterness and belligerence, which increases her distress and jeopardizes her social support system. In between these endpoints is a woman who is struggling in her relationship with God, hoping to find some explanation for why this has happened to her. The pastor wisely encourages her to share her grief – both over the loss of her baby and the loss of her relationship with God – with Him, rather than dogmatically demanding an acceptance she would not be able to muster, leaving her abandoned again. For the last two women, a new understanding of God might need to be forged, one in which good fortune or tragedy is not a reward or punishment for one's behavior or an expression of God's inscrutable will. For a more in-depth discussion on spirituality in fertility counseling, please see Chapter 8.

A client's search for meaning can be facilitated, first, by not getting in the way. It certainly isn't our job to impose or suggest or reconcile an answer to the frequent contradictions and conflicts between the tragedy that brought them to this crisis and the values they hold. We can, however, normalize how common, often necessary and worthy this searching is, which is in stark contrast to the frequent admonitions by family and friends to stop "obsessing" and not to keep going over something that has no answer. Taking a genuine interest in their searching, despite its inevitable blind alleys and getting lost along the way, dignifies a basic human trait of trying to make sense of one of the worst tragedies imaginable.

Continuing the Bond

So much of reproductive loss entails a prospective loss of that child as a person in the future and what the parenting relationship would be like. The inability to get to know that child and the cutting short of an actual parenting relationship makes reproductive loss such an empty, profound and pervasive death – a passing life with so few memories upon which to grieve and a totally blank future upon who would be loved. Many parents may ease these unbearable losses by experiencing an ongoing connection with their child. Although there are not quantitative studies that demonstrate such a continued bond supports resilience, the qualitative literature and clinical experience bolster this claim.

Rituals can play a crucial role by celebrating a child's entrance into the world and grieving the loss of life, as both provide the rudiments of that child's identity, enhancing the ability for him or her to be remembered. The child's emotional embodiment within the family can be achieved through a visible active presence in rituals and symbols, holding a place in the family and sharing lifelong impressions, as few as they may be [14]. On a more spiritual plane, the ongoing bond with one's child is reinforced by a religious community and beliefs sustaining such parental connections beyond death [15]. Several examples will illustrate the range of ways parents maintain a more permanent bond with their child.

One deeply religious evangelical mother took great comfort visiting her daughter at the cemetery. The close physical proximity to her grave resulted in her often feeling her spiritual presence. Sometimes, when the wind whistles through nearby trees, she thought she could hear her daughter calling to her and she could respond in kind. Each birthday she could celebrate by her grave, participating in her maturing though separated from her daughter who is in heaven.

A father excitedly brought in and showed me a copy of the memorial service they just had for his son. The couple, not being religious, took quotes and favorite poems to represent and remember what he meant to them. He delighted in the timeless form of a pinwheel as a symbolic expression of the anticipated endless nature of his love for him.

Paradoxically, in the midst of the parents' acute grief over their baby who just died, there may be an expression of delight to see for the first time their beautiful child, the family resemblance, and the details of her body. Just as with healthy babies, this more complicated bonding at birth with the deceased child establishes the connection between the much loved but unseen prenatal baby and the postpartum actual child. Memorabilia from birth, such as foot and hand prints and first photos may be too painful to view initially as objects documenting what was lost, yet over time may become more positive reminders of the continuation of

that relationship. This may take a literal form, as in the first anecdote where the mother experiences at the gravesite the actual presence and connection with her baby, or it may assume a more symbolic, often secular tie, as in the second anecdote. It should be the parents' choice how to embody that connection (or not) and the therapist's role to bear witness to that expression, not judging whether it is real or not but supporting the meaningfulness of that bond to them. By gently encouraging but not pressuring the bereaved mother to bring in such memorabilia, this facilitates the baby taking on a social existence which is recognized by others beyond the immediate family. Birthdays are often celebrated as markers for the fantasized developing child and ongoing parenting relationship, or experienced as opportunities for there to be actual contact with the child via dreams, sensory connection of some kind, etc.

Continuing the bond may be more challenging for earlier reproductive losses, such as miscarriages and ectopic pregnancies, for infertility and the more stigmatized losses such as elective abortion, pregnancy termination for fetal anomaly and relinquishing a child for adoption. Personhood of the baby may not have been established, a prerequisite to bonding, or the mother may have internalized societal shame and humiliation judging her as not being worthy of having such a connection due to having "chosen" this loss. This ignores the dire circumstances that usually precede that action. Even when infertility results in no actual baby to grieve, disappointment and a sense of failure may eventually be resurrected as prospective parental pride for how hard they tried, allowing the parents to honor and grieve the fantasized wished-for son or daughter. All parents should be entitled to remember and sustain (or not) their relationship with their deceased or absent baby whatever the situation. It is the therapist's responsibility to honor parental defining of that relationship, not to mandate or judge it, recognizing that maintaining a tie may represent in many instances not unresolved grief but the best way to affirm a crucial parental identity, facilitating a richer, albeit at times sadder life.

Secure Attachments

The capacity to sustain secure attachments can promote resilience in multiple ways. It is a biopsychosocial achievement advancing overall well-being. Biologically, secure attachments have been associated with lower stress and cortisol levels, improved self-regulation, better integration of brain hemispheres (through the corpus callosum) and less anxiety [3]. Psychologically, the securely attached child develops a working model of the world in which s/he is effective and competent, promoting self-esteem. Socially, secure attachment provides a template for interpersonal ties. Establishing a dependable sense of trust and safety in early parental relationships can facilitate intimacy in other close ties, while tolerating separation through an internalization of security when the attachment figure is physically unavailable.

These attributes of secure attachment can foster resilience by addressing the challenges of coping with reproductive loss. A strong social support system, within the marriage as well as with family and friends, is a key predictor of a more resilient and benign response to reproductive loss [16]. Secure attachment directly strengthens those social ties and support network as well as increases frustration tolerance when friends and family inevitably disappoint expectations, ensuring less disruption of those relationships. Improved self-regulation can result in greater mastery of strong feelings which enables a fuller expression of grief, thereby reducing the likelihood of being overwhelmed by such feelings leading to trauma. Finally, a stable sense of self-worth can moderate and make more manageable the virtually universal expression of maternal self-blame after reproductive loss.

Insecure attachments predicated on insensitive, neglectful or abusive parenting are not easily undone. However, when a therapist takes an active, empathic and psychologically attuned stance, building up a sense of trust and reliability can gradually enable the bereaved to accrue sufficient benefits of a secure attachment. The continuity and regularity of therapy hours becomes an arena for gradually establishing a new, more secure attachment. Over time, this may generalize to other relationships, improving marital ties and fostering a richer system of social support. The more deeply entrenched the attachment system of the bereaved is in avoidant and anxious modes, the longer it will take for this component of resilience to be realized. Many clients with these insecure attachments often do not come in with grief being their presenting problem, complaining instead about how hurtful and unhelpful one's partner, friends or family have been to them. Their painfully disappointing social ties in the past must be given a voice before they can take some responsibility for their current genesis, making it possible to better empathize with others through learning their impact on them. It may take much time for a more positively stable attachment to be consolidated, during

which time their reproductive losses begin to take center stage.

Positive Emotions in Life

Maintaining one's optimism and positive spirit in the midst of grieving a tragic loss can be one definition of resilience. Positive affect can buffer stressors, with an appreciation of one's strengths and accomplishments bolstering one's self-esteem, leading to a sense of confidence in being able to master adversity [1,3]. When tragedy strikes, it is common to bewail one's fate, as if one has been singled out for punishment. Sustaining positive feelings often engenders the opposite response, that of gratitude and appreciation of what good there is in one's life.

While often believed to be primarily inherited, in fact positive emotions are more associated with daily life experiences and person-specific environment fit [3]. Thus, interventions may be able to impact the expression of positive feelings. Perhaps the most comprehensive and evidence-based approach to improve self-worth and counter depression, by transforming negative attitudes to more positive emotions and happiness, is the Positive Psychology movement pioneered by Martin Seligman and colleagues [17]. Interventions demonstrating sustained positive benefits in mood and happiness include documenting and appreciating positive events in one's life on a daily basis, journaling one's accomplishments as well as applying one's strengths in a new way, and expressing gratitude to someone never thanked [18]. By quieting the ever-present barrage of anxious and guilty thinking, through focusing on the immediacy of the present and tuning out the past and future, meditation can be a productive method to reduce negativism in favor of a more compassionate stance to oneself.

Many of the tools discussed increase a sense of well-being by promoting a positive emotional reaction incompatible with troubling thoughts. Humor often takes some threatening or anxiety-provoking feeling or topic, such as death, sex or aggression, and through irony or mockery defang it by evoking laughter. You can't laugh and cry at the same time unless the joke is so funny it brings you to tears. Humor not only defuses the original anxiety, but offers at least momentary relief from suffering by looking at it from a distance, enabling a more playful perspective to the world in general. It is very encouraging when a couple in the midst of grief over multiple miscarriages can joke about the unusual name given to their baby, which was based on the city where the pregnancy was conceived. There is a place for the therapist to join in on a joke given by the couple, or even introduce humor on one's own, so long as there is ample evidence based on accurate empathy that a lightening of the mood is wanted by them. In the context of seemingly unremitting sorrow, humor can say it doesn't always have to be like this, pleasure in life will not be gone forever. For those whose grief abates sooner than expected, it can be very comforting to be reassured about this being normal and they need not feel guilty as they begin to feel happier again.

Post-traumatic Growth

The prior components reference what is likely to soften the loss initially, while post-traumatic (or post-loss) growth indexes positive outcomes that flow from the loss experience. The same factor (such as close marital ties) may both reduce loss-related stress as one goes through bereavement and be augmented (or not) as a result of the loss. In this section, we will consider only post-loss benefits after the death. The research on post-loss growth following infertility is meager and inconclusive, while the larger literature on post-loss growth following reproductive loss is quite similar to the post-traumatic growth studies of other losses. For that reason and for the sake of simplicity I will combine reproductive with other loss studies.

Post-loss growth is often overlooked in examining reactions to loss because studies are often designed to discover liabilities rather than assets. There is also the common, though inaccurate, belief that significant distress cannot co-exist with hard-fought victories following a terrible loss. There is usually tremendous disappointment when a woman loses a term birth, after experiencing many miscarriages. Despite her sadness and grief, that woman can feel profound pride in finally becoming a mother, transforming her identity in the process.

Some of the primary areas of growth following a major loss are developing greater closeness with others (especially one's partner), an increased capacity to cope with adversity, enhanced religious faith and spirituality, a greater appreciation of life, and a newfound altruism designed to prevent or soften the blow of this loss happening to others [2,19]. These benefits representing post-loss growth are the "flip sides" of attributes that portend and often embody a poorer outcome. Bereaved parents often become substantially closer as a couple, having survived this together versus the estrangement that precedes and follows such a loss. While many women feel intense vulnerability and would not risk another

pregnancy loss, believing that would destroy them, others feel having endured this, they could take anything life throws at them. Sometimes the same woman can feel both at different times. To comprehend two of life's most inscrutable challenges – that of birth and death – colliding together, a new and deeper understanding of God may emerge. Or a deep disillusionment due to such a tragic outcome may lead one's previously solid religious commitments to unravel. Similarly, the precariousness of life learned after such a loss may lead to a fuller appreciation of life, resulting in a more intense engagement with the world and all that is in it. Or resulting bitterness may provoke a withdrawal from others.

A few examples of post-loss growth in action might be useful. A couple dealing with almost a decade of infertility and unsuccessful treatments must face some difficult decisions of what to do next. The husband wants to continue and his wife hopes they adopt. Through sharing their feelings, she deeply appreciates his ability to empathize with her suffering due to painful and humiliating medical treatment, and she understands in a more complete way how important it is for him to parent a biological child, having lost his father at five due to cancer. They compromise and agree to one last IVF attempt and if not successful to move towards adoption.

An obstetrician loses her own twins at birth, blaming herself mercilessly while rationally knowing she had nothing to do with it. Her husband and parents worry about her somber mood, her anxiety and her loss of all the things that give her pleasure, except with her own two young children with whom she is still her old self. Before her losses, she was thinking of cutting back on her job, not finding the work as meaningful as it used to be. Her family hoped she would follow through with that and allow herself more time to relax. After returning to work, she felt a new thrill in delivering babies that she hadn't felt since residency. Each new birth, each new life became a miracle for her. She continues to work full-time and her family backs off, seeing her earlier symptoms considerably lessen as a newfound happiness appears.

Putting It All Together

For explanatory purposes, the components of resilience were distinguished and discussed separately to more precisely describe the impact of each. In the actual world, they form a mosaic, a unique patterning of the resources a couple or individual has, to meet the challenge of reproductive loss. It would take too long to catalogue all the possible combinations of sources of resilience, but in this section, I will give a sample of the more common clusters.

A model of hardiness has been applied to perinatal bereavement, defining the key ingredients as having a sense of personal control, an active orientation and making sense of the situation [20]. This appears to be an abbreviated version of my model. How important each factor is will determine what predominates in post-loss growth (e.g., whether hardiness is more behaviorally expressed through active orientation, affectively driven by taking control or having positive emotions, or more cognitively derived by a search for meaning).

Some ingredients of resilience naturally cluster together because they may be subsumed under a common categorization. For example, active coping, positive emotions and post-traumatic growth all typically involve a behavioral orientation which propels change post-loss into future maturation or self-actualization. A more social orientation to resilience might be rooted in a healthy foundation of empathic relatedness embodied in a secure attachment. The world becomes coherent when an attachment figure instils dependability in the social sphere, which may enhance one's sense of meaning in life in the larger world. Being able to continue one's bond with the deceased baby may be predicated both on the need to find meaning in such a tragic and unbearable situation and the stability of secure attachments facilitating connectedness which spans the division between the living and the dead.

Finally, a brief clinical example might illustrate how these factors can function together. A couple in their early thirties receive the terrible news that their baby has Trisomy 18 (an often-fatal disorder where there are usually severe handicaps). After educating themselves about the likely devastating impact of this condition on their baby, and the profound effects this would have on their family, they quickly decide to terminate the pregnancy (applying active coping). With limited grief, they felt grateful they had this option (positive emotions including gratitude). Before the termination, she unexpectedly delivers and having seen the baby who survived two minutes they decide to change course (taking control in positive emotions), naming the baby and incorporating her into their family (making meaning of the loss and continuing the bond). Their ability to integrate their initial intense disappointment with the pleasure of having an actual baby they got to see, speaks to their capacity to manage ambivalence – that is maintaining stable ties to others despite inevitable mixed feelings (secure attachment). They talk to their older kids frequently about their deceased sister and get themselves matching tattoos with her name on their arm (continuing bonds). Every year on the anniversary of her birth/death they hold a fund-raiser in her honor to benefit research on Trisomy-18, using their altruism to make sure that something tangibly positive would come from this loss (continuing bonds, post-loss growth and making meaning).

Some Concluding Clinical Thoughts

The therapist or counselor must resist the temptation to try to apply these elements of resilience in a manualized model of effective healing. As already discussed, there is too much variability among individuals to apply a specific combination of factors for all. Ultimately, it is the troubles, conflicts, and maladaptive coping with which the therapist must empathically understand, no matter what is one's theoretical approach. Hopefully, these components will help broaden and even challenge one's usual emphasis on disturbed outcomes. The grief-seeking therapist may regard a discussion of coping as defensive and less relevant, although when coping is effective it may be a mainstay of resilience. On the other hand, a therapist proposing active denial in the midst of someone's intense grieving may be grossly insensitive to the client's need to grieve in the moment, rather than suppress that sadness as so many families and friends are wont to recommend. The need to make meaning of this tragedy is not idle speculation but, when sought, it may be a profound transformative activity to be respected, for it may alter one's goals, values and place in the world. Maintaining a meaningful and sometimes visceral continuation of the bond with one's baby is usually not a maladaptive failure "to get back to the real world" but a normal expression of the irrepressible motivation to parent, even beyond death. When cases get stuck, it can be helpful to have the concept of insecure attachment as a potential cause of the difficulty, taking in what the therapist has to offer. Maintaining positive emotions is such an important reminder that psychopathology should not have the final word in defining a client. Finally, post-loss growth emphasizes the potentially positive legacy of reproductive loss. Working with resilience clinically, if applied broadly, does not have to be only seen as separating the haves from the have-nots, but carefully identifying and nurturing the sources of strength in all our clients.

References

1. Bonanno GA. Loss, trauma and human resilience: have we underestimated the human capacity to thrive after extremely aversive events? *Psych Trauma: Theory Res Pract Policy* 2008;**8**:101–113.

2. Tedeschi RG, Calhoun LG. Beyond the concept of recovery: growth and the experience of loss. *Death Studies* 2007;**32**:27–39.

3. Rutten BP, Hammels C, Geschwind N, et al. Resilience in mental health: linking psychological and neurobiological perspectives. *Acta Psychiatrica Scandinavica* 2013;**128**:3–20.

4. Ridenour AF, Yorgason JB, Peterson B. The infertility resilience model: assessing individual, couple, and external predictive factors. *Contemp Fam Ther* 2009;**31**:34–51.

5. Price SK. Stepping back to gain perspective: pregnancy loss history, depression, and parenting capacity in the early childhood longitudinal study, birth cohort (ECLS-B). *Death Studies* 2008;**32**:97–122.

6. Diamond, Kezur D, Meyers M, et al. *Couple Therapy for Infertility*. New York, NY: Guilford Press, 1999.

7. Leon IG. Understanding and treating infertility: psychoanalytic considerations. *J Am Acad Psa Dynam Psycho* 2010;**38**:47–76.

8. Stroebe M, Schut H. The dual process model of coping with bereavement: a decade on. *Omega* 2010;**61**:273–289.

9. Janoff-Bulman R. *Shattered Assumptions: Toward a New Psychology of Trauma*. New York, NY: The Free Press, 1992.

10. Neimeyer R. Searching for the meaning of meaning: grief therapy and the process of reconstruction. *Death Studies* 2000;**24**:541–558.

11. Uren, Wastell C. Attachment and meaning-making in perinatal bereavement. *Death Studies* 2002;**26**:279–308.

12. Frosch DJ, Shakespeare-Finch J. Grief, traumatic stress, and posttraumatic growth in women who have experienced pregnancy loss. *Psychol Trauma: Theory Pract Policy* 2017;**9**:425–433.

13. Brin D. The use of rituals in grieving for a miscarriage or stillborn. *Women and Therapy* 2004;**27**:123–132.

14. Cote-Arsenault D. Weaving babies lost in pregnancy into the fabric of the family. *J Fam Nurs* 2003;**9**:23–37.

15. Klass D. *The Spiritual Lives of Bereaved Parents*. Philadelphia, MA: Brunner/Mazel, 1999.

16. Lasker J, Toedter L. Predicting outcomes after pregnancy loss: results from studies using the perinatal grief scale. *Ill Crisis Loss* 2000;**8**:350–372.

17. Seligman ME, Csikszentmihalyi M. Positive psychology: an introduction. *Amer Psychol* 2000;**55**:5–14.

18. Seligman ME, Steen TA, Park N, et al. Positive psychology progress: empirical validation of interventions. *Amer Psychol* 2005;**60**:410–421.

19. Lathrop A, Van deVusse L. Continuity and change in mothers' narratives of perinatal hospice. *J Perinat Neonat Nurs* 2011;**25**:21–31.

20. Lang A, Goulet C, Aita M, et al. Weathering the storm of perinatal bereavement via hardiness. *Death Studies* 2001;**25**:497–512.

Chapter 20

Reproductive Trauma and PTSD: On the Battlefield of Fertility Counseling

Janet Jaffe

Introduction

The alarm goes off; the coffee maker goes on. Whatever your morning routine, you expect today to be similar to yesterday, and tomorrow to be very much like today. And while there may be differences in the details of each day, the routine will probably stay the same. Although we may complain about being stuck in a rut, these unconscious expectations bring great comfort in being able to predict what is coming next.

Trauma occurs when the ability to envisage our future and feel safe in the world is no longer possible. While trauma is often a one-time horrific occurrence – a car accident, a school shooting, an earthquake – it can also be chronic in nature. Indeed, like a soldier on the battlefield, it can be protracted and feel never-ending, leaving deep psychological wounds. Reproductive trauma can encompass both types of anguish: the frightening and painful loss of a miscarriage, with massive bleeding and the potential need for surgery, or the seemingly endless cycle of hope and despair during fertility treatments. Sadly for our patients, it is not uncommon to experience both infertility and pregnancy loss. Indeed, women who have suffered the dual experience of pregnancy loss and childlessness report the highest levels of distress [1]. This chapter not only explores the trauma that occurs in reproductive patients, but also how we, as fertility counselors, cope with being on the battlefield with them. Whether we are in the middle of our own reproductive journey or have experienced reproductive trauma in the past, the intense pain our patients feel has an impact on us. The consciousness of our own reactions is invaluable in nurturing therapeutic relationships and in helping our patients heal.

What Is Reproductive Trauma?

The Diagnostic and Statistical Manual of Mental Disorders (DSM-V) defines trauma in terms of post-traumatic stress disorder (PTSD) as the "exposure to actual or threatened death, serious injury or sexual violence" [2]. The distress caused by PTSD is considerable: flashbacks, depression, anxiety, sleep disturbance, irritability and social isolation are some of the common indications. In examining PTSD in reproductive patients, a triad of symptoms has been described: (a) persistent retriggering (i.e., seeing other pregnant women, a return to the doctor's office); (b) avoidant behavior (disengaging from friends, avoiding baby showers); (c) hyper-arousal (high states of anxiety, feeling unable to let down one's guard) [3].

The trauma that is typically associated with PTSD is caused by an *external* event, which rocks one's world. While many reproductive patients have features of PTSD, a broader definition of trauma more adequately captures their experience: an event, but likely more than one, which overwhelmingly shatters core beliefs and assumptions [4]. Thinking about trauma in this way, one can understand it coming from an *internal* source. One's sense of self in the context of today as well as into the future gets turned upside-down. It's as if a rug has been pulled out from underneath; everything that was once in place is suddenly flying up in the air, and the ability to predict where it will land is impossible. Infertility and pregnancy loss cause the disintegration, not just of a would-be pregnancy, but also of one's entire inner narrative of how the world is and how the world should be. Without the ability to foresee how one's hopes and dreams of creating a family will come to pass, patients are left with questions about their sense of self, their purpose, relationships and the very meaning of life: clearly not minor concerns.

To better understand reproductive trauma, it can help to examine the significance of one's underlying, usually unconscious, reproductive story and one's set of core beliefs [5,6]. Reproductive stories begin in childhood, as we ourselves are parented. We observe our caregivers and integrate ideas about what it means to be part of a family, and what it might be like to be an adult and possibly have a family of our own someday. Everyone has a reproductive story, whether we consciously want children or not. This early narrative and the assumptions we believe will unfold are deep in our core and form the foundation of our sense of self. It is when the story goes off course, when we can't have children how or when we want to, that we feel the profound sense of trauma and loss.

Core Beliefs: About Pregnancy, about Ourselves

Everyone Can Get Pregnant

What are some of the common core beliefs of pregnancy? One of the most widespread assumptions: everyone can do it. Reproduction and the biological imperative of pro-creation are fundamental convictions across cultures. There is an underlying belief that after years of trying *not* to conceive, conception will happen as soon as one stops birth control. This is important for fertility counselors to take note of because even after the very first month of trying without success, many clients feel traumatized. A shadow of a doubt may now hover over their inner narrative of potency. This intensifies with each subsequent month, until it is no longer a shadow that hangs overhead, but a dark cloud of depression, anxiety and sense of doom. By the time they arrive at a clinic or fertility counselor's office, after months and months of trying, they are deep within an emotional storm.

I Am Strong and in Control

Feeling healthy, strong and in control, how could a pregnancy not easily occur? With fertility issues or pregnancy loss, the betrayal of one's body, the fact that it is not doing what it is meant to do, can be devastating. While a miscarriage, for example, can happen if there is a genetic flaw in the gametes, from a psychological perspective fertility patients jump to the conclusion that they are damaged goods. The part becomes the whole: it is not a cell that has caused a loss, but rather one's entirety that is to blame. The disintegration of belief in one's body adds to the trauma. An otherwise healthy person seeking out fertility treatment may feel dehumanized by becoming a patient. Removing one's clothing to don a flimsy medical gown and exposing one's most private parts, often to a stranger, is traumatizing to us all.

Added to self-blame is the assumption that fertility issues are caused by stress. The unwanted advice administered by well-meaning family or friends to *just relax* adds insult to

injury, and reinforces the belief that stress causes fertility problems. Thus, patients erroneously believe they are causing their own infertility and have control of its outcome. Early explanations of reproductive problems were based on psychogenic theory: the belief was that reproductive difficulties were caused by a woman's ambivalence about becoming a mother because of unresolved emotional issues with her own mother [7]. Medical advances in reproductive medicine have generally discredited psychogenic theory, however, in a recent survey, about 30% of patients believed that emotional stress caused infertility and miscarriage. Nearly 70% of participants believed that stress would negatively impact fertility treatment. A surprisingly low percentage (less than 25%) felt stress had no impact on fertility at all, suggesting that patients assume they are to blame [8]. There is no doubt that fertility problems and pregnancy loss *cause* stress but is the opposite true? As will be discussed in the *Case Studies* volume associated with this chapter, perhaps the key is helping people debunk this myth to reduce their stress and help them feel in control again.

Good Things Happen to Good People

Deeply embedded in all of us is the sense of right and wrong; whatever one's religious or spiritual convictions, these belief systems get challenged when fertility and pregnancy loss occur. The struggle between belief and doubt may rock one's basic foundations: good happens to the righteous while bad things happen to the immoral. Perhaps one person will reconcile this by becoming more pious: *I'm not being devout enough,* while another may have faith that *God has a plan for me; I am being tested.* Additionally challenging is how a person resolves the use of reproductive medicine with one's religious practice. Important for the fertility counselor is to understand what role religion plays in each client's inner world, and how it may help or hinder in managing a crisis [9].

Whatever one's religion or belief system, the idea that good things happen to good people is deeply rooted in us all (think about Santa Claus rewarding good behavior). The flip side, if something isn't going right, there has to be a reason for it; the negative outcome must be warranted. The emotional response to how clients make meaning out of the "bad" things is at the crux of our work. As fertility counselors, we hear the self-blame or blame of one's partner all the time: *What did I do to deserve this? Does he work out too much (or not enough)? Did she party too much in college? Was it the diet soda I drank?* Rationally we can reassure our clients that they have done nothing wrong; there is no scorecard keeping a tally of our hypothetical infractions.

Finding something or someone to blame, a reason for fertility issues or a miscarriage, might paradoxically feel comforting rather than having no explanation at all.

Blame can echo loudly, particularly if there has been a history of trauma. A victim of sexual abuse, a survivor of an unstable family of origin, drug abuse or sexual promiscuity can all contribute to the self-narrative that one is undeserving to have a child. Medical examinations for fertility treatment can trigger PTSD in abuse victims. One fertility specialist, in his initial meeting with a patient, declared that *he* could get her pregnant. While she understood he meant he could help, it sparked flashbacks and panic about a rape she experienced in college.

Especially painful is the potential for self-reproach around a previously unwanted pregnancy, whether the baby was relinquished for adoption, or the pregnancy was terminated with an induced abortion. Feelings that may have been resolved at the time can re-emerge, bringing forth doubts about prior decisions. While having an abortion does not generally increase fertility problems or pregnancy complications [10], patients may feel that they have lost their only chance at becoming a parent, or that they are being punished for earlier choices.

Life Is Fair

An assumption that life is fair, in spite of all the inequities in our society and in the world at large, is linked with the notion that "you get what you deserve." It is a harsh and simplistic way of looking at others, without taking into account the entirety of a situation. Blaming the victim, whether it is in the case of rape, poverty, race or ethnicity, is undeniably a part of our culture. It's important to note that while reproductive trauma and loss knows no boundaries, treatment is generally available only to a privileged group. Those with means and/or good health insurance are able to seek medical attention when faced with reproductive trauma [11].

Blaming the victim is often directed outward. The belief that *it can't happen to me because I am not like them* is a way of distancing oneself from trauma. When it comes to pregnancy, however, all bets are off. Here again self-blame can be harshly punitive. The psychological loss of not being able to believe in the fairness of life creates additional damage to the self.

I Can Achieve What I Set Out to Do if I Just Work Hard Enough

Many of us believe at some core unconscious level, that if we strive for a reasonable goal, we'll be able to attain it.

The old proverb: *If at first you don't succeed, try, try again* implies that if you keep at it, all will turn out well. If only this were true in our reproductive lives.

Our possible selves – defined as what we would like to become (the hoped-for-self), or what we are afraid of becoming (the feared-self) – is an essential link between our sense of self and motivation [12]. It can be fascinating to hear children describe what they want to be when they grow up; the number of options is seemingly endless. If a child wants to be a baseball star, he/she/they may beg to play T-Ball. Possible selves are dynamic in nature, which change and grow over time. The young athlete may move on to new interests, as what is attainable gets redefined; likewise, multiple possible selves (*I want to play the cello* **and** *study biology*) can exist simultaneously.

The possible-self-as-parent is deeply rooted in our core. In fact, parenthood has been rated as one of the most important facets of future possible selves [13]. Embedded in one's reproductive story, as possible-self-as-parent, is the assumption that one will become pregnant easily and have a healthy child. The feared version might worry about infertility, miscarriage or a child with disabilities. Parenthood, unlike other hoped for futures, is not something that one can study more to pass an exam, practice more to make the team, concentrate on more to accomplish one's goal. In other words, it is not something one can attain by working harder at it. Trauma occurs when the feared possible self becomes a reality, but also because the core belief that working hard guarantees success is shattered.

I'm on Par with My Peers

A common hoped-for wish in the reproductive story is: *my friends and I will all have babies at the same time!* It can feel like an additional trauma and loss when fertility patients are left behind in the timeline of having children. One client portrayed it as waiting for the invitation to come; all dressed up but nowhere to go. Another described the anxiety she had every time she opened social media, expecting yet another announcement showing off yet another baby bump.

The narcissistic blow in feeling out of the loop can be profound. Rather than having a supportive network, reproductive clients find themselves isolated and alone. Parents-to-be are in limbo: as soon as they start trying to have a baby, their psychological state changes. They become *psychological parents* way before they are parents in a physical sense. It is normal for both men and women to have fantasies about the perfect child they will produce;

additionally, assumptions about their new role as parents and the subsequent changes in their relationships with family and friends feel palpable. With reproductive trauma, however, this normal developmental shift is just out of reach. Self-worth plummets, and with it the loss of status that having a child can bring. One client remarked: *I may be 34 years old but I still feel like I'm sitting at the kid's table.* Another wondered about going to baby showers: *Is there still space for me?* The injury to the self, the impact on relationships and feeling as if the ground is no longer solid adds to the chronic sense of trauma.

Getting Off the Battlefield

As fertility counselors, not only do we need to recognize the trauma and multiple losses that our clients experience, we need to help them process it and heal. While there are numerous strategies to doing therapy, coming from an understanding of a patient's core belief system, and how it has failed, allows us a unique perspective into their experience. As will be demonstrated in the corresponding *Case Studies* chapter, careful listening to the narrative of their hopes, dreams and deep expectations of pregnancy and parenthood provides us with an opportunity to challenge some pre-conceived notions. Additionally, we can help them rewrite their story to create new and different outcomes.

Using a combination of concepts from cognitive-behavioral and narrative therapies, in addition to enabling clients to process grief and loss, is an effective way to treat reproductive patients. Keep in mind the disequilibrium they feel: their core beliefs have been shattered (the rug pulled out), they are frightened (everything is flying in the air) and their coping mechanisms have been overwhelmed (when and where is everything going to land?).

Grief Work

It goes without saying that fertility counselors need to listen to their client's story. What are the crises that are devastating them right now? Why are they seeking support at this time? Have they just had disturbing news from their reproductive endocrinologist? Are they at a point where their family building options are diminishing? In the initial sessions, it is likely that clients will have an outpouring of grief. The loss of a child or the loss of the possibility of having a child can shake the very foundations of one's sense of self. The degree to which the current situation misaligns with their assumptions and original story, and the measure to which they have

attached to their baby or dreams of their baby, is comparable to the intensity of the grief.

Reproductive losses are complicated to grieve. At a time when parents anticipate the creation of a new life, they instead experience a death: of an actual baby (as in a miscarriage or stillbirth) or an imagined one (as in a failed IVF cycle). Regardless of the loss, there are few if any rituals to help process pregnancy demise. In fact, parents are often given the advice to *move on* or *don't dwell on it.* This well-meaning effort to comfort misses the mark and often yields the opposite effect. Rather than help, it minimizes and invalidates the deep emotions that parents are feeling [14]. As one client put it: *It makes me feel dismissed and a little crazy; like I'm not supposed to have the feelings I am having! I can't even get grieving right!* Having her emotional state undermined further reduced her self-esteem, already diminished by her loss.

As therapists, we should never assume that all losses are equal; for example, one woman may feel relief knowing she needs an egg donor (*I can take some action and move forward*), while another may be panic-stricken (*Will this really be my baby?*). Similarly, each person will have a unique reaction and coping style to loss. Commonly held gender differences suggest that women process grief through tears and a need to talk, while men focus on their thoughts, take action and avoid emotional displays. Stroebe and Schut, while recognizing gender differences, proposed a dual-process model in understanding how people cope with grief [15]. They postulated that everyone balances degrees of loss-orientation (rumination on the loss, expression of feelings) and loss-restoration (acceptance, rebuilding one's life). For reproductive patients there is a seesaw-like balance between their current state of loss, while simultaneously looking toward the future. The fluctuation of their affect makes clear the need for reproductive counselors to be present and hear their story, without judgment or advice, and to remind patients that there is no one "right way" to grieve.

Cognitive–Behavioral Therapy

Cognitive–behavioral therapy (CBT) is a well-established therapeutic approach for treating depression and anxiety. In general, CBT combines an examination of peoples' adverse thoughts, core beliefs and assumptions, and challenges patients to approach adversity and trauma from a different framework. Not only are ideas about one's self questioned, but strategies to alter behavior are put into action. Applying CBT tactics to reproductive traumas, with special attention to the therapeutic dyad, can help patients manage their affect, reframe negative beliefs about themselves and engage in adaptive behavior [16].

As previously discussed, core beliefs related to pregnancy and parenthood are a central component in defining one's adult self. When the transition to parenthood meets with hardship and one's reproductive story is thrown off track, CBT can be applied to understand the activation of a generalized negative self-assessment. The particular loss of a pregnancy or a would-be pregnancy (based in physiology) develops into a global pessimistic appraisal of one's self (a psychological function) with thoughts such as: *I am not worthy; I can't do anything right.* There is a difference in acknowledging knowing something is wrong with a body part versus believing that they are a complete failure. Cognitive restructuring, a feature of CBT, challenges negative thought patterns in order to modify them. It can be thought of as an untangling of the knotty thoughts people hold on to when trying to make sense out of painful, traumatic situations.

When assumptions are shattered, basic trust in the world is ruptured. Working with reproductive clients on cognitive restructuring, it is necessary to consider the particular assumptions about pregnancy and parenting that have been destroyed. For example, if a woman thinks she has done something to cause or deserve a pregnancy loss, the therapist can explore her beliefs, and guide her in a gentle and thoughtful way to see faults in her logic. The effort here is to have the client become less self-critical and judgmental by replacing negative appraisals with different ways of thinking about the loss. The attempt is to replace self-loathing with self-loving.

One adaptive approach is to find benefit in the traumatic experience. The reproductive trauma can actually be a catalyst for new goals. Posttraumatic growth will be discussed later in the chapter, but cognitive reframing can promote positive experiences that would not have otherwise occurred. Adoptive parents, for example, often state how fortunate they feel: *We would never have known this child if not for our struggles with infertility.* This kind of restructuring can reassert control and change previous held assumptions about the way things should be.

Narrative Therapy

Narrative therapy is based on the idea that people define themselves and make meaning of their life through their life stories. Narrative identity provides an opportunity for people to make sense of their past (the story of how they arrived and where they are now) and their future (the story of where they hope to be) [17]. A significant chapter

of one's narrative identity involves parenthood, one's parental identity and reproductive story [5,6]. Of particular interest to fertility counselors is what happens when the lived experience of trauma contradicts with the patient's reproductive story.

Research on narrative therapy suggests a two-step process to resolve adverse life experiences: (1) examination of the negative event in depth; and (2) formulation of a new, alternative story [17]. In psychotherapy, fertility counselors are in the position to both hear the story and encourage clients to re-story their lives. In other words, help patients process their grief and loss, examine the assumptions that have fueled their story and have created false narratives, and rewrite the story in a way that is meaningful and constructive.

Isolation is a common occurrence for reproductive patients. So often no one outside of the medical staff or a few select people even knows what is going on. Here's a trauma, possibly the biggest event that is happening in a person's life, and the need to keep it secret prevails. Being able to tell one's story, however, to the right people and as often as necessary, reduces shame and isolation. Psychotherapy is a natural arena for the recounting of these painful stories, and studies suggest that the telling of them leads to psychological growth [17]. A note here: sometimes clients are hesitant to bring up the darkest parts of their story; the parts that they ruminate on in the middle of the night and that bring the most shame or fear. These are the details that need to be befriended and not reviled. Asking about details, what hurt physically, what they saw, what they tried to do but couldn't – and listening without judgment is what we do. Our acceptance of these dark stories allows for healing.

In working with clients, it can be helpful for them to think of a story's structure: a beginning, middle and end. When our services are sought, patients are in the middle of their reproductive story, dealing with traumatic and emotionally fraught circumstances. The meaning of the reproductive trauma and loss, the significance of the attachment to their assumptions about pregnancy and parenting, and the overwhelming sense of helplessness patients feel, complicates their ability to regain their footing. It may feel to them that they will be stuck here – in the middle – forever. One of the intrinsic messages that narrative therapy conveys, however, is that stories are not static. They are part of a creative process that can be edited, revised and thus a variety of endings can be considered. As therapy progresses, one can observe a shift in the vulnerability and despair that patients initially express to a sense of control over their future. An exercise in "trying on" different endings to their story – whether it's doing another round of IVF, exploring adoption or considering remaining childfree – allows patients to see beyond their current trauma. It can help remind them that they have a choice in all this; they are in charge of the path they want to pursue.

Whatever the theoretical base of one's psychotherapy practice, the goal is the same: listening to the story, processing emotionally charged content, and guiding the client with support and compassion to a deeper understanding of the self. As will be discussed in the next section, when patients are able to resolve traumatic events into something positive, and make constructive meaning out of these events, their lives can grow in rich and unanticipated ways.

Post-traumatic Growth

Posttraumatic growth (PTG) is the ability to convert a traumatic experience into something constructive and meaningful. From adversity, it is possible to gain an increased appreciation for life, with gratitude for meaningful relationships and for one's own fortitude [18]. It is not unusual for priorities to change after a traumatic experience; things that might have been upsetting in the past now take a backburner to what is really important. A positive awakening can occur: people find themselves not taking life for granted as they discover joy and pleasure in daily living.

While painfully challenging one's fundamental assumptions, the experience of trauma – whether it's a single event or an ongoing chronic battle – can also be a time of enormous change and growth. It can serve as a catalyst for self-improvement and setting new goals. It's not as if the pain from the trauma and loss vanishes, but the attempts at restructuring one's fundamental assumptions lead to affective and psychological change. A study, which investigated PTG and pregnancy loss, measured the disruption to women's core beliefs. The findings suggested that the greatest PTG occurred in participant's appreciation of life, recognition of their personal strength, and their ability to have increased empathy for others [19].

Tedeschi and Calhoun discuss the importance of both the crafting of narratives as well as cognitive processing in the development of PTG. Highlighting the benefits of support groups, in particular a bereaved parents' group, they suggest that telling one's story of trauma to others provides a basis for validation, understanding and intimacy. It allows for the cognitive processing of one's traumatic experience to occur, along with the revising of assumptions [18]. Support for reproductive patients through individual or group therapy can help them change perspective on their negative self-evaluation and reconsider their life story from a different perspective. Finding purpose after reproductive trauma is key. Growth occurs by reforming a coherent and meaningful narrative that integrates and makes sense of one's loss [20].

From a clinical perspective, there are many ways in which reproductive patients leave the battlefield and heal from their wounds – whether they go on to have children or not. Clients have spoken about the growth in their sensitivity and empathy for others. One woman realized that she never really listened before: *I was always in a rush to get onto the next task without really taking the time to assess the present. Now I slow myself down and really focus on what's in front of me.* Other people have used their reproductive trauma to reassess their life: they may decide to change careers, go back to school, concentrate on their health, focus on what they enjoy. Many times, clients will start a session by saying: *I always wanted to . . .* and realize that they can. Likewise, PTG can be seen in patients who want to "give back." One couple made memory boxes to bring to the hospital where their daughter was stillborn. Another woman took to social media to educate the community as to what to say, and what not to say, when someone is struggling to conceive. My own story evolved from climbing out of the trenches of fertility treatment and pregnancy loss to become a psychologist, and devote my career to helping reproductive patients survive this battle. Without hesitancy, I can say it has proven to be both positive and meaningful for me!

The Counselor's Personal Battlefield: The Need for Self-Care

Not only are we fertility counselors, we are also human beings; thus, we too have reproductive stories that may have veered off course. Whether in the midst of a crisis or having long resolved it, the nature and course of our story has an impact on the clinical work we do. Self-awareness is key in this process: if the wound is fresh, or if we are in the middle of a traumatic experience, it may affect our objectivity. What is critical is focusing foremost on the needs of the patient, while at the same time taking care of our self. Using our own life experience in the service of the client is the goal; this can greatly enhance the therapeutic alliance and deepen the healing process.

Because fertility counselors have a reproductive story of their own, exposure to their patients' experiences of trauma and loss can be especially overwhelming. The nature of this work entails listening repeatedly to accounts of disappointment, in client's self-assessment and in their relationships, hearing descriptions of their psychological and physical pain, and reports of their sadness and loss. It is difficult, if not impossible, not to be affected when the client's world has come crushing down; it is that much more intense if the therapist can relate to it on a personal level. Having a shared experience may increase therapeutic understanding, but it may also tap into the therapist's grief and vulnerability. The impulse to do something to ease the client's pain is reflexive – just listening may not feel like enough. The helplessness that the fertility therapist feels echoes the state that the client is in.

Vicarious trauma is a term used to describe the effects that a client's distress has on the healthcare professional. It's as if some of the patient's traumatic experience has rubbed off. Hearing the details of an ectopic pregnancy, seeing photographs of a baby who was stillborn, listening to the anguish of a failed IVF cycle: these are the traumas that we, as fertility counselors, endure. The impact of these traumas can negatively transform the therapist, especially if they have experienced a similar reproductive event [21]. Another phenomenon that fertility therapists are exposed to is *compassion fatigue*. This refers to the cumulative effects of overexposure to clients' suffering. Therapists may feel worn out and drained, they may become irritable, depressed and be less available to process their clients' concerns. In essence, the definition of compassion fatigue is a therapist who has become tired of caring [22]. While compassion fatigue can occur in any helping profession,

the issues raised by reproductive clients can feel particularly draining.

Self-care is essential for the fertility counselor, especially if they are in the middle of their own fertility struggles or if they are pregnant (see also Chapter 24). It's particularly important for therapists to self-assess on a regular basis: *Do I feel more drained at the end of a day than usual? Am I burning out? Is a particular patient irritating me? Can I stay neutral?* Questions such as these can indicate therapeutic decisions. For example, perhaps it is too disturbing to work with a patient who is dealing with a pregnancy loss while the therapist is pregnant herself. Therapists' reactions – or countertransference – are a part of every clinical encounter and can be used constructively to enhance one's understanding of the client. It can also serve as a kind of alarm system: advising the therapist when to seek consultation or supervision on a case. Listening to one's own feelings is crucial in self-care. Table 20.1 compares compassion fatigue, vicarious trauma and countertransference; while there is overlap among these phenomena, it's important to understand how they differ, as each requires different forms of self-care.

In general, our own self-care requires finding a balance between work, play, exercise and rest. Knowing what is personally re-energizing – whether it's socializing with friends or family, taking a yoga class, getting outdoors or any other rejuvenating activity – makes a great difference in our attitude. Equally important is finding a balance in the actual workday itself. This may mean building in breaks during the day, or not scheduling back-to-back clients who are particularly challenging. Simple things that we might take for granted – like making sure to hydrate and eat – are critical to our well-being. Clinical supervision and peer support is also an essential

Table 20.1 Compassion fatigue, vicarious trauma and countertransference

Compassion fatigue	Vicarious trauma	Countertransference
Based on caring for those who are suffering	Based on developing trauma secondary to a client's trauma	Based on interaction between the client's world and the therapist's inner feelings
Cumulative experience of care-giving	Related to the client's traumatic experiences	Pervasive to all clients
General exhaustion; feeling burnt out	Reaction to a specific client's trauma	Challenging but not exhausting
Can interfere with clinical work	Can interfere with clinical work	Can be used as a tool to enhance clinical work
Self-care: Need to rejuvenate (yoga, meditation, exercise, be in nature, social support, supervision/consultation)	Self-Care: In addition to compassion fatigue suggestions, limit number of trauma clients	Self-care: Self-reflection to better understand clients; supervision; one's own psychotherapy

component of self-care. Being aware of our own inner struggles and taking care of our self can enable us to meet patients with clarity.

Summary

The analogy of being on a battlefield is apt for reproductive trauma. Unlike a soldier, however, who is trained to approach combat, reproductive patients are unprepared for the emotional distress caused by infertility and/or pregnancy loss. The basic, core assumptions about pregnancy and parenthood have been shattered. Getting off this particular battlefield is not easy – emotions may linger for longer than expected. Our role, as fertility counselors, is to help our clients rebuild their sense of self, reduce their shame and guilt and find routes to a meaningful future, whether they are able to go on to have children or not. Similarly, awareness of our own reproductive story, which may have brought us into this field, is always present and needs to be recognized in the work we do. The corresponding chapter in the *Case Studies* volume will weave together the theories discussed here with illustrations from clinical cases on how reproductive clients cope with and survive this trauma.

References

1. Schwerdtfeger KL, Shreffler KM. Trauma of pregnancy loss and infertility for mothers and involuntary childless women in the contemporary United States. *J Loss Trauma* 2009;**14** (3):211–227.

2. American Psychiatric Association. *Diagnostic and Statistical Manual of Mental Disorders*, 5th ed. Arlington, VA: American Psychiatric Association, 2013.

3. Bartlik B, Greene K, Graf M, Sharma G, Melnick H. Examining PTSD as a complication of infertility. *Medscape General Medicine* 1997 (online). Available from: www .medscape.com/viewarticle/719243 [last accessed June 16, 2022].

4. Cann A, Calhoun LG, Tedeschi RG, et al. The Core Beliefs Inventory: a brief measure of disruption in the assumptive world. *Anxiety Stress Coping* 2010;**23**(1):19–34.

5. Jaffe J, Diamond MO. *Reproductive Trauma: Psychotherapy with Infertility and Pregnancy Loss Clients*. Washington, DC: American Psychological Association, 2011.

6. Jaffe J. Reproductive trauma: psychotherapy for pregnancy loss and infertility clients from a reproductive story perspective. *Psychotherapy* 2017;**54**(4):380–385.

7. Leon IG. *When a Baby Dies*. New Haven, CT: Yale University Press, 1990.

8. Negris O, Lawson A, Brown D, et al. Emotional stress and reproduction: what do fertility patients believe? *J Assist Reprod Genet* 2021 (online). https://doi.org/10.1007/s10815-021-02079-3.

9. Dombo EI, Flood M. Spirituality in fertility counseling. In: Covington SN, Ed. *Fertility Counseling: Clinical Guide and Case Studies*. Cambridge: Cambridge University Press, 2015, 74–84.

10. American College of Obstetricians & Gynecologists. Are there any long-term health effects from having an abortion? *Patient FAQ Induced Abortion*. 2015. Available from: www.acog.org/womens-health/faqs/induced-abortion [last accessed June 16, 2022].

11. Owen CM, Goldstein EH, Clayton JA, Segars JH. Racial and ethnic health disparities in reproductive medicine: an evidence-based overview. *Semin Reprod Med* 2013;**31** (5):317–324.

12. Markus H, Nurius P. Possible selves. *Am Psychologist* 1986;**41**:954–969.

13. Hooker K, Fiese BH, Jenkins L, Morfei MZ, Schwagler J. Possible selves among parents of infants and preschoolers. *Develop Psychol* 1996;**32**:542–550.

14. Markin RD. An introduction to the special section of psychotherapy for pregnancy loss: review of issues, clinical applications and future research direction. *Psychotherapy* 2017;**54**(4):367–372.

15. Stroebe M, Schut H. The dual process model of coping with bereavement: rationale and description. *Death Studies* 1999;**23**:197–224.

16. Wenzel A. Cognitive behavioral therapy for pregnancy loss. *Psychotherapy* 2017;**54**(4):400–405.

17. McAdams DP, McLean KC. Narrative identity. *Curr Directions Psychological Sci* 2013;**22**(3):233–238.

18. Tedeschi RG, Calhoun LG. Posttraumatic growth: conceptual foundations and empirical evidence. *Psychol Inq* 2004;**15**(1):1–18.

19. Krosch DJ, Shakespeare-Finch J. Grief, traumatic stress, and posttraumatic growth in women who have experienced pregnancy loss. *Psychol Trauma: Theory Res Pract Policy* 2017;**9**(4):425–433.

20. Rosner M. Recovery from Traumatic Loss: A Study of Women Living Without Children after Infertility. Doctorate in Social Work (DSW) Dissertations. 2012. Available from: https://repository.upenn.edu/edisserta tions_sp2/20 [last accessed June 16, 2022].

21. Trippany RL, Kress VEW, Wilcoxon SA. What counselors should know when working with trauma survivors. *J Couns Dev* 2004;**82**:31–37.

22. Berzoff J, Kita E. Compassion fatigue and countertransference: two different concepts. *Clin Soc Work J* 2010;**38**:341–349.

Pregnancy Loss Counseling

Irving Leon

This chapter will guide therapists in dealing with the range of the most frequent reproductive losses, including miscarriage, ectopic pregnancy, stillbirth, infant death and pregnancy termination for fetal anomaly. Working with infertility will be considered only in the context of having additional reproductive losses. We will explore many of the common themes in dealing with these losses, while never losing sight of how individualized a loss is for each woman or man, each couple and each family. The reader is directed elsewhere for a more general description of the nature of and differentiation among the range of reproductive losses [1,2].

Cultural differences can have a profound effect on how these losses are experienced and grieved. Space constraints limit the thorough discussion that ethnic, religious gender and national differences deserve. These differences influence when a loss is defined as a baby or something else; how publicly or privately grieving is allowed expression; the stigmatizing or normalizing function of mental health intervention; feminine, masculine as well as LGBTQ models of grieving; and so forth, which significantly contribute to the emotional impact of these losses around the world. Practitioners who work with particular sub-groups are advised to become familiar with their different orientations to these losses. However, one should never assume an individual simply represents (i.e., caricatures) the norms of a larger group. It never hurts, and usually helps, when a clinician asks questions in an open, curious and respectful manner in order to better understand the impact of those cultural factors on those particular parents.

Before examining therapeutic interventions for reproductive loss, reviewing the unique features of this kind of loss is necessary [1,2]. These losses feel less real than the death of a person one has known in the "outside world." Grieving is more challenging without the rich store of memories upon which grief is based. Thus, while reproductive loss involves "prospective" grieving for the life and relationship projected into the future, other grieving is retrospective, based on painfully remembering the

interactions with and images of the lost loved one. Accustomed to only understanding retrospective grieving, well-intentioned family and friends frequently minimize these losses, telling the bereaved couple to "forget," "move on," and "just have another child." They do not realize that encouraging remembering these losses helps the bereaved to gradually return to embracing the living and future, and not remain "stuck" in the past. Because the unborn baby often represents the best parts of oneself, defying mortality by projecting oneself into a new future life, a pregnancy loss is a tremendous assault on one's self-worth. If there are no other children, it may also block the normal transition into a crucial stage of adult development, that of parenthood. Finally, as cherished as the unborn baby is, his/her identity is nebulous, making it quite common for past, unresolved grief to merge with the baby, making this loss even more profound. All of these unique aspects of reproductive loss will be discussed and illustrated in this chapter. Too often, paternal grief is overlooked and will occasionally be examined here. However, space constraints lead me to focus on the impact these losses have on mothers.

Models of Counseling and Psychotherapy

A variety of therapeutic approaches are available to treat reproductive loss. While psychodynamic versions are oriented to an examination of the client's emotional and cognitive experience, they tend to be eclectic and not traditionally psychoanalytic. They focus on resolving current repercussions from the loss, not seeking broader characterological change via transference interpretation, and build on the power of the therapeutic alliance with a highly interactive give and take. Each has its own particular emphasis. Jaffe and Diamond [3] follow a developmental perspective, contrasting one's "reproductive story" (anticipated life, especially family-to-be, narrative) with the unexpected subsequent losses in order to resolve traumatic grief. Covington [4] often employs cognitive behavioral techniques of creating mementoes, planning memorial activities and advocating self-care activities in providing a place to safely grieve these losses. Leon [5] considers the therapist's empathy as the critical healing agent in fostering a secure attachment, enabling the client to concurrently grieve, process trauma and repair self-esteem.

Cognitive behavioral therapies (CBT) are oriented towards exposure to (and extinction of) stimuli provoking anxious and/or grief-related reactions; increased engagement with others through behavioral activation; and a cognitive re-structuring and mindfulness which shifts negative, more depressive ideas towards more benign and affirmative responses [6]. With a sample size of 228, Kersting et al. [7] reported very impressive, significant reductions in grief, depression and PTSD following a pregnancy loss when CBT was administered over the Internet with individualized therapist responses to client writing assignments.

Differential diagnosis appears to be especially important in deciding upon psychopharmacologic treatment. Antidepressant medications are unneeded or ineffective in dealing with, respectively, normal or complicated (prolonged) grief. However, antidepressants were found to be very helpful in treating grief-related major depression – with symptoms no different from nonbereavement major depression – especially when combined with a supportive and individually tailored psychotherapy. Guidelines for working with pregnancy loss are summarized in Table 21.1 and will be discussed at length throughout this chapter.

Table 21.1 Guidelines for working with pregnancy loss

- The first session is usually the client telling their story. Listening fosters understanding.
- Take several sessions to acquire history and establish rapport.
- Give and get feedback to promote collaboration.
- Acknowledge longer term issues, even if they are not the focus of the work.
- Do not medicate grief. Reserve medications for major depression and other disorders.
- Be flexible. Individualize therapy.
- Include the partner whenever feasible.
- Be aware of maternal versus paternal differences in grieving.
- Empathy is more critical than insight.
- Work with past dynamics as they influence current issues.
- Respect, highlight and support strengths.
- Making meaning of this loss – "why did it happen?" and "what good can come from it?" – may subdue trauma.
- Tune into sub-cultural differences in grieving.
- Acknowledge and appropriately challenge stigmatization.

Key Components in Treating Pregnancy Loss

Flexibility

A cornerstone in working with pregnancy loss is flexibility. As Covington describes her practice, "I advise, analyze, educate, advocate, console and support while employing a variety of treatment modalities" [4, p. 204]. Ideological purity should take a far back seat to therapeutic efficacy. How directive and structured one is should be determined by the needs for crisis intervention (if the loss is very recent) and not a preset, one size fits all treatment plan. Similarly, the length of therapy should be customized. Three or four sessions may be sufficient for a more normative counseling: A mother with a young child was initially shocked and dismayed by her miscarriage at 9 weeks. Given a license to grieve by her therapist that had been derailed by family and friends, she readily obtained closure once she decided to honor her loss by constructing a life lesson session on pregnancy loss for her middle school health students. Grief counseling (not specifically applied to reproductive loss here) may do more harm than good when universally administered to those with normal bereavement.

However, when earlier, especially depressive, problems associated with emotional neglect and insecure attachment intervene, a longer therapy is usually necessary to more painstakingly establish a safer tie. A chronically depressed 35-year-old woman entered therapy in the midst of losing her preterm twins. Intertwined with the deep grief of losing them, she mourned the absence of emotionally available parents. Now, as in the past, her relentlessly upbeat and grief-avoiding parents would hear none of her sadness. Over the course of 5 years of weekly therapy, she was able to grieve the loss of her children, forge on to give birth to a healthy child whose pregnancy she was understandably convinced would end unsuccessfully, and with much less anxiety and despair have a relatively calm fourth healthy pregnancy. The therapist's consistently empathic and emotionally available stance provided a solid chamber to contain her, at times, seemingly bottomless despair. Very fulfilled over having the relationship with her sons that she never had with her parents, her depression has subsided considerably.

Many such extended treatments involve incipient prolonged or complicated grief which, while having elements of depression and PTSD, can be clearly distinguished from those conditions, even if that diagnosis is only provisionally accepted in DSM-V. As many as 25%

of bereaved women go on to have more chronic difficulties [8], with the majority not in fact following the "normal" model of a steady decline in grief, but instead some variant [9]. Because in the midst of such a recent loss, it often is not possible, clinically, to know how quickly emotional problems are likely to be resolved, it can be critical to be flexibly attuned to new issues as they arise and not be rigidly harnessed to a standardized treatment manual for all clients. An initial consultation of about three to four sessions enables getting to know the woman as a whole person, including her childhood, adolescence and young adulthood, not simply as a victim of a traumatic loss. Discussing extended feedback and recommendations at that point may provide a clearer sense of direction, as well as establishing a collaborative relationship, which is indispensable for change. Earlier, perhaps more chronic, issues may be identified and handled, if at all, or flagged for later, after the pregnancy loss has been sufficiently grieved.

Boundary and confidentiality concerns often mitigate against concurrent individual and conjoint work by the same therapist in general psychotherapy. However, with reproductive loss absent, such multimodal work is often effective with earlier, significant individual and marital problems. Typically (though not inevitably) the mother's more enduring, deeper and self-blaming grief than her partner's is given additional time individually, while tensions created by those differences may be worked through in conjoint sessions. It is neither necessary nor natural to expect men and women to grieve equivalently for these losses, particularly because the loss is so much more personal and immediate for the woman, it being within her body. It is crucial, however, that those differences be acknowledged and respected. Men especially need to be able to support, not reject, and join in – when honestly felt – their partner's grief. He may need to be told by his partner that sharing his grief will not burden her, but bring them closer, as often happens following this loss. A bereaved father will rarely come to therapy for pregnancy loss of his own accord, but is quite willing to participate to help his partner. Usually that motivation is sufficient for him to meaningfully engage in the therapy. Conjoint sessions are usually not as critical for pregnancy loss as they are for infertility because the course of medical treatments, multiple stressors and marital decisions that need to be made are so much greater for the latter.

Rarely do I feel it is helpful to directly include children in the therapeutic work. That may inadvertently reinforce a parent's sense of failure after such a loss by usurping a parenting function. It is better to empower parents by coaching them on addressing a child's concerns based on their own intimate knowledge of their children (for a more thorough discussion of dealing with sibling issues, see reference [10]).

Strengths

A more detailed discussion of building on client strengths can be found in Chapter 19. Most clinical consultations focus on client weaknesses, vulnerabilities, problems and ultimately, psychopathology. No evaluation is complete without an understanding of the crucial assets, traits and values which are a foundation of the Positive Psychology movement [11]. Empirical research indicates that by building on clients' positive emotions, promoting their exceptional strengths in engaging in their pursuits and creating meaning through their primary activities can be a powerful triad in reducing depression [12]. Clinically, the therapist needs to identify and echo her strengths, providing that as feedback during the consultation, and an integral part of genuinely and positively supporting past personal resources as a way to meet the rigors of grieving. Finally, there is also a place to respect and sometimes encourage the legitimate need to have breaks from grieving and "come up for air."

Empathy

Empathizing with the client's experience in general and grief in particular engenders healing. In a meta-study of all psychotherapy, empathy is a moderately strong predictor of therapeutic success [13]. The utter sense of feeling abandoned among all kinds of bereavement may make empathy critical in facilitating grief. Grieving pregnancy loss may make therapeutic empathy even more indispensable due to the usual minimization, avoidance and solutions others often apply to this loss if not personally familiar with it. Empathy is a key ingredient appreciated in medical care for perinatal loss [14]. If we understand one form of empathy as being intuitively attuned to what kinds of statements or emotional expressions would be helpful or hurtful, empathy can occupy an important self-monitoring function for the therapist.

Empathy embodies three arenas [13]. By taking the other's perspective, it fosters a cognitive sense of understanding what the client is experiencing, promoting feeling heard. There is an emotional resonance felt within the therapist for the client, enabling the client to feel less alone. Finally, authentic caring actions and providing realistic reassurance help the client to be genuinely cared for, aiding in the regulation of distress.

Ironically, while empathy is often belittled for its soft, soggy, unscientific connotations, its neurological credentials are impressive. Empathy is a mammalian trait rooted in the brain's mirror neurons which are activated by another's actions and emotions. The three different empathic processes described above have been associated with different areas of brain function, including, respectively, temporal cortex, limbic system and orbitofrontal cortex [13]. The client's affective experience of feeling understood, appreciated and cared for takes precedence over the cognitive aspects of insight and interpretation. Empathy is at the crossroads of several overlapping clinical models: the client-centered approach of Carl Rogers [15], which cites empathy as a crucial ingredient in a therapeutic relationship; Kohut's self-psychology [16], using empathy as the crucial tool to accessing the client's experience; and an attachment model of psychotherapy [17] which, in part, through empathic attunement, can provide a form of a secure attachment from which many of the therapeutic tasks of integrating trauma, grieving the loss and repairing self-esteem may be resolved.

Our empathic failures are inevitable and potentially therapeutic. It enables the therapy to be truly collaborative, with the therapist's willingness to acknowledge mistaken understandings (without being willy-nilly or pleading mea culpa about it) and the client feeling more empowered in defining her own experience. It may promote resilience by fostering adaptation to an empathically imperfect world. A 35-year-old woman was able to confront and readily forgive her doctor's empathic failure of not expressing condolences over her son's death once he more openly demonstrated by tears how much the loss meant to him. It was a powerful lesson to both, demonstrating to her that she could help effect the support she needed in her medical environment, and it made clear to him that completely avoiding his own sadness and grief does no good for his patients.

At the outset, clients may be encouraged to share when inevitable misunderstandings occur. We may be more susceptible to empathic errors when we expect clients to follow our prior clinical experience and/or what "the literature" suggests, rather than their own path. Our own personal (especially pregnancy) losses may facilitate empathy, while ironically encourage empathic mistakes when we expectantly project our personal loss experience onto our clients. As wisely noted, "Empathy should always be offered with humility and held lightly, ready to be corrected" [13, p. 48].

It is an ongoing, evolving inter-subjective feedback loop, not a static, one-way expression of therapeutic sensitivity.

Therapeutic Tasks in Treating Reproductive Loss

Most clients dealing with these losses will need to address most of the following issues, yet each client will have her particular emphasis, combination and texture of problems. These tasks are also very inter-related, distinguished here for didactic purposes while naturally occurring together.

Processing Trauma

After briefly reviewing the consultation process, I typically begin the first session by asking, "Where would you like to begin?" This is an invitation to tell the story of usually traumatic losses. For many, it began years back with the diagnosis and treatment of infertility, telling you the other crucial related issues and events leading up to the specific loss. Asking this question also empowers the mother to construct her own narrative, replacing the utter helplessness of loss with a greater sense of control by telling her story. Typically, the details become more painstakingly specific, indicating the tell-tale imprinting of trauma on the mind, leading up to the shock and tears at the moment of loss. More traumatized and less trusting clients may not initially be able to tell their story with full intensity. Constructing a narrative, done over time with many repetitions, becomes an important, active way of processing a traumatic loss, that in one's utter helplessness and initial shock felt beyond assimilation. Re-living the loss makes it more real. Many a mother will note, even 3 months later, she still can't believe it happened.

Therapeutic empathy and responsiveness lead to the client feeling less isolated and more supported, allowing the traumatic emotions and memories to be processed. It offers a "holding" environment in which the client feels safe with the therapist, solidifying the bond felt between them. This explains why the psychologically healthy client almost always reports feeling much better after the first session. The emotionally overwhelming residues of the traumatic experience may be primed in later sessions by asking what continues to be the most difficult, painful or unforgettable aspects. Inquiring into what has helped the most may reveal what sources of strength and resilience can be mobilized, whether internal (e.g., fortitude,

215

sense of humor), interpersonal (e.g., connection with others, emotional intelligence) or spiritual (e.g., faith in God, hope).

Cognitive–behavioral therapy similarly emphasizes the importance of exposure to the most traumatizing stimuli in order to extinguish the anxiety response [7]. However, if the CB therapist is not empathically attuned to what might re-traumatize the client, certain exposure practices (e.g., going to the baby section at Target) may be exactly what is recommended to be *avoided* in the early work because it is just too painful. Interestingly, qualitative results from a CBT study indicated that one of the most helpful aspects of the intervention was "having an empathic, nonjudgmental person to talk to about their emotions and experiences around the loss" [18, p. 172].

These losses may be traumatizing not only due to anxiety-producing, affective overstimulation, but because of "shattered assumptions" [19] of the world being viewed as safe, just and predictable. Schemas defining our security in the world undergo massive cognitive disruption, sometimes uprooting the foundations of religious beliefs. Reassuring cornerstones, often of one's religious faith, (e.g., "If I am good and work hard, my just rewards will follow") are now replaced by disorganizing, confusing questions of "What did I do to deserve this?" A crucial task of resolving these traumatic losses is making meaning and sense of what happened, assimilating what one can to one's existing beliefs, and gradually modifying those schemas accommodating to the new harsh reality [20]. Multiple schemas are often simultaneously violated. Not only is one's basic safety in the world eradicated by this loss, but the prior confidence in modern medicine and dependability of friends being sources of support and understanding may be casualties as well.

It is not the therapist's job to prophetically resurrect the client's infrastructure of meaning. But by articulating the areas of disrepair, encouraging a process of making sense of this loss, and, crucially, offering an emotional climate of respect, patience, understanding and confidence in her finding, not alone, her way through this, usually allows the client to adaptively integrate past and current good in her life with the current tragedy. A new, more realistic and sober view of the world can co-exist with a renewed, though wary, confidence.

Both forms of trauma may besiege the bereaved, singly or in combination, and sometimes revives earlier traumatic events. A 32-year-old woman expressed muted grief at her son's premature birth and death, avoiding his name and thinking about him. It soon became evident that she was emotionally repeating the secrecy of a rape at 14 about which she never told her neglectful parents. Once this earlier trauma could be processed in re-telling what happened, reducing her shame and self-blame, she was better able to more emotionally grieve her son's death, with less dissociative-like detachment. An understandable, lingering sense of vulnerability from the earlier rape could be challenged and modified by appreciating her capacity for assertiveness as an attorney.

Traumatic residues are normal and to be expected in the pregnancy following a prior loss. Anticipating another shocking death, re-living cues of the last pregnancy, and detaching oneself from the much-wanted child as one lives in a state of low-level hyper-vigilant anxiety keeps her "one step in and one step out" of that difficult pregnancy [21]. One woman who endured multiple pregnancy losses was so convinced she would lose another one that she guiltily acknowledged wishing it would happen already, finding it intolerable to endure the wracking helplessness, defining how traumatic those losses were. Her husband was troubled by her seeming indifference to the pregnancy defined as "it." Yet, once she gave birth to a healthy girl, her attachment quickly blossomed. In this situation, support figures – medical, mental health, family and friends – need to empathically and patiently accept her anxiety and responses as understandable, based on her earlier loss(es), not trying to minimize or "talk her out of it," but instead encouraging additional ultrasounds if that relieves anxiety and maintains an air of quiet hopefulness.

Husbands are very susceptible to these traumatic repercussions, often feeling like helpless bystanders to their wives' bodily injuries. One man was always able to comfort and reassure his anxious wife, until his firm guarantee that their baby would be OK was shattered by a stillbirth. No longer could he maintain the aura of being her protector, requiring a slow process of accepting the limitations of his sense of power. Too often men are left out of the grieving process, asked by family and friends how their wife is doing, with no acknowledgment of their own sadness and hurt. Cultural prohibitions against men expressing grief (i.e., viewed as weakness) may make it more acceptable for him to show anger rather than loss. Often, he may show more grief by vicariously sharing with his wife's tears.

Defining the Loss

A crucial therapeutic task is helping the couple appreciate what or who has exactly been lost. My own clinical work indicates that there is a typical sequence of experiencing an ongoing pregnancy, first as a fetus, then as a baby, often (but not always) culminating as a son or daughter, usually in the last trimester. Couples vary considerably in how rapidly they progress through that sequence in any particular pregnancy. Both the nature of the loss and the degree of maternal fetal attachment will determine the intensity and nature of the grief reaction. Typically, the termination of an unwanted pregnancy (i.e., elective abortion) experienced as a fetus with very limited maternal fetal attachment will not evoke significant grief [22], in contrast to a later termination for fetal anomaly of a much-wanted pregnancy, akin to grieving a spontaneous perinatal loss. A miscarriage may be experienced as a devastating, shocking blow to a woman's feminine potential and/or the loss of a baby as well, depending upon whether personhood has been conferred in viewing it as the loss of a baby. Because the pregnancy is within the woman, she is more likely to experience a deeper attachment, with an earlier sense of it being a baby than her male partner, generally resulting in deeper and more prolonged grief with a greater degree of felt failure.

Listening carefully to whether the bereaved parent refers to the child by name, as a baby or something else usually indicates where the loss is on the trajectory of personhood. One may ask more specifically if it was felt as the loss of a baby or something else, if the clinician is unclear.

Clinical experience along with anthropological and research data suggest three factors impact maternal fetal attachment and development of personhood. Societal expectation of a healthy pregnancy and baby in the developed world accelerates the establishment of babyhood and promotes maternal fetal attachment. Conversely in the developing world, such as in Tanzania, with a very high perinatal mortality rate, babies born with visible defects are often not considered humans, and miscarriages and stillbirths not worthy of mourning [23]. Similarly, the normative frequency of pregnancy loss among Irish Catholic women at the turn of the twentieth century resulted in such losses usually not deeply grieved, being instead, "just one of those things" [24, p. 189].

Motivation to parent is another important factor influencing maternal–fetal attachment and development of personhood. When there is no desire to parent a child, whether in elective abortion [22] or relinquishing a child

by a third-party surrogate [25], there is little maternal–fetal attachment or resulting grief. Analogously, psychosocial factors which mitigate focusing one's energies and hopes on the pregnancy, such as lack of family support, emotional disturbance including depression, anxiety and substance usage, are significantly associated with less maternal–fetal attachment [26].

Finally, increased interaction with the fetus/baby accelerates both the experience of personhood and maternal–fetal attachment. Perinatal loss often results in a deeper and more prolonged grief than losses earlier in the pregnancy, with quickening usually marking a more profound sense of the baby being separate from the mother [26]. Similarly, the magnified, increasingly refined image of the fetus in ultrasound often accelerates the experience of personhood and maternal–fetal attachment [26]. Over the past 30 years, with improved technology and greater usage of ultrasound, women are much more likely, in my clinical experience, to view a miscarriage after the first 8-week ultrasound as the more personal death of her baby, not solely the loss of a pregnancy.

Of course, these models are intended as guidelines to understanding the variability of response to different pregnancy losses. Clinical acumen best determines what such a loss will mean to a particular woman at the time in her life. A 38-year-old woman experienced the termination of her pregnancy with baby who had Down's syndrome as the deeply disappointing loss of a potential, not actual, child, a "pre-human creature." Reporting neither guilt nor regret about her decision, she was readily able to share her sadness, feeling minimal grief, and was soon ready to attempt another pregnancy, concerned about her advancing age. A 42-year-old woman expressed a deep and lonely grief for the entirely unexpected ectopic pregnancy following a history of successful infertility treatments and birth of twins 6 years earlier. Her prior history of reproductive frustration heightened this loss, felt as that of a baby, much to the chagrin of her relieved family who did not believe having more children made sense.

Facilitating Grieving

Grieving the loss of the baby is generally what is most equated with counseling for perinatal loss. This unique form of grieving entails transforming the loss of a baby into the death of a specific, named son or daughter. There is a two-step process of establishing the identity of the baby and then constructing the memories of interaction, which is the raw material of grieving. Much of this may be accomplished in the hospital with seeing and holding the baby, making a memory box with mementoes, and so forth. A controversial study by Hughes and colleagues [27] challenged the value of such contact, reporting increased anxiety, depression and PTSD either during the subsequent pregnancy or 1 year after the next birth. However, the vast majority of qualitative and quantitative studies (i.e., 21 out of 23) report parents endorsing the preference and positive meanings of having contact with their deceased child after birth [28]. Psychotherapy can continue that process as well (see Table 21.1 for a useful reference of interventions to facilitate grieving), especially since a brief hospital stay laden with traumatic shock usually deters much overt grieving. Imparting a child an identity also enables the rituals around memorials and remembering, which help to make sense and meaning of such a loss, increasingly understood as an important ingredient in adaptation to loss [20]. It is quite striking and poignant to observe during a therapy hour in the midst of the sadness of grief, the paradoxical pleasure parents may demonstrate of the love and pride they felt in the time together with their child. One father especially appreciated taking a video of his very premature son's movements soon after birth, documenting his brief life.

Because so much of grieving perinatal loss is projected prospectively into the future, anniversaries and birthdays often take on great importance in missing what might have been. "Weaving babies lost in pregnancy into the fabric of the family" [29, p. 23] through rituals, symbols, a visible presence and other means enables a continuing bond with one's child that is now recognized as a normative adaptation to this loss [30], rather than a defense against resolving grief. Some parents state a need to briefly take their baby home to create memories of his/her place concretely in the family. One mother planned a family picnic by the grave of her deceased son on his birthday as a way of celebrating his brief life. A special song, memory or dream may conjure up the spiritual presence of and connection to the baby. While we need to encourage and validate parents' own actions that sustain their unique everlasting, ongoing parental relationship with their child, it can sometimes be useful to offer what memorializing activities that have helped other parents. Remembering such a young loss is so important due to others not knowing him and the constant fear of that child being forgotten.

For some parents an earlier, unresolved loss or trauma becomes fused with a current perinatal death, extending and complicating the therapy. The earlier loss must be identified and often grieved to some degree in its own right, before reconciliation with the perinatal loss can be achieved. A 35-year-old woman relentlessly grieved the intrauterine fetal demise of her 16-week pregnancy, month after month, with no relief. It was only when she was able to discuss in considerable detail the suicide of her psychotic, bipolar father (which was a family secret) and openly grieve the loss of him that she was able to more effectively relinquish the loss of her daughter. A 32-year-old father reported increasing anxiety about the safety of his 2-year-old son and his distancing from the family following several miscarriages. Being able to explore in greater depth traumatizing sexual abuse when he was 4 years old significantly alleviated his anxious reactions.

Sometimes grieving is more diffuse, not of a son or daughter but of a sense of failed parenthood or reproductive capacity, especially with an earlier miscarriage or pregnancy terminated for fetal anomaly. Not following the parental path one expected [3] entails prospective grieving of a loss of one's future and identity, analogous to not parenting the deceased child one loves. There may also be significant losses associated with pregnancy demise. A 40-year-old woman did not grieve the loss of a baby due to an elective abortion at 16, but sorrowfully missed the relationship with her boyfriend, the only figure at that time who genuinely cared for her, and who faded from her life soon after.

Grieving does not occur in an interpersonal vacuum. The empathic support, sharing of sadness and crying at a funeral powerfully facilitates grieving. Similarly, and more deeply, a secure attachment with a therapist enables an open expression of multifacetted parental grief embodying sadness, rage, despair, loneliness and so forth. Such emotional support for grieving perinatal loss may be painfully missing due to the tendency of family and friends to quickly minimize or avoid discussing the death. The heightened yearning of the recently pregnant woman for maternal nurturance is a normal regression in preparing to empathically care for the vulnerable infant. This also makes the need of the newly bereaved mother for empathic understanding so critical.

Repairing the Self

Pregnancy loss is almost inevitably a major if not devastating blow to the self. The multiple strands of the "bio-psycho-social" foundations of the self are challenged.

One's helplessness in the face of identity being shaken can be traumatizing.

Pregnancy loss shatters a basic bodily function, that of reproduction. A young woman in her mid-twenties called her miscarriage not so much the death of a baby but a "loss of invincibility." The sense of omnipotence and immortality through projecting one's genes into the next generation is dismantled, sometimes permanently. Shame, commonly felt after any bodily malfunction, can be intense, along with feeling defective.

Psychologically, pregnancy loss assaults a woman's self-worth in general, and gender identity in particular. Even when a woman rationally understands she did nothing wrong and everything right to ensure the health of her baby, there is a virtually ubiquitous tendency to emotionally blame herself and feel the resulting guilt. A very successful Latina business-woman in her mid-thirties relentlessly attacked herself for not going to the hospital sooner when she felt unusual pains at 20 weeks, even though she was told by the hospital to wait and see if it got better by morning. Her baby was prematurely born that dreadful night. Her motto in life, that she could fix anything she set her mind to, was left shattered.

There are multiple interventions to keep in mind in addressing these biological and psychological assaults on the self. For many, simply identifying these multiple injuries is therapeutic, broadening her understanding that more has been taken away than solely the loss of her baby. Amid the self-blaming and bashing, having someone take the time to understand her pain conveys the sense that she matters. Different strategies will work for different women. Understanding what medically caused the loss will go a significant way for some in subduing irrational self-blame and guilt. For others, blaming oneself – if specifically designed to be able to avoid another such traumatic loss – may in fact improve mood and sense of competence by increasing one's sense of control. This seemed to work effectively for the busi-nesswoman, serving to preserve a sense of control over the future rather than being left with her shredded self-confidence. Reinforcing other areas of self-esteem in one's life – that of career, parent (if one has surviving children of course), marriage, etc. – can significantly ameliorate, over time, one's wounded self-worth. When prior infertility has taken its toll, simply becoming preg-nant can be validated as a legitimate boost to one's self-esteem.

Cognitive–behavioral therapy techniques may be useful in addressing unrealistic self-blame. Cognitive re-appraisal [6] directly challenges the irrational under-pinnings of these beliefs as well as recognizes what has been gained in adapting to these losses. This may be done, respectively, by having the client "put her thoughts on trial, and weigh the evidence" [31, p. 528] or consider "The Gifts," [4, p. 209] given by the lost baby, such as greater marital closeness, gratitude for the good in life, etc. When applying these techniques, one needs to be very careful in timing them not too soon, when in the midst of intense sorrow, or in any way justifying this loss as something positive. Once again, accurate empathy will guide when, how and ultimately if those interventions are made, directed by the client and not a manual.

Interactions in one's social world can be a critical determinant of the depletion or sustenance of self-worth. A 42-year-old woman became intolerably infuriated by the lack of acknowledgement and minimi-zation of the loss of her 16-week-old twins by her extended family. When attempts to encourage more empathic responses failed, recommending avoidance of them – typically not the best alternative – in this case seemed warranted.

Finally, when pregnancy loss occurs before parent-ing a live child, there can be tremendous disruption in one's psychosocial adult development, interfering with attaining "generativity." One not only experiences estrangement from family-forming peers, but feels out of synch with one's own life plan and vision of the future. Men can profoundly feel such frustration when these losses prevent entering fatherhood. Empathically identifying the source of this social and personal isolation, as well as supporting steps to real-ize other important developmental goals (e.g., career aspirations) and for now finding alternatives to paren-tal wishes (e.g., mentoring) can be important thera-peutic tasks.

Preserving Social Connections

Due to the vulnerability of social isolation and the increased probability of feeling one's loss has been mis-understood and minimized by others, maintaining sup-portive social ties, especially conjoint, is significantly related to a quicker adaptation to this loss [32]. Just as was the case in defining optimal therapist and health provider support, empathy in its multiple ingredients (i.e., comforting, listening, being nonjudgmental, etc.) registered as the most helpful form of support that could be provided by family and friends. Support groups have emerged as a particularly valuable resource offering a safe place to share one's loss and feel validated, whether meeting face-to-face or over the Internet.

While a therapist's empathy with the inevitably painful and tactless comments the bereaved will receive is necessary, when clinically feasible it can be helpful to underscore family and friends' desire to be helpful, even when they fail to do that. Modeling ways to nonaggressively but assertively confront repeatedly hurtful remarks ("I know you mean well but when you say that, it doesn't help me") is often necessary, along with educating family and friends as to what actions will be healing. If the offending family member or friend persists, limiting contact for now may be the best solution. Finally, in recommending support groups as a useful adjunct to therapy, it is important that be conveyed as supplementing, not replacing, the work (and support) in therapy, lest the bereaved feel rejected.

Weathering Termination

While termination varies among clients in this kind of work, it tends towards brevity. In brief therapy it may be announced that session, though in longer work I encourage at least several sessions to allow for a usual expression of some loss over ending, especially meaningful as it is loss which brought them in. Because traumatizing helplessness is usually such a critical ingredient in the loss, I am reluctant to challenge what may feel like a rushed exit. Even if you may wish for a more planned departure (in part, perhaps, to deal with one's own sense of loss in ending), it may be most important for the client to feel in control of *this* loss compared to the last traumatizing one. Sometimes ending soon becomes an understandable desire to put this loss behind them, especially if a ticking biological clock has them thinking of a subsequent pregnancy before it is too late.

A more maladaptive, shockingly sudden termination may be unconsciously designed to provoke the abandonment the parents have felt by their loss, which may be re-activated by interruptions in the therapy. Parents of a stillbirth many years prior suddenly announced their decision to end therapy in the final minutes of their first appointment following my 3-week summer vacation after having worked productively for over a year. The better approach, I believe, is not to metaphorically slam the door on their way out, but to express one's disappointment in not having more time to say goodbye, while letting them know the door is open

should they choose to return (a message I convey in all terminations).

The Special Case of Pregnancy Termination for Fetal Anomaly

Pregnancy termination for fetal anomaly (PTFA) is a unique loss. It is often inaccurately associated with elective abortion, though the former is ending the pregnancy of a much-wanted unhealthy fetus/baby while abortion is ending the life of an unwanted presumably healthy fetus/baby. PTFA is a much more frequent loss than most people realize, with an estimated incidence of 1.7–2.8% of all pregnancies, [33], about double or more the frequency of perinatal loss, which is about 1% of all pregnancies.

A Very Stigmatized Loss

The loss experience of PTFA is shrouded by abortion stigma. Societal condemnation of abortion in the US has led to much controversy in this area, with most research in PTFA being historically done in Europe, few guides available to therapists working with couples dealing with PTFA, and conference presenters often being told to avoid discussing this loss. The dynamics of stigmatization – the denigrated action being unspeakable, leading to secrecy and estrangement from others – culminates with that condemnation being internalized, usually leading to guilt and especially shame. Rejected by the Pro-life movement for ending a pregnancy and alienated from the Pro-Choice faction which is very reluctant to view their loss as a baby and not a fetus, the couple often feels extremely isolated from others, ironically "in no man's land" [34, p. 133]. It is appropriate for the therapist to identify that stigmatization when it appears and ally with the couple against it, encouraging a telling of the whole story, thereby challenging the secrecy and shame that make it unspeakable. Despite the reality of social deprecation of abortion, in my experience most family and friends are likely to react more often with understanding and compassion, with the couple's expectation of denunciation being more a product of the projection of one's guilt than the danger of reproach.

In order to appreciate the greater complications of PTFA compared to other reproductive losses, I will discuss the additional tasks confronting couples making this decision [35], represented in Table 21.2.

Table 21.2 Additional tasks confronting couples choosing pregnancy termination for fetal anomaly

1. Challenge abortion stigma.
2. Address traumatic impact of learning of the fetal anomaly.
3. Educate oneself about nature and consequences of the anomaly.
4. Determine what and who has been lost.
5. Assess resources and limits of parenting an impaired infant.
6. Decide whether to terminate or continue the pregnancy.
7. Decide which termination procedure is used.
8. Endure the termination experience.
9. Decide who should be told what narrative.
10. Manage the legacy of PTFA.

The recent US Supreme Court overturning of Roe v Wade will no doubt change in some profound ways the experience of PTFA. However, until more clinical data is accumulated, it will not be possible to know precisely what that will be. It appears likely that the stigma and resulting shame associated with all pregnancy terminations will be amplified due to their increased illegality in many states. Defining the loss as a fetus or baby will probably be made more complicated resulting from external pressure to define personhood to all pregnancies. Prohibitions against all terminations may limit or entirely prevent deciding not to continue the pregnancy. Termination procedures will likely be more dictated by legal requirements rather than solely medical considerations and personal choice. These are but a few of the ways making terminations illegal will likely exacerbate the challenges and psychological turmoil for couples who might choose PTFA.

Absorbing the Impact of Learning About the Anomaly

Learning the bad news of the medical situation can be traumatizing. One never imagined oneself getting such bad news or having to make such a decision [36]. Emotional and cognitive challenges must be addressed at virtually the same time. On the emotional side, the shocking news must be processed while the couple sets upon the intellectual job of learning all they can about their fetus/baby's condition in order to make an informed decision. While they begin the process of emotionally grieving the loss of the healthy child they anticipated, they must construct a coherent narrative of what is happening, to make sense of it. With the window of having a choice ever narrowing, a woman needed to decide within a week whether to terminate her pregnancy of a baby diagnosed with Down's syndrome. What appeared to be a pathologic

self-punitive paralysis of spending many weeks obsessively reviewing her choice after the termination, later became understood as a necessary process of validating a decision that had to be made too soon for her psyche to absorb. It is the therapist's job to help articulate and normalize the many intense and mixed emotions the couple feels. Even if learning the devastating news occurred some weeks or months ago, their shock, denial, tearful grieving, anxiety about the future, etc. can come back full force as a means of processing the loss and allowing the therapist to empathically understand what they are going through. It can be explained that these intense feelings and confusion is not their feared belief that they are going crazy, but the understandable reaction to beginning perhaps the most difficult situation they have ever been in. If the news was given recently and they are in the process of deciding what to do, it is important (and much appreciated) to meet with them as soon as possible and as often as necessary to resolve this crisis.

Deciding What or Who Has Been Lost

Pregnancy termination for fetal anomaly is perhaps the most variably experienced loss, within and between couples. The sense of what has been lost is often fluid, not statically determined once and for all. Frequently – especially if the anomaly is detected early in the pregnancy, being unseen and gender unknown – it is viewed as the loss of a potential child, clearly not a person. Some others who choose to view the body uncomfortably consider the loss an "it," somewhat less than a baby, but more than simply a potential being. Increasingly I have found that over the course of our work more and more choose (their decision, not my agenda) to transform that loss into the more personal death of their child, often a named son or daughter. Psychologically speaking, no one but the couple can decide what or who was lost and what that loss means to them.

Parents who choose to embody their loss as a baby, son or daughter, may endure great guilt in ending their child's life, though the availability of having mementoes, memories and rituals may allow them to grieve their loss, much like a perinatal death. The couple who does not view their loss as that of their child may be spared the guilt of ending their child's life, but many grapple with a different sort of guilt, of not allowing their fetus to come into existence and not being worthy of grieving. It is of course not the therapist's role to manipulate them in a particular direction but to reflect their opinions and convictions, assuring them there is no "right" or "wrong" answer to how the fetus/baby should be viewed and the kind of grief that follows.

Deciding Whether to Continue or Terminate the Pregnancy

It is crucial that the therapist be neutral in the active decision-making process. However, this should not be misinterpreted as emotional detachment. Quite the contrary, this is a time when the therapist must convey his/her empathic awareness of how profoundly difficult it is to make such a monumental decision with limited, often ambiguous information in such a short time. McCoyd [37] offers a useful decision-making model that many couples intuitively apply to some degree: they acquire sufficient medical information to assess the needs and demands of the disabled child, balancing them against a psychosocial, practical inventory of their family's strengths, challenges, resources, emotional limitations and financial situation. This is not intended as an algorithm that spits out the "right" answer based on quantifying variables. Instead, it is potentially a useful heuristic tool that facilitates a discussion between the couple. Instead, one's gut feelings may be most influential in decision-making, although those visceral feelings should be articulated as much as possible to clarify discussion. For most parents who choose to terminate, the concern about the baby suffering is a paramount consideration.

Some couples choose, for many different reasons, to continue the pregnancy with a serious fetal anomaly. For those given a fatal fetal diagnosis, continuing the pregnancy can prepare them to grieve, much like a spontaneous perinatal loss, with the customary rituals and mementoes which can make that child a family member. For others who are likely to have their child survive, they must balance their anticipated parenting of an impaired infant with the grief of losing the healthy child they imagined and cherished. For many it is less an emphatic decision to continue the pregnancy, but an emotional inability to terminate. This may be based on religious reasons, where choosing to terminate is intolerably "playing God," not only in making decisions of life and death over the child, but to determine existentially whether that being is human. Others are unwilling to accord doctors the certainty of their diagnosis, as skepticism of the medical prognosis leads to the decision to leave the outcome up to God instead. Finally, for those who are dealing with infertility, this pregnancy might be their last, if not their best, opportunity for being parents, finding it too painfully dystonic to decide to end a life when they have been so dedicated to creating one. For them, their being bereaved parents may offer some solace than never being parents at all.

The therapist working with the couple should review with them their expectations of the pregnancy and postpartum to aid their planning while being mindful of not indirectly questioning or judging their decision. Perhaps the most difficult obstacle they will encounter will be the readiness of the vast majority of their support and caregiving networks – medical professionals, family and friends – to try to persuade them to terminate the pregnancy instead, believing that will spare them the pain of further loss or the burdens of parenting a severely impaired child. Such well-meaning recommendations overlook the reality that losses are inevitable here and facilitating the couple making their choice may mitigate a traumatizing sense of helplessness, supporting their right to know and decide what is best for them.

Once the decision has been made, I believe the therapist must be able to support that choice unless it appears likely to seriously damage the well-being of one of the partners or the couple. Pointing out the mental health consequences of such a decision are made on psychological, not moral grounds. For example, a man pushing his wife to terminate a pregnancy she can't bear to end or his leaving it up to her alone to make the decision since the pregnancy is in her body both deny the importance of it being a joint decision that is discussed together, even if they don't see eye to eye on it. To do this work effectively, I believe it is necessary for the therapist to be able to support either a decision to terminate or continue the pregnancy. Even after the decision has been firmly made, the parents may bewail "the right decision couldn't hurt this much" [38, p. 40]. It can be explained that some decisions have extremely awful options, where sometimes the best choice is to select that which is least intolerable. For some, making such a decision is unacceptable, believing it is playing God. For others, it is such a horrible choice that the only thing worse would be not having that choice at all.

Going through the termination procedure is usually the most difficult aspect of PTFA. Knowing exactly when the fetus has died can sharpen feelings of guilt and hubris. Partner support is extremely helpful, reminding the woman that this was a joint decision, not her sole responsibility. Tuning out by listening on headphones to music or whatever will get her as mentally far away from the procedure as possible can be adaptive coping and not solely denial as it may superficially appear.

Deciding Who to Tell What

While couples in the Western world typically share with family and friends their spontaneous pregnancy loss, no such assumptions are made for PTFA. Commonly, a usually inaccurate fear of others' condemnation leads the couple to say as little as possible about the circumstances of the pregnancy demise, often omitting to tell all it involved termination. While this is a decision they of course need to decide for themselves, there are several problems with this approach. First, this is hard to do successfully as the whole story has a way of getting out. Second, the secrecy often increases over time feelings of shame by keeping the truth unspeakable. Third, it can seriously diminish the healing power of others' support, both by discrediting the support given when deception is involved ("They wouldn't be so compassionate if they knew what I did") and preventing the additional empathic understanding of how difficult it must have been to have to make such a decision. While there are exceptions of course, most family and friends respect this is their decision to make and whatever the couple choose will be supported.

In order to diminish shame bred on secrecy, I usually encourage couples to share the whole story with someone they expect will be understanding. A therapist's acceptance and compassion usually help reduce the stigma associated with PTFA as well, making it more possible to share the story with others. The therapist may be the only one who has been told the complete story, bearing witness to this tragic loss, justifying its telling being as long and unrushed as needed. For those couples who came in to facilitate decision-making and chose to terminate, it almost always makes sense to meet in a session post-procedure to provide support and offer additional meetings as needed.

The Legacy of Pregnancy Termination for Fetal Anomaly

Pregnancy termination for fetal anomaly resides in the shadows because it is a stigmatized, taboo loss, not to be spoken of, but unable to be forgotten. While the decision made is rarely regretted, the guilt it generates may never be completely silenced. Traumatic scars may remain, but for most the loss can be reconciled. Feeling one has killed one's baby is balanced by the belief one spared that child a life of suffering.

Conclusions

The more experience I gain in working with pregnancy loss, the less of a sense I have of knowing the answers. Despite commonalities in reactions, profound individual differences persist. A couple shared a common deep Christian faith in grappling with the neonatal loss of their son due to an extremely rare metabolic disorder. While the father was furious with God for not hearing his prayers, the mother was at peace with Him, knowing her son was whole, resting in heaven.

One is likely to stay on the right track by listening to what the bereaved has to say, feeling what they are going through, asking questions about what may be omitted in their account, empowering them to be as much as possible the authors of their experience, and providing guidance when they feel lost.

References

1. Covington SN. Pregnancy loss. In Covington S, Burns L, Eds. *Infertility Counseling: A Comprehensive Handbook for Clinicians*, 2nd ed. Cambridge: Cambridge University Press, 2006, 290–304.

2. Leon IG. Understanding pregnancy loss: helping families cope. *Postgrad OB & GYN* 1999;**19**:1–7.

3. Jaffe J, Diamond MO. *Reproductive Trauma: Psychotherapy with Infertility and Pregnancy Loss Clients*. Washington, DC: American Psychological Association, 2011.

4. Covington SN. Miscarriage and stillbirth. In Rosen A, Rosen J, Eds. *Frozen Dreams: Psychodynamic Dimensions of Infertility and Assisted Reproduction*. Hillsdale, NJ: Analytic Press, 2005, 197–218.

5. Leon IG. Understanding and treating infertility: psychoanalytic considerations. *J Am Acad Psa Dyn Psychiatr* 2010;**38**:47–76.

6. Wenzel A. Cognitive behavioral therapy for pregnancy loss. *Psychotherapy* 2017;**54**:400–405.

7. Kersting A, Dolemeyer R, Steinbeg J, et al. Brief internet-based intervention reduces post-traumatic stress and prolonged grief in parents after the loss of a child during pregnancy: a randomized controlled trial. *Psychother Psychosom* 2013;**82**:372–381.

8. Bennett SM, Litz BT, Maguen S, et al. An exploratory study of the psychological impact and clinical care of perinatal loss. *J Loss Trauma* 2008;**13**:485–510.

9. Lin SX, Lasker JN. Patterns of grief reaction after pregnancy loss. *Amer J Orthopsychiatr* 1996;**66**:262–271.

10. Leon IG. *When a Baby Dies: Psychotherapy for Pregnancy and Newborn Loss*. New Haven, CT: Yale University Press, 1990.

11. Seligman MEP, Csikszentmihalyi M. Positive psychology, an introduction. *Amer Psychol* 2000;**55**:5–14.

12. Seligman MEP, Rashid T, Parks A. Positive psychotherapy. *Amer Psychol* 2006;**61**:774–778.

13. Elliott R, Bohart AC, Watson J, et al. Empathy. *Psychotherapy* 2011;**48**:43–49.

14. Gold KJ. Navigating care after a baby dies: a systematic review of parent experiences with health providers. *J Perinat* 2007;**27**:230–237.

15. Rogers C. *A Way of Being*. Boston, MA: Houghton Mifflin, 1950.

16. Kohut H. *How Does Analysis Cure?* Chicago, IL: University of Chicago Press, 1984.

17. Sable P. *Attachment and Adult Psychotherapy*. Northvale, NJ: Jason Aronson, 2000.

18. Bennett SM, Ehrenreich-May J, Litz BT, et al. Development and preliminary evaluation of a cognitive-behavioral intervention for perinatal grief. *Cog Behav Pract* 2012;**19**:161–173.

19. Janoff-Bulman R. *Shattered Assumptions: Towards a New Psychology of Trauma*. New York, NY: Macmillan, 1992.

20. Neimeyer RA. Searching for the meaning of meaning: grief therapy and the process of reconstruction. *Death Studies* 2000;**24**:541–558.

21. Cote-Arsenault D, Marshall R. One foot in – one foot out: weathering the storm of pregnancy after perinatal loss. *Res in Nurs Heal* 2000;**23**:473–485.

22. Cameron S. Induced abortion and psychological sequelae. *Best Prac Res Clin OB GYN* 2010;**24**:657–665.

23. Wembah-Rashid JAR. Explaining pregnancy loss in matrilineal southeast Tanzania. In: Cecil R, Ed. *The Anthropology of Pregnancy Loss*. Oxford: Berg, 1996, 75–93.

24. Cecil R. Memories of pregnancy loss: recollections of elderly women in Northern Island. In: Cecil R, Ed. *The Anthropology of Pregnancy Loss*. Oxford: Berg, 1996, 179–196.

25. Hanafin H. Surrogacy and gestational carrier participants. In Covington S, Burns L, Eds. *Infertility Counseling: A Comprehensive Handbook for Clinicians*, 2nd ed. Cambridge: Cambridge University Press, 2006, 370–386.

26. Alhusen JL. A literature update on maternal-fetal attachment. *J Ob Gyn Neonat Nurs* 2008;**37**:315–328.

27. Hughes P, Turton P, Hooper E, et al. Assessment of guidelines for good practice in psychosocial care of mothers after stillbirth: a cohort study. *Lancet* 2002;**360**:114–118.

28. Kingdon C, Givens J, O'Donell E, et al. Seeing and holding baby: systematic review of clinical management and parental outcomes following stillbirth. *Birth* 2015;**42**:206–218.

29. Cote-Arsenault D. Weaving babies lost in pregnancy into the fabric of the family. *J Fam Nurs* 2003;**9**:23–37.

30. Klass D. *The Spiritual Lives of Bereaved Parents*. Philadelphia, PA: Brunner Mazel, 1999.

31. Davis CG, Wortman CB, Lehman DR, et al. Searching for meaning in loss: are clinical assumptions correct? *Death Studies* 2000;**24**:497–540.

32. Lasker JN, Toedter LJ. Predicting outcomes after pregnancy loss: results from studies using the Perinatal Grief Scale. *Illness, Crisis & Loss* 2000;**8**:350–372.

33. Coleman PK. Diagnosis of fetal anomaly and the increased maternal toll associated with pregnancy termination. *Issues Law & Med* 2015;**30**:3–23.

34. McCoyd J. Women in no man's land: the abortion debate in the USA and women terminating desired pregnancies due to foetal anomaly. *Brit J Soc Wrk* 2010;**40**:133–153.

35. Leon IG. Empathic psychotherapy for pregnancy termination for fetal anomaly. *Psychotherapy* 2017;**54**:394–399.

36. Sandelowski M, Barroso J. The travesty of choosing after positive prenatal diagnosis. *J Obstet Gyn Neon Nurs* 2005;**34**:307–318

37. McCoyd J. "I'm not a saint": burden assessment as an unrecognized factor in prenatal decision making. *Qual Hlth Res* 2008;**18**:1489–1500.

38. McCoyd J. Pregnancy interrupted: loss of a desired pregnancy after diagnosis of fetal anomaly. *J Psychosom Ob Gyn* 2007;**28**:37–48.

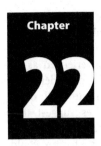

"A Little Bit Pregnant": Counseling for Recurrent Pregnancy Loss

Rayna D. Markin

Samantha: A Case of Recurrent Pregnancy Loss

Yesterday, I got up early with the sun, and I told myself, "Samantha, today is a new day and this is a new pregnancy, time to put the negativity and fears behind you." I felt good, a little hopeful. I even dared to look in the mirror and admire my growing baby bump. I got dressed, worked out, made breakfast, took a long leisurely walk with the dog. Then, I came back inside from walking the dog and noticed that my orchids, you know the ones I've been growing from tiny seeds, were dead. I lost it. I melted down onto the floor and started sobbing uncontrollably. It was like this tidal wave of sadness just hit me and knocked me off my feet, but I was also so angry. I took that plant that I had dedicated so much time to growing and nurturing, and I threw it across the room. The pot hit the wall and shattered, and that only made me feel worse. Like, what have I done? I did everything right! I watered it, tended to the soil, made sure the temperature and amount of sunlight were perfect, and it still died! It felt so unfair. I realized in that moment just how scared I am that I am going to lose another baby, how much the fear has impacted every fiber of my being for so long. I hardly remember what it is like to live without that fear. It is terrifying to me that I could do everything right and still have another miscarriage. I don't know if I can go through another loss. I don't know how I would survive it. I can't continue to live like this, feeling danger around every corner, checking for blood compulsively every time I go to the bathroom, holding my breath before every doctor's appointment, feeling the sting every time someone says, "congratulations, you must be so excited for the baby," and feeling so angry, like "isn't that nice for you that you assume there is going to be a baby." I tell myself not to care, not to think about the future or this pregnancy as real, not to get my hopes up. But the truth is, I do care, my hopes are up, and I think about it all the time. I'm so used to feeling half pregnant, like this isn't really real, that I think allowing myself to relax a little and feel, well,

more than just a little bit pregnant for a second, terrified me. I feel like I'm going crazy, can you help me?[1]

Samantha seeks counseling desperate for help with feelings and experiences all too common for women struggling with recurrent pregnancy loss (RPL). Repeatedly cycling between fleeting flashes of relief and silent hope upon a positive pregnancy test, and devastating moments of pure anguish upon yet another loss, takes an emotional, mental and physical toll on Samantha. She feels exhausted and emptied, emotionally raw and fragile, and like a shell of the person she used to be. When not pregnant, Samantha is "obsessed" with getting pregnant again, only to live in a state of chronic hypervigilance and anxiety over the possibility of another miscarriage when pregnant. Each loss leaves behind a new layer of grief, with no time to process it before the next cycle or pregnancy occurs. Each pregnancy, rather than being the hoped-for time of joy and excitement for the future, feels like a reminder of all that Samantha has lost, and like a ticking time bomb that any moment could go off, leaving behind in its wake even more death and devastation. For Samantha, pregnancy no longer equals a healthy baby and she is envious of other pregnant women who remain innocent and unaware of the possibility of loss.

Despite all this, somehow, Samantha functions in everyday life. She goes to work, does the laundry and pays the mortgage. However, to cope, she emotionally and mentally distances herself from each pregnancy, rarely thinking of the baby as real or herself as a mother. Feeling chronically unsafe in her own body and perpetually on-guard for signs of another loss, Samantha puts all the mental energy she has left into surviving, rather than feeling and processing the trauma and loss that has compounded inside her. To allow the cascade of emotions to pour out of her would feel like

---

The addenda referred to in this chapter are available for download at www.cambridge.org/covington-clinical-guide

---

[1] All clinical examples are based on an amalgamation of clinical experiences and thus no one person can be identified.

too much to bear while trying to make it through each day. When Samantha finally seeks counseling and asks you for help, she is further along in her pregnancy than ever before. She finds it more difficult to avoid thinking about the baby as real or her hopes and dreams for the future, which makes her more fearful than ever of another loss. To help Samantha, and patients like her, this chapter will first review literature on the experiences of women and of their partners going through RPL, and subsequently offer specific clinical guidance.

The Psychological Impact of Recurrent Pregnancy Loss

The American Society for Reproductive Medicine (ASRM) defines RPL as the failure of two or more clinical pregnancies [1]. RPL can further be separated into *primary RPL*, for patients who have never had a successful or viable pregnancy, and *secondary RPL*, for patients with a history of at least one live birth before the pregnancy losses. About 1% to 3% of all couples in their reproductive years will experience RPL, which has been shown to have a significant psychological impact on women and their partners (for review, see [2]).

Psychological Symptoms: The Woman's Perspective

Recurrent pregnancy loss encompasses a series of stressful life events that undoubtedly have a tremendous impact on a woman's psychological and emotional well-being [2]. However, most of the existing literature concerning the psychological consequences of miscarriage rely on studies investigating women with single early-term pregnancy loss. These studies suggest that feelings of grief after a miscarriage are comparable to other kinds of severe losses and will often abate within 6–12 months [2], although grief following a miscarriage is often non-linear and can extend for years after the loss [3]. Depressive symptoms have been found to occur in 20% to 55%, and anxiety in 20% to 40%, of women who have suffered such a loss. These women are also at an increased risk for posttraumatic stress disorder and obsessive compulsive disorder [2].

The intense and often long-lasting psychological consequences reported after a single early-term loss increase in severity with the number of pregnancy losses and in cases of primary RPL [2]. The few studies that do exist on RPL specifically suggest that affected women are at increased risk for anxiety, depression, grief, guilt and anger [2]. In particular, single women going through infertility

treatment and RPL may feel isolated, alone in their grief, and unsupported, and may be particularly at risk for experiencing depression and anxiety. Furthermore, perhaps because pregnancy loss is often experienced as an attack on one's sense of self, self-esteem, and gender identity [4], it is not surprising that women with RPL often report low self-esteem [2]. These studies suggest that women who experience recurrent loss often have several areas of concern that counseling or psychotherapy could address, including grief and loss, posttraumatic stress-like symptoms, depression and anxiety and low self-esteem.

Psychological Symptoms: The Man's/Partner's Perspective and the Impact on the Couple

While most studies have examined the psychological consequences of pregnancy loss on women, a few studies involving male partners and single perinatal loss suggest that men often feel helpless, anxious, depressed, angry, guilty, lonely and preoccupied with thoughts of the loss, albeit to a lesser degree than their female partners [2]. One would expect these reactions to intensify with multiple pregnancy losses. A few studies have looked at the impact of RPL on men and on the couple as a unit in heterosexual relationships. These studies suggest that while men, compared to their female partners, are at a lower risk for anxiety and depression after RPL, they still often experience severe emotional consequences [2]. For instance, in a recent study and review by Voss and colleagues [2] looking at couples experiencing RPL, men and women were at significant risk for relatively high levels of anxiety, depression and poor social support. However, women were at somewhat higher risk for depression and anxiety and men for poor social support. Many men feel the burden of responsibility to support their partner, leading to the suppression of their own feelings and needs, as well as delayed grieving. It is less socially acceptable for men to display feelings of sadness and loss, especially within the context of paternal grief, which is typically not recognized in society [2].

These societal factors can lead to the male partner suppressing his feelings of grief and loss, while simultaneously attempting to "fix" his female partner's sadness and distress. While men tend to use more problem-solving and active coping strategies to deal with grief and loss, women typically want a place to share their sadness and receive emotional validation and support. These different ways of coping with and communicating about grief can cause conflict in relationships. Women often feel alone in their grief, neglected and/or dismissed, while men often feel helpless, rejected and emotionally overwhelmed [5]. These couples come to feel like adversaries just when they need each other's support and understanding the most. Fertility counselors should help couples to understand one another's style of coping with grief and how to best support one another through the grieving process [4,5]. Improving the couple's relationship satisfaction can decrease depression and increase social support for men and women [2].

Psychological Symptoms: The Experience of Loss for Lesbian Couples

Mary and Sharon are two cisgender women in a committed partner relationship. Though Sharon was diagnosed with primary infertility, the couple decided that Sharon would undergo IVF and carry their baby, as being pregnant was a lifelong dream of hers, whereas this was not the case for Mary. Sharon endured four rounds of IVF, which resulted in four pregnancies that were each miscarried during the first trimester. Because family, friends and medical professionals focused solely on Sharon, who grieved deeply after each miscarriage and felt a great deal of anxiety when pregnant again, Mary felt as if her experience of loss was invisible. Moreover, Mary felt generally excluded from both the process of conception and that of loss. She reported a constant "coming out" process at the fertility clinic, as nurses, medical staff and doctors repeatedly asked if she was a friend or sister of Sharon's, which invalidated Mary's role as a second mother. Mary felt further sidelined when the doctor would not even allow her in the examining room during Sharon's three dilation and curettages (D&Cs). Mary was never legally recognized as the babies' second mother, and she mourned never getting the chance to legally adopt their child. Yet, Mary felt guilty communicating her feelings to Sharon since she did not have to undergo the invasive medical procedures that Sharon did, nor experience the physical losses. Lastly, insensitive comments from family members like, *at least it wasn't really your baby that was lost*, were particularly hurtful and invalidating. Sharon also dealt with insensitive comments from friends and family, who asked why Mary didn't just carry their baby since Mary did not have any infertility issues, which invalidated Sharon's dream of carrying a child.

Mary and Sharon's story exemplifies how the grief of lesbian parents is often disenfranchised, or not socially acknowledged or validated, and misunderstood within a heteronormative society. To become pregnant in the first place, LGBTQ parents are often forced to navigate a heteronormative system that does not leave room for their experience and invalidates them as parents [6]. When a pregnancy is lost, lack of understanding and validation makes it even harder for these couples to have their grief and loss acknowledged, understood and supported. While there is a general lack of research on the experience of RPL for same sex couples, reflecting the invisible status of these grieving parents in society, one study of interviews with six bereaved lesbian mothers found that they experienced "double disenfranchisement," since not only did they experience a dearth of support for their experiences with loss, but they also avoided support services that require them to explain or justify their family [7]. It is important for fertility counselors working with lesbian couples to be aware of their own heteronormative biases, and to explicitly acknowledge and validate past emotional injuries caused by heteronormative or homophobic systems and individuals. Lastly, fertility counselors should help each partner to acknowledge and validate the other's personal struggles with RPL.

The Psychological Experience of Pregnancies After a Loss

Because women living with RPL repeatedly vacillate between suffering another miscarriage and coping with subsequent pregnancies, it is important for fertility counselors to understand a woman's experience of pregnancy after loss (PAL). Women who are PAL typically report a lack of support and understanding, as family and friends often expect them to be joyful upon a new pregnancy and are surprised when they continue to mourn the loss of a prior pregnancy when pregnant again [8]. On the contrary, pregnancies after loss are frequently characterized by perinatal grief and posttraumatic stress symptoms, depression, anxiety and prenatal attachment problems (for review, see [9]).

Pregnancy Loss as a Trauma and the Impact on Subsequent Pregnancies

Pregnancy loss is a traumatic loss, or *reproductive trauma*, for a woman's trust in her body and in the world as a fundamentally safe and just place has been broken [9]. In general, *traumatic loss* involves an abrupt or unexpected loss that is so devastating that it overwhelms or surpasses the mind's usual ways of coping with distress and of making sense of the world (for review, see [10]). RPL exposes parents to ongoing traumatic loss, which no parent expects when starting out on their reproductive journey, and which challenges these parents to make sense of a world in which such bad things can repeatedly happen. In a continued state of shock and devastation, it is difficult for these parents to process their feelings at the time of each loss and to make sense of events and their reactions. Unprocessed feelings of grief and loss therefore compound after each miscarriage, the sum of which may overwhelm a parent's typical way of coping.

Chronic Hypervigilance and Intrusive Thoughts and Images

Later pregnancies are often reminiscent of those that were previously lost and can trigger posttraumatic stress reactions, specifically chronic hypervigilance for signs of another potential loss, and/or psychological intrusion of unwanted thoughts and images related to prior losses [8]. Like a veteran home from war, these parents often anticipate danger around every corner and are chronically on "high-alert" for signs of another potential loss. Their chronic hypervigilance leaves them constantly anxious, on-guard and emotionally and behaviorally dysregulated. These patients often proscribe almost magical-like power to their own behaviors to either prevent or cause another miscarriage, leading them to anxiously scrutinize everything they do as possible threats to the pregnancy. Moreover, they are frequently haunted by unwanted images and thoughts related to past losses that loop through their mind like a videotape on repeat. Consistent with this, about 21% of women pregnant after loss meet posttraumatic stress disorder (PTSD) criteria [11] (see also Chapter 20).

Importantly, for women who are pregnant and suffer from RPL, the trauma of loss lives not only in the past (as is typical with *post*traumatic stress reactions), but also in the present, as these women and their partners experience ongoing loss and stressful life events. The fact that traumatic events are often still occurring in the present makes it challenging for RPL patients to reflect on prior traumatic events as a set of memories that occurred in the past but are no longer a current threat, which typically helps to process trauma and regulate emotional arousal in other types of posttraumatic stress reactions. Because past and present are not well differentiated, when these patients recall memories of past traumatic reproductive losses, they may feel all the emotions experienced at the time, as if these events were occurring in the moment, and become affectively overwhelmed [12], particularly when these events, or ones like them, *are* occurring again in the moment, such as in the case of recurrent miscarriage.

Pregnancy-related Anxiety

Pregnancy-related anxiety, or the fear of yet another loss, has been shown to characterize PAL [13], and can be understood as a "normal" reaction to the trauma of one or more prior pregnancy losses [14]. Anxiety, or chronic hypervigilance to signs of potential danger or threat, is a classic reaction to traumatic events and a criterion of PTSD in the *Diagnostic and Statistical Manual of Mental Disorders* (DSM-V). Within the context of PAL, anxiety is the mind's way of trying to exert control in an uncontrollable situation, through alerting the mother to any and all potential signs of threat, in the hope that if the mother is always on guard for signs of another loss, then she can prevent it from happening. Because of this, those experiencing PAL tend to anticipate threats related to fetal health, fetal loss, childbirth and parenting and newborn care [15]. Chronic hypervigilance and pregnancy-related anxiety go hand-in-hand, as chronic hypervigilance keeps parents in a constant state of arousal and anxiety, wherein all mental efforts go toward avoiding potential traumatic loss in the future, rather than processing feelings and experiences related to actual traumatic losses from the past.

Counseling for pregnancy-related anxiety should help the patient to process underlying and unresolved feelings of trauma and loss. When treatment focuses solely on behavioral strategies to regulate pregnancy-related anxiety, then the underlying trauma and loss remain unresolved. In conjunction with the long-term goal of processing trauma and loss, in the short-term, cognitive–behavioral and other strategies can be used to help regulate pregnancy-related anxiety. Perhaps more than any one technique or strategy, however, the patient's anxiety can be regulated within a warm, empathic and emotionally containing therapeutic relationship, both by the medical professional and the fertility counselor. Often, the therapist's nonverbals and soothing tone of voice help to regulate the patient's anxiety more than what the therapist says or does. Interventions for regulating pregnancy-related anxiety are summarized in Table 22.1.

Emotional Cushioning

Leon [4] calls the phenomenon wherein women pregnant after loss anticipate yet another traumatic death, relive cues of the last pregnancy and detach from oneself and from one's much desired child, as *traumatic residues*. Similarly, according to the theory of emotional cushioning, women PAL fear another potential loss, and thus, to

Table 22.1 Interventions for regulating pregnancy-related anxiety

Type of intervention	Examples of intervention
Cognitive–Behavioral and/or supportive care	• Meditation • Mindfulness • Encouraging the patient to think of the pregnancy in terms of hours or days, rather than weeks or trimesters • Increasing checkups, ultrasounds and the checking of blood levels • Encouraging the patient to work with the same doctor throughout the first trimester
Relational	• A warm, empathic and emotionally containing therapeutic relationship • Empathize with underlying feelings of PRA, mainly lack of control and basic safety • Identify and empathize with undifferentiated feelings that manifest as anxiety, such as grief and loss or anger • Therapist's nonverbals and soothing tone of voice

varying degrees, protect their emotions by avoiding pre-natal bonding [16]. Women PAL are less likely to engage in reverie about the baby, try not to think too deeply about the pregnancy or the baby as real, focus on the physical or concrete aspects of the pregnancy, and report less strong prenatal bonds [17]. For RPL patients, this is often evident in the mother's desire to delay sharing the news of the pregnancy with others until well into halfway through the pregnancy or even later. Consistent with this, Gaudet at al. [18] found that pregnant women with prior perinatal loss reported significantly higher scores of grief, depression and anxiety as compared to a control group, and that these symptoms predicted lower prenatal attach-ment scores. Interestingly, pregnancy-related anxiety and emotional cushioning positively correlate [16], suggest-ing that it is not that these women are not bonded or attached to the unborn baby, but that they avoid approaching this bond for fear of yet another traumatic loss [14].

Markin [14] understands emotional cushioning, or the mother's tendency to turn away from or disavow her internal subjective experiences concerning the pregnancy or unborn baby, and her imagined relationship to the unborn baby, as an effort to cope with trauma and loss. In general, when the amount of stress engendered by one or more traumatic events (such as RPL) exceeds the patient's ability to cope, then the mind, in order to survive, will split off the emotions from the experience [12]. Overwhelmed, the mind cannot tolerate, process or think about the emotions related to the trauma in an organized and coherent manner [12]. In the context of emotional cushioning during PAL, the mother, to varying degrees, is believed to avoid her feelings and fantasies related to the unborn baby because, to approach these subjective experi-ences would also mean approaching traumatic affects

associated with prior losses that are deemed too unbeara-ble to acknowledge. The clinical implication of this being that, while some emotional cushioning during PAL is likely a normal and adaptive coping strategy, more severe and long-lasting emotional cushioning suggests underly-ing and unresolved trauma and loss that needs to be processed and worked through [14]. In essence, as human beings, we do not have the luxury of turning off intense negative emotions without also turning off positive ones, and so the mother's capacity to tolerate and process traumatic affects associated with past losses is directly tied to her ability to acknowledge positive emotions related to her current pregnancy and relationship to her future baby.

Interventions Following Recurrent Pregnancy Loss and Pregnancy After Loss

Interventions for perinatal loss are typically brief and target immediate symptom relief following a loss, before the woman is pregnant again. For instance, one study found that emotional distress, depression and anxiety significantly decreased over the course of an open trial of cognitive-behavioral therapy for women who had recurrent miscarriages [19]. Yet, perinatal grief is often delayed, elevates during subsequent pregnancies and potentially impacts the attachment relationship with the next baby (for reviews, see [8,9]).

In a rare empirical study of psychotherapy for PAL, Markin and McCarthy [8] conducted an evidence-based case study examining the process and outcome of 22 pre-natal sessions and one post-partum follow-up session of psychodynamic therapy for a woman pregnant after RPL. Their results suggest that the patient experienced reliable and clinically significant change on all pregnancy-specific measures, including pregnancy-related anxiety, perinatal grief, trauma and prenatal attachment. However, general symptoms of depression and anxiety were variable and highly volatile over time. Qualitative analyses from exit interviews conducted with the therapist and patient suggested that therapist empathy and validation were helpful in promoting change on pregnancy-specific symptoms, whereas ruptures in the therapeutic alliance may have been associated with a lack of change on general psychiatric symptoms. Although the results of one case study cannot be generalized to other therapy dyads, these results warrant future research on the effectiveness of psychodynamic therapy for pregnancies after RPL and on the therapeutic relationship as an important change mechanism.

Clinical Guidance: A Relational Perspective to Counseling for Recurrent Pregnancy Loss

The following clinical guidance is offered in the context of counseling for patients suffering from RPL. Rather than a specific set of techniques, direction is offered on how an empathic therapeutic relationship can help these patients to process trauma and loss, and to mitigate associated symptoms of emotional cushioning and pregnancy-related anxiety. Furthermore, guidance on the establishment of the therapeutic alliance in couples counseling as a vehicle to increase shared purpose and co-investment in the therapeutic process and help the couple to grieve together, are suggested.

Empathy and the Processing of Trauma and Loss

Empathy, a consistent predictor of therapy outcome [20], is a multidimensional construct that includes cognitive and/or affective types of understanding [20]. *Cognitive empathy* involves seeing the world from another person's perspective, while *affective empathy* involves the therapist emotionally resonating and joining with the patient's sadness or affective experience more broadly [20,21]. An empathic therapy relationship is proposed to help RPL patients to process their multiple experiences of trauma and loss through: (a) building narrative coherence, and (b) providing a safe base from which they can process traumatic affects and grieve [22].

Cognitive Empathy and Narrative Coherence

Cognitive empathy is believed to facilitate the processing of trauma and loss through fostering *narrative coherence* [22]. In the trauma literature, narrative coherence, or narratives

with more complexity, elaboration and articulation, is associated with fewer symptoms of posttraumatic stress and anxiety and the successful treatment of traumatic stress symptoms (for review, see [22]). Although these studies have looked at other types of traumatic events and not pregnancy loss specifically, Engelhard et al. [23] found that a lack of a sense of coherence is a significant risk factor for poor maternal outcomes after perinatal loss. Though narrative coherence appears important to the processing of traumatic events, RPL patients often enter therapy with a chaotic and disorganized narrative of the multitude of adverse events that they have experienced and need help making sense out of a senseless situation. The details of their reproductive story [9] have been violated and each page torn apart. Fertility counselors need to help these clients to revise their reproductive story into a coherent and meaningful narrative.

For RPL patients, just the act of telling their reproductive story can be a disorganizing and overwhelming one. The patient repeatedly telling his or her complex story of RPL to an understanding and supportive therapist, and the therapist reflecting back and articulating an accurate understanding of the patient's thoughts, reactions and feelings, may be the primary mechanism through which narrative coherence is enhanced, helping to resolve trauma and loss [4,21,22). Through the therapist's moment-to-moment empathic attunement to the patient's ongoing experience, the therapist helps to make sense of and clarify the patient's reactions, elaborating upon and clarifying her reproductive narrative. The patient actively participates in clarifying his or her internal experience, validating or modifying the therapist's understanding [4,21,22]. Essentially, the patient articulates a reproductive story characterized by greater narrative coherence, as she modifies and integrates the therapist's empathic understanding of traumatic events.

Affective Empathy and Processing Traumatic Affect

Emotional resonance and connection in the therapeutic relationship provide a holding environment in which the therapist can share and co-regulate the patient's feelings of trauma and loss. This kind of emotional holding environment helps the patient to feel less alone and facilitates grieving (4,21,22). The therapist acts as a secure attachment figure, providing a safe base to which the patient can return for comfort, safety and understanding when feelings and experiences become too overwhelming or painful [4]. This is necessary because, as patients recount their story of recurrent traumatic loss to the therapist, they often become overwhelmed by the unprocessed traumatic affects associated with each event, which were too overwhelming to process at the time (4,21,22). The therapist intuitively recognizing and emotionally joining with the patient's feelings of grief and loss, allow the therapist to vicariously be there with her during each loss to comfort, understand and co-regulate her affective experience [4,22].

Empathy as a Tool for Working with Emotional Cushioning and Pregnancy-related Anxiety

Cognitive empathy can be used to normalize emotional cushioning as an understandable reaction to trauma and loss. Empathy into the meaning and function of emotional cushioning helps the patient to understand her reluctance to bond to the unborn baby, not as a sign that she does not care or love her child, but, as a way of coping with the fear of yet another loss. As the therapist and patient work together to craft an empathic understanding of what past experiences of trauma and loss have meant to the patient, she may be better able to differentiate in her mind past pregnancies from the current one, making it feel safer to approach her bond to the current fetus/baby. Sometimes, just the therapist empathizing with the patient's need to distance herself from the unborn baby as a self-protective mechanism, and all the pain that lies underneath the numbing and mental distancing, is enough to help her feel safer to approach the unborn baby and pregnancy as real. Affective empathy, or emotionally resonating with the patient's feelings of trauma and loss, lessens the need for emotional cushioning and creates emotional space for feelings of both attachment and loss. In other words, the therapist joining with the patient's sadness, emotionally containing and soothing her overwhelming experiences, helps her to feel less alone and overwhelmed, and safer to approach the bond to her unborn baby.

Similarly, cognitive empathy can be used to help patients make sense of and regulate pregnancy-related anxiety, through understanding it as a function of trauma. This often involves the therapist reflecting to the patient that, of course, when so many bad things happen to us, we are left feeling unsafe and as if more bad things could happen at any moment. We often feel out of control and do not want to be caught off guard by more devastating events ever again. In other words, the therapist should empathize with feelings underling the anxiety, usually lack of control and of basic safety. Relatedly, pregnancy-related anxiety can be thought of as the sum total of undifferentiated and unprocessed affects associated with past traumatic events. The

therapist's empathic understanding of what experiences with RPL have meant to the patient helps to tease apart, identify and understand each affective experience, disentangling the jumble of feelings inside that when tangled together manifest as anxiety. Emotionally resonating with the patient's affective experience helps to co-regulate and sooth her fears and anxieties, making room for underlying feelings of grief and loss, anger and often shame to emerge.

The Therapeutic Alliance in Couples Counseling

The therapeutic alliance is the collaborative aspect of the therapeutic relationship, or the degree to which the therapist and client agree on the tasks and goals of therapy and have a safe and trusting bond (see [24]). In couples counseling, each person forms a personal alliance with the therapist, but also observes the unfolding alliance between the therapist and his or her partner, and, the couple as a unit forms an alliance with the therapist. A *split alliance* refers to an imbalance among these multiple alliances, wherein person X's alliance is stronger than person Y's alliance. Studies show that stronger alliances are associated with better outcomes, whereas split alliances are associated with poorer outcomes in couples counseling [24] (see also Chapter 4).

There is often a pull for the therapist to align more with the partner who physically lost the pregnancy/baby, and, in heterosexual couples, with the female partner who most often initiates treatment, while her male partner agrees to come to "support" her. To avoid such split alliances, the therapist should define the treatment goals and tasks in such a way that both partners within the couple can "sign on" or "join in" as co-investors in the therapeutic process [24]. This requires the therapist to align with and empathically connect to each partner within the couple. For instance, the therapist should emphasize that despite differences in how each partner copes with grief, each is grieving and in emotional pain. Each feels alone in his or her distress, and yet wants comfort and understanding from the other. The treatment goals can then be defined in terms of helping each partner to respect the other's way of coping with grief so that they can approach the pain of loss together, rather than feeling so alone in their distress [22]. Similarly, the therapist can make interventions to increase "shared purpose" and "validate common struggles" [24]; emphasizing, for example, that while each partner might have a different way of grieving, both are struggling to grieve [22]. As seen in the case example above of Mary and Sharon, in same sex couples, while each partner may have a different experience of grief and loss, both are struggling to grieve within a heteronormative society that often misunderstands and invalidates their experience as parents.

Conclusion: Back to the Case of Samantha

Like other trauma survivors, Samantha first came into counseling feeling fundamentally out of control and help-less; so, she did what most human beings would do in that situation. She tried to control *everything* and feel *nothing*. Her desire to control everything fueled her constant worries about the health of her unborn baby. Samantha feared that if she put her guard down for even just one second then she would miss that next bad thing running right toward her, causing her to lose yet another pregnancy and feel even more grief and loss. Overwhelmed by the intensity of her emotions, she distanced herself from her feelings and from her unborn baby, who she so desperately wanted, all so she could get a break from the intense and chaotic feelings swirling inside of her and function in everyday life. Yet, no matter how hard Samantha tried to push down her feelings and pretend they weren't there, the pain somehow managed to live on, for grief is the one thing that never really dies. Though painful, it was not until Samantha stopped trying so hard to distance herself from her feelings about her current pregnancy and past losses that she could begin to heal. In therapy, Samantha, for the first time, talked about all the traumatic events of the past few years while trying to conceive. As her fertility counselor empathically understood what these experiences have meant to her, Samantha began to feel understandable and less alone. She still worries about the health of the baby, but this anxiety has begun to feel more manageable. Sometimes, Samantha still feels a little bit pregnant, a little anxious, a little sad or angry, and, other times, she feels a little closer to the unborn baby, and a little hopeful about her future as a mother; the point being, that she now feels a little bit safer to feel just a little bit more.

References

1. American Society for Reproductive Medicine. Evaluation and treatment of recurrent pregnancy loss: a committee opinion. *Fertil Steril* 2012;**98**(5):1103–1111.

2. Voss P, Schick M, Langer L, et al. Recurrent pregnancy loss: a shared stressor–couple-orientated psychological research findings. *Fertil Steril* 2020;**114**(6):1288–1296.

3. Lin SX, Lasker JN. Patterns of grief reaction after pregnancy loss. *Am J Orthopsychiatry* 1996;**66**(2):262–271.

4. Leon IG. Pregnancy and loss counseling. In: Covington SN, Ed. *Fertility Counseling: Clinical Guide and Case Studies*. Cambridge: Cambridge University Press, 2015, p. 226–238.

5. Peterson B. Fertility counseling for couples. In: Covington SN, Ed. *Fertility Counseling: Clinical Guide and Case Studies*. Cambridge: Cambridge University Press, 2015, p. 60–73.

6. Holley S. Pasch L. Counseling lesbian, gay, bisexual and transgender patients. In: Covington SN, Ed. *Fertility Counseling: Clinical Guide and Case Studies*. Cambridge: Cambridge University Press, 2015, p. 180–196.

7. Cacciatore J, Raffo Z. An exploration of lesbian maternal bereavement. *Social Work* 2011;**56**(2):169–177.

8. Markin RD, McCarthy KS. The process and outcome of psychodynamic psychotherapy for pregnancy after loss: a case study analysis. *Psychotherapy* 2020;**57**(2):273–288.

9. Diamond DJ, Diamond MO. Understanding and treating the psychosocial consequences of pregnancy loss. In Wenzel A, Ed. *Oxford Handbook of Perinatal Psychology*. New York, NY: Oxford University Press, 2016, pp. 487–523.

10. Neria Y, Litz BT. Bereavement by traumatic means: the complex synergy of trauma and grief. *J Loss Trauma* 2004;**9**(1):73–87.

11. Turton P, Hughes P, Evans CD, Fainman D. Incidence, correlates and predictors of post-traumatic stress disorder in the pregnancy after stillbirth. *Br J Psychiatry* 2001;**178**(6):556–560.

12. Herman J. Trauma and recovery: the aftermath of violence from domestic abuse to political terror. New York, NY: HarperCollins, 1992.

13. Côté-Arsenault D, Mahlangu N. Impact of perinatal loss on the subsequent pregnancy self: women's experiences. *J Obstet Gynecol Neonatal Nurs* 1999;**28**(3):274–282.

14. Markin RD. "Ghosts" in the womb: a mentalizing approach to understanding and treating prenatal attachment disturbances during pregnancies after loss. *Psychotherapy* 2018;**55**(3):275–288.

15. Bayrampour H, Ali E, McNeil DA, Benzies K, MacQueen G, Tough S. Pregnancy-related anxiety: a concept analysis. *Int J Nurs Stud* 2016;**55**:115–130.

16. Côté-Arsenault D, Donato K. Emotional cushioning in pregnancy after perinatal loss. *J Reprod Infant Psychol* 2011;**29**(1):81–92.

17. Côté-Arsenault D, Donato KL, Earl SS. Watching & worrying: early pregnancy after loss experiences. *Am J Maternal Child Nurs* 2006;**31**(6):356–363.

18. Gaudet C, Séjourné N, Camborieux L, Rogers R, Chabrol H. Pregnancy after perinatal loss: association of

grief, anxiety and attachment. *J Reprod Infant Psychol* 2010;**28**(3):240–251.

19. Nakano Y, Akechi T, Furukawa TA, Sugiura-Ogasawara M. Cognitive behavior therapy for psychological distress in patients with recurrent miscarriage. *Psychol Res Behav Manage* 2013;**6**:37–43. http://dx.doi.org/10.2147/PRBM .S44327

20. Elliott R, Bohart AC, Watson JC, Murphy D. Therapist empathy and client outcome: an updated meta-analysis. *Psychotherapy* 2018;**55**(4):399–410.

21. Leon IG. Empathic psychotherapy for pregnancy termination for fetal anomaly. *Psychotherapy* 2017;**54**(4):394–399.

22. Markin R. *Clinical Application of Evidence-Based Relationship Principles in Psychotherapy for Pregnancy Loss.* Oxford: Oxford University Press, in preparation.

23. Engelhard IM, van den Hout MA, Vlaeyen JW. The sense of coherence in early pregnancy and crisis support and posttraumatic stress after pregnancy loss: a prospective study. *Behav Med* 2003;**29**(2):80–84.

24. Friedlander ML, Escudero V, Welmers-van de Poll MJ, Heatherington L. Alliances in couples and family therapy. In: Norcross J, Lambert M, Eds. *Psychotherapy Relationships That Work: Volume 1: Evidence-Based Therapist Contributions.* New York, NY: Oxford University Press, 2019, p. 117–166.

Pregnancy and Postpartum Adjustment in Fertility Counseling

Teni Davoudian and Laura Covington

Introduction

The complex emotional journey associated with reproduction does not end with a positive pregnancy test. When experiencing infertility, patients often believe that their stressors will resolve once there is a baby in their arms. Yet, pregnancy and the birth of an infant are times of transition and uncertainty for parents. In addition to adapting to social, occupational and relational changes that accompany parenthood, carrying parents[1] also face biological changes that can impact their mental health. While fertility counselors may not provide care to patients during the latter stages of pregnancy or postpartum, their knowledge of the psychological issues associated with reproduction can help mitigate the impact of mental health problems among the perinatal[2] population.

The specialty psychological services required by the American Society for Reproductive Medicine (ASRM) allow fertility counselors the unique opportunity to care for prenatal patients who may not otherwise meet with or have access to a mental health professional. Education regarding perinatal mood and anxiety disorders (PMADs) can be provided to patients during third-party consults, psychological screenings and support groups (in addition to psychotherapy sessions). This chapter explores topics to consider when providing care to patients receiving fertility treatment prior to, during and following pregnancy.

Mental health disorders experienced during the perinatal period, such as generalized anxiety disorder (GAD),

---

The addenda referred to in this chapter are available for download at www.cambridge.org/covington-clinical-guide

[1] We will use feminine terms such as "woman," "she" and "her" to describe a patient, but we recognize that not all patients may identify with these feminine terms.

[2] Medical definitions of the perinatal period may differ. From a mental health perspective and the purpose of this chapter, pregnancy through the first year postpartum are considered perinatal. When we refer to perinatal, this will include pregnancy and postpartum. If specific, we will indicate pregnancy, antenatal or postpartum.

obsessive compulsive disorder (OCD), panic disorders, posttraumatic stress disorder (PTSD), major depressive disorder (MDD), bipolar disorder and psychosis, are collectively referred to as perinatal mood and anxiety disorders (PMADs). These disorders are highly prevalent, yet underdiagnosed and undertreated [1,2]. Parents across the globe, regardless of their ethnicity, socioeconomic status, relationship status and reproductive history can develop PMADs [3]. The presence of an infant or fetus creates unique considerations when identifying, treating and managing PMADs.

Noncarrying parents, including adoptive parents and parents who have children via gestational surrogacy, can experience postpartum adjustment that places them at risk for anxiety and depression, albeit there is limited research on this topic [4]. Regardless of their reproductive histories, parents are often expected to immediately develop new parenting skills, such as soothing, swaddling, bathing and feeding a newborn, with little (if any) lived-experience of caring for an infant. Parenting is one of the most important jobs in life, but many parents are equipped with little to no training.

While caring for an infant presents challenges for many parents, there are important biological and hormonal differences between carrying and noncarrying parents. Carrying parents often face unique stressors, such as postpartum pain, difficulties breastfeeding, rapid hormonal fluctuations and sleep deprivation while trying to care for their infant. The first three months after birth, referred to as *fourth trimester,* can be particularly demanding, as parents and infants are adjusting to one another with a mutual need for connection (particularly when breastfeeding).

Risk Factors

The perinatal period is now recognized as a window of vulnerability for the development or exacerbation of psychopathology. The transition to motherhood is marked by unprecedented biopsychosocial changes [3]. Biological theories on the pathophysiology of PMADs suggest that

Table 23.1 Biopsychosocial risk factors for perinatal mood and anxiety disorders

Biological risks	Obstetrical risks	Psychological risks	Social/demographic risks
Perinatal hormonal fluctuations Family history of PMADs Changes in hypothalamic–pituitary–adrenal axis	Gestational diabetes Hyperemesis gravidarum Fetal anomaly Previous pregnancy loss(es) Pre-eclampsia Major obstetric hemorrhage NICU stay	Personal history of psychopathology History of physical and/or sexual trauma Maternal personality traits, such as perfectionism Premenstrual dysphoric disorder Previous episode(s) of PMADs Significant postpartum sleep disturbances	Younger maternal age Lower maternal education level Low socioeconomic support Parents from chronically disadvantaged communities, such as Black, Hispanic, BIPOC and LGBTQ+ Intimate partner violence Insufficient paid parental leave in the United States Insufficient emotional, informational and instrumental support

the neurologic, immunologic and endocrine alterations associated with pregnancy and postpartum can impair maternal mental health [3]. From a psychological standpoint, one of the most robust predictors of PMADs is a history of psychopathology [5,6]. While an exhaustive review of the determinants of psychopathology during the perinatal period is beyond the scope of this chapter, common risk factors are summarized in Table 23.1 [2,3,5,6].

Perinatal Anxiety Disorders Spectrum

Much like assisted reproduction, pregnancy and parenthood are often fraught with unpredictability. Anxiety disorders are prevalent during the perinatal period. While perinatal depression has gained recognition among medical associations and the media, perinatal anxiety disorders are largely underrecognized and undertreated [5,6]. Women who experience postpartum anxiety without depressive symptoms often feel misunderstood and unsupported by their healthcare professionals and family members, whose main concern is typically postpartum depression. While all anxiety disorders, such as panic disorder, social anxiety disorder and phobias can emerge or worsen during the perinatal period [6], this chapter will focus on the most prevalent perinatal anxiety disorders.

Generalized Anxiety Disorder

Parents with generalized anxiety disorder (GAD) consistently experience excessive, uncontrollable worry that negatively impacts their social, academic or occupational functioning. Accurately diagnosing antenatal GAD is complicated given the shared symptoms of pregnancy and GAD, such as fatigue, irritability, difficulties concentrating and sleep disturbances. The use of validated psychological assessments, such as General Anxiety Disorder-7 (GAD-7), in conjunction with

a clinical interview that examines the frequency, severity and the rationality of the pregnant person's cognitive processes can help differentiate anxiety disorders from expected side effects of pregnancy. During the postpartum period, mothers who have difficulties sleeping, when given the chance to do so, should be assessed, as they may be experiencing clinically significant anxiety or other mental health issues. The course of perinatal GAD symptomatology is currently unclear [5]. While some studies suggest that GAD steadily increases throughout pregnancy and peaks following childbirth, others have found that GAD is prevalent during the first trimester of pregnancy (perhaps partially due to fetal viability concerns) and immediately postpartum, with periods of low anxiety in between [5].

Generalized anxiety disorder and MDD are highly comorbid during the perinatal period. Women with overlapping depression and anxiety experience more anger, sleep disturbances and relationship discord when compared to women with only perinatal depression or only perinatal anxiety [7]. Longitudinal research comparing women with only postpartum depression or GAD, with women who have co-occurring postpartum depression and anxiety, found that comorbidity predicts longer symptom duration of both disorders [6].

Obsessive Compulsive Disorder

The perinatal period can precipitate onset or exacerbate underlying symptoms of obsessive compulsive disorder (OCD) among women [6]. For those who develop OCD following the birth of their child, the onset of symptoms occurs rapidly, typically within 2–4 weeks postpartum. Mothers report experiencing recurrent, intrusive, unwanted thoughts and images of harm befalling their child via contamination, accidents and deliberate actions.

Most women with perinatal OCD have intrusive thoughts of themselves harming their child. For example, mothers may have intrusive thoughts of images of dropping their child, leaving their child in a hot car or drowning their child during baths. These obsessions are ego-dystonic, cause significant stress and often lead mothers to engage in avoidance behaviors, including staying away from their child out of fear of harming the child. Women with perinatal OCD are not typically at increased risk of harming themselves or others.

Perinatal Post-traumatic Stress Disorder

Nearly half of women in the United States (US) find their labor and delivery experience to be emotionally traumatic [8]. Approximately 3–15% of women go on to develop perinatal PTSD. One of the most robust obstetrical predictors of perinatal PTSD is the use of forceps during delivery. Perinatal PTSD mirrors the symptoms experienced as a result of nonreproductive traumas. Fertility counselors should assess for evasion tactics of mothers with perinatal PTSD. Avoidance of appointments at the medical facility where the reproductive trauma occurred is common. This avoidance can compromise the timeliness and quality of medical care received by postpartum individuals. Mothers with perinatal PTSD may report that their infant triggers flashbacks, hypervigilance and other symptoms of PTSD. For some women, their child serves as a consistent reminder of the emotional and medical traumas that the mother and/or infant endured during labor, delivery and immediately postpartum.

The most distressing memories, flashbacks and cognitions reported by women with perinatal PTSD are connected to interpersonal events that took place prior to, during or shortly after the reproductive trauma occurred. For example, traumatized mothers may focus on feeling abandoned or ignored by their obstetrics team or support person(s). If left untreated, these interpersonal betrayals experienced during a reproductive trauma can extend into the postpartum period and impair relationships at a time during which social support is vital.

Given the close connection between assisted reproduction and reproductive losses/traumas, it is important for fertility counselors to screen for symptoms of PTSD. Patients undergoing assisted reproduction may have untreated or unresolved trauma from previous reproductive loss(es). For those who are experiencing secondary infertility, fertility counselors should inquire about possible emotional and/or medical traumas that may have occurred during labor, delivery or postpartum.

Perinatal Depression

One out of seven women meet diagnostic criteria for MDD during pregnancy and postpartum. The prevalence of perinatal depression is significantly higher among women from ethnic minority and marginalized communities [2]. Similar to GAD, symptoms of MDD, such as changes in appetite, sleep disturbances and loss of energy, mirror common pregnancy symptoms. Factors that are strongly linked to perinatal depression include consistent low self-esteem, difficulties accessing pleasure, substance use, poor compliance to medical recommendations and suicidal ideation.

Approximately 14% of perinatal women express suicidal ideation [9]. Women are more likely to die by suicide during pregnancy than postpartum. However, suicide is still one of the leading causes of maternal mortality during the postpartum period. Women who die by suicide during the perinatal period utilize more irreversible and violent methods when compared to non-perinatal women. Given that untreated and undertreated mental illness (including anxiety disorders) increase risk of perinatal suicidal ideation and acts, all perinatal persons should be asked about suicidal thoughts, intentions and plans.

In order to determine the level of psychological or psychiatric care that is appropriate for newly postpartum mothers with depression, it is important for mental health professionals to accurately decipher postpartum depression from "baby blues." Unlike postpartum depression, the symptoms of postpartum baby blues are mild, transient and resolve in response to increased support and self-care [2,3]. Symptoms typically peak within 4–5 days postpartum. Rapid hormonal fluctuations, lactation and fatigue are believed to contribute to this brief mood disturbance. While postpartum blues should not be pathologized, women exhibiting such symptoms should be assessed on an ongoing basis, as postpartum blues can progress into MDD. The factors that differentiate baby blues from postpartum depression are summarized in Table 23.2 [2,3].

Bipolar Disorder and Postpartum Psychosis

Approximately 1–2/1,000 childbearing women will experience postpartum psychosis [2,3]. The strongest predictors of postpartum psychosis are history of bipolar disorder and past episode(s) of postpartum psychosis. The overwhelmingly vast majority of women who develop postpartum psychosis have unrecognized or undertreated bipolar disorder, rather than a premorbid psychotic disorder. Some individuals with bipolar disorder or a previous episode of postpartum psychosis may choose to forego pregnancy and pursue gestational surrogacy in order to preserve their mental health postpartum. Symptoms of postpartum psychosis develop a few days to 4 weeks following childbirth. Individuals with postpartum psychosis experience decreased need for sleep, auditory or visual hallucinations, confusion, labile mood, elation, disorganized cognitive processes, bizarre behaviors, suicidal and infanticidal ideation/intent/plans. They perceive their suicidal and homicidal thoughts to be acceptable and ego-syntonic.

Women with postpartum psychosis often lack insight into their symptoms and have difficulties recognizing the marked changes in their behaviors and cognitions following childbirth. They may screen negative on self-report questionnaires assessing depression, anxiety or PTSD. Seeking corroborating information from the postpartum person's spouse, family members or close friends can help mental health professionals gain a better understanding of their patient's baseline mood, personality and functioning.

Table 23.2 Postpartum blues versus postpartum depression

	Postpartum blues	Postpartum depression
Prevalence	50–85%	10–15%
Course	Transient, symptoms taper off by 2–3 weeks postpartum	Symptoms persist for at least 2 weeks
Symptoms	Feeling overwhelmed, uncertain, irritable, mood swings, lonely	Consistent sadness, worthlessness, lowered self-esteem, hopelessness, lack of interest in baby, suicidal ideation
Functionality	Mother still able to care for child and, to some extent, herself	Symptoms interfere with ability to care for self and child
Recovery	Spontaneous, for some, and with support, rest and good nutrition, baby blues resolve without professional psychological intervention(s)	Symptoms persist despite support, rest and nutrition

Postpartum psychosis can be life-threatening to mothers and their child(ren). It is a psychiatric emergency that necessitates an immediate evaluation by a psychiatrist and/or emergency medicine department. A medical assessment is typically conducted to rule out organic factors that may be causing onset of symptoms, such as neurological issues or infectious diseases. Psychiatric hospitalization is often required for women with postpartum psychosis.

It is widely recognized that psychiatric care during pregnancy serves as a strong protective factor against new onset or recurring postpartum psychosis. Fertility counselors can contribute to the prophylactic mental health care of women who are at high risk of postpartum psychosis, by assessing for possible bipolar or psychotic disorders among women undergoing assisted reproduction. By providing psychoeducation regarding PMADs and strongly recommending prenatal psychiatric intervention, fertility counselors can help save the lives of prenatal women and their children. The clinical differences and similarities between postpartum psychosis and OCD are presented in Table 23.3 [2,3,6].

Infertility and Perinatal Mood and Anxiety Disorders

Fertility counselors often care for patients who recently experienced a miscarriage. Following pregnancy loss, hormones such as human chorionic gonadotropin (HCG), estrogen and progesterone rapidly decrease. While endocrine disturbances that occur following the birth of a full-term are more pronounced and impactful, hormonal fluctuations associated with miscarriage can impact mood and anxiety [10]. As a result, fertility counselors should consider post-miscarriage hormonal shifts as an aspect of the psychological fallout of pregnancy loss.

Parents from all backgrounds are susceptible to PMADs, even those who highly desired having a child. However, due to the intentional nature of growing the family, parents who have undergone fertility treatments may believe that they cannot openly discuss any emotional challenges they face during the perinatal period and, instead, should only hold gratitude for becoming pregnant or having a live birth. Patients who utilized assisted reproductive technology (ART) may find comfort in hearing that they are just as entitled to have mixed or difficult feelings during the perinatal period as those who conceive spontaneously. Fertility counselors can help patients explore the concept of simultaneously holding several complex (and possibly contradictory) emotions.

Table 23.3 Postpartum obsessive compulsive disorder versus psychosis: differences and similarities

	Postpartum OCD	Postpartum psychosis
Cognitions	Intrusive thoughts that cause distress (Ego-dystonic)	Aggressive thoughts without guilt or distress (ego-syntonic)
Prominent symptoms	Anxiety, hypervigilance Fear of acting on or thinking the thoughts Avoidance or rituals	Confusion, agitation Hearing voices or seeing things that other people do not see Bizarre or violent behaviors
Mental health history	Personal or familial history of anxiety No history of violence, over controlled	Personal or familial history of bipolar disorder History of impulsivity, violence
Screening	May screen negative for depression	May screen negative for depression

Prevalence rates of perinatal depression and anxiety do not significantly differ between women with medically assisted conception versus spontaneous conception [11]. In fact, women who conceive with medical assistance may be less likely to develop PMADs than women with unplanned pregnancies. While research suggests that infertility and ART are not independent risks for PMADs [12,13], certain factors associated with but not specific to ART, such as multiparity, obstetrical complications (e.g. preterm birth, cesarean section, preeclampsia), reproductive traumas, strained relationship with intimate partner and idealization of parenting, can increase possibility of PMADs. The emotional burdens and stress associated with undergoing fertility treatments may also lead to the development or exacerbation of mental health issues, as parents enter the perinatal period. In order to gain a deeper understanding of patient's susceptibility to PMADS, fertility counselors should assess mental health history prior to and concurrent with fertility treatments.

Fertility counselors should also consider exploring ART's impacts on their patient's perspective and fantasies of pregnancy, birth and parenting [14]. These perspectives and expectations can influence postpartum adjustment. Fertility counselors can help patients explore expectations for birth, acknowledging the possibility of various interventions, and helping to restructure the goal of birth as a "healthy mother and healthy baby." Postpartum, mental health professionals often shift their focus to the parent–infant relationship. Grief related to expectations versus the realities associated with how pregnancy was achieved, childbirth and postpartum may also be a focus of treatment.

Research is lacking regarding the use of gamete donation and surrogacy in relation to PMADs. Data on general psychological adjustment suggests parents and families who have utilized third-party reproduction are psychologically well-adjusted [15]. While parenting at an advanced age, which is common among egg donor recipients, is not a recognized risk factor of PMADs in and of itself, the obstetrical complications associated with advanced maternal age (e.g., cesarean section, preterm birth, blood pressure issues, preeclampsia, gestational diabetes) may increase risk of PMADs [16].

Fertility counselors have the opportunity to provide education on PMADs and explore patients' expectations of pregnancy and parenthood following successful ART. Normalization of mixed feelings and disappointment related to parenthood, despite one's reproductive history, is an important aspect of counseling: *What did I get myself into? I don't have time to sleep or see friends. This isn't what I imagined!* Some patients may also benefit from discussing ways to cultivate or re-build social support networks as they enter the perinatal period.

Breastfeeding

Studies examining the relationship between breastfeeding and postpartum mental health have yielded inconsistent results. While some research suggests that breastfeeding may protect against postpartum depression, other studies show that women who do not intend to breastfeed are at higher risk of postpartum depression when they go on to breastfeed [17]. Also, women who plan to exclusively breastfeed and, subsequently, experience difficulty with latching and milk production, may have worse mental health outcomes than women who are receptive to using formula. The beneficial mental health effects of breastfeeding can vary across time and appear to be strongest at 8 weeks postpartum and weaken thereafter [18]. Overall, the effects of breastfeeding on maternal depression are heterogeneous and impacted by breastfeeding intentions and women's expectations versus lived-experiences with breastfeeding. Unmet expectations can strongly influence the experience, implications and adjustment to breastfeeding.

Breastfeeding may come easily for some, but certain physiological factors can impact the breastfeeding experience. Little research exists regarding IVF and breastfeeding outcomes. Yet, there are many contributing biological and psychological factors that may lead to difficulties breastfeeding after infertility. With an increased risk of cesarean section, premature delivery and multiple births in IVF, challenges around breastfeeding may arise. While IVF can increase rates of depression, anxiety and decreased confidence, if the birthing and breastfeeding experiences also do not go as envisioned, it can increase parenting insecurities. A lack of self-confidence can make the breastfeeding experience more challenging and possibly lead to a cessation of breastfeeding [19].

While breastfeeding is considered to be a choice, it is important to acknowledge the immense psychological pressure placed on mothers to exclusively breastfeed. The acceptability of formula feeding may be influenced by many factors (demographic, socioeconomic, cultural, etc.), yet the overwhelming societal and medical messaging appears to support the "breast is best" movement. From the moment an infant is born in a hospital, medical professionals may assume that breastfeeding is desired and place the baby to mother's breast directly after delivery. Consulting a doctor and lactation consultant is helpful in addressing any physical issues that may arise and help to improve confidence. However, every doctor and lactation consultant has varying views and opinions on breastfeeding. It may be useful to interview practitioners to find one who is open to supporting the mother in exploring their options. Some healthcare professionals may put an enormous amount of pressure on a mother to breastfeed, which may make the experience even harder. The use of family and social supports can also influence the breastfeeding experience due to varying views. The supports can help to normalize and problem solve around breastfeeding challenges, but they may also provide additional pressure and stress.

When possible, mental health professionals should initiate the conversation about breastfeeding while the mother is pregnant. Psychotherapists can help patients explore the peer pressures, social stigmas and imaging that the mother might have been exposed to regarding breastfeeding. Mental health professionals can also help patients develop cognitive flexibility when it comes to the ways in which they feed their child. For example, some mothers breastfeed but also allow themselves and others to bottle-feed the baby. This may involve encouraging mothers to give themselves permission to stop breastfeeding. It is important for psychotherapists to provide education on the various feeding options that may be available to mothers, while also respecting patient autonomy.

The support provided to mothers to start or continue breastfeeding must be balanced with the psychological implications of doing so. The mental health of mothers can have a far greater impact on their infant than the presence or absence of breastmilk. Self-compassion and self-care are also ways to support a baby, such as acknowledging this is a time of transition, getting enough sleep, going for a walk and eating healthy meals. Should a mother decide that stopping breastfeeding is in her and her baby's best interest, gradual weaning may be important. Abrupt discontinuing breastfeeding may bring forth hormonal fluctuations that can increase anxiety and depression [19]. Addendum 23.1 provides a handout to review with a mother (including history of breastfeeding) to help her have a voice in the decision to breastfeed. Ensuring the health of mothers and their infants is not a one size fits all model, and breastfeeding does not always result in the healthiest outcomes. Fertility and perinatal mental health counselors may be the only professionals who encourage patients to explore alternatives to exclusively breastfeeding and acknowledge the positive benefits of supplementing.

Implications of Untreated Perinatal Mood and Anxiety Disorders

Women who do not receive appropriate treatment for PMADs often face adverse obstetrical, neonatal and parenting outcomes [2,7]. Untreated mental illness during pregnancy is associated with negative maternal health behaviors, such as inadequate or excessive weight gain, poor nutrition, reduced participation in prenatal visits and substance use [3,7]. Obstetrical complications including preeclampsia, low birth weight, preterm birth and miscarriage are also correlates of untreated PMADs.

Lack of appropriate treatment for perinatal mental illness can have intergenerational consequences. Longitudinal studies suggest that children born to mothers with uncontrolled/poorly controlled PMADs experience disorganized sleep patterns, high levels of reactivity, difficulties regulating attention and increased impulsivity [2]. These neurodevelopmental issues not only negatively impact the offspring but can also impair maternal–fetal bonding. Parental behaviors, such as psychological unavailability (associated with depression) or hyperreactivity (linked to anxiety) can also

239

hinder the emotional bond between parents and their infant [6]. It is important to note, however, that not every person with PMADs experiences significant difficulties parenting. It should not be assumed that PMADs automatically leads to poor parenting practices.

Screening and Monitoring Instruments

Routine screening of PMADs is recommended by public health organizations across the globe, such as the World Health Organization, International Marcé Society for Perinatal Mental Health and the American College of Obstetricians and Gynecologists. Self-report measures validated for use during pregnancy and postpartum, such as the Edinburgh Postnatal Depression Scale (EPDS, available in 18 languages)[3] and Patient Health Questionnaire-9 (PHQ-9, translated into 49 languages)[4] are available for free on the Internet and screen for perinatal depression. Healthcare professionals should pay close attention to questions related to suicidality. If suicidal ideation is endorsed, further assessment of the perinatal person's mental health should be conducted in order to determine risk factors, mitigating variables, acuity and the appropriate level of mental health care. Anxiety can be screened via GAD-7, which has been validated for use within the perinatal population (translated into 9 languages).[5]

There are no known self-report questionnaires specifically for perinatal OCD, PTSD and bipolar disorder. Perinatal mental health professionals often utilize the Yale-Brown Obsessive Compulsive Scale (Y-BOCS)[6] to assess for perinatal OCD and gain a better understanding of obsessional content [6]. To help differentiate bipolar from unipolar depression, the Composite International Diagnostic Interview 3.0 (CIDI-3)[7] can be utilized. The Posttraumatic Stress Disorder Checklist for DSM-V (PCL-5)[8] is a useful tool when screening for perinatal PTSD as well as PTSD related to other traumas [8].

It is important to note that mental health diagnoses cannot be made by simply relying on the results of self-report questionnaires. However, perinatal individuals who screen positive for any mental illness should be referred to psychological and/or psychiatric follow-up care. Motivated by the desire to have healthy relationships with their offspring, some parents are particularly willing to engage in psychotherapy during the perinatal period [2].

While specialty perinatal mental health care is not available or affordable in various parts of the world, medical clinicians, such as Ob/Gyns and primary care professionals may have access to psychiatry helplines that provide nonpsychiatrist prescribers with guidance in prescribing psychotropic medications for PMADs. For example, Postpartum Support International (PSI)[9] provides a no-cost psychiatric consult line to medical professionals. Patients who are more interested in non-pharmacological interventions can also be directed to PSI, which provides free support groups and individual perinatal mental health treatment in 53 countries.

Diversity Considerations

Understanding cultural considerations that might be impacting the perinatal experience is another element to assess for when working with a patient. Being mindful of various cultures, races, ethnicities, sexual orientation and gender identification can address other needs. Difficulties finding culturally sensitive care through fertility treatment, pregnancy and delivery can be a barrier to receiving care and a risk factor for PMADs among diverse populations. Healthcare professionals should be aware of the pictures displayed, staff members represented and language utilized in their clinic.

Individuals from chronically disadvantaged and underserved populations (e.g., black, indigenous and people of color (BIPOC)) may be more likely to have experienced traumatic events in their lives due to societal oppression and stigma. History of trauma, in turn, increases the likelihood of experiencing PMADs. Disenfranchised populations may be less likely to seek mental health treatment due to oppression. Because the evaluating screening tools may not accurately screen low-income, women of color (or other ethnic minorities), research suggests that it may be prudent to have a lower cut-off score for women of color [20].

---

[3] The EPDS can be found at: www.fresno.ucsf.edu/pediatrics/downloads/edinburghscale.pdf.

[4] The PHQ-9 can be found at www.apa.org/depression-guideline/patient-health-questionnaire.pdf.

[5] The GAD-7 can be found at www.uofmhealth.org/health-library/abn2339.

[6] The Y-BOCS can be found at https://iocdf.org/wp-content/uploads/2016/04/04-Y-BOCS-w-Checklist.pdf.

[7] The CIDI-3 can be found at: www.oregon.gov/oha/HPA/DSI-Pharmacy/SiteAssets/Lists/MHCAGRecs/EditForm/OHA-3670B-MHCAG-Final.pdf.

[8] The PCL-5 can be found at www.ptsd.va.gov/professional/assessment/adult-sr/ptsd-checklist.asp#obtain.

[9] More information about PSI can be found at www.postpartum.net.

Military families are another subgroup who may be at increased risk for developing PMADs. The reasons are multiple, as they face unique stressors added to the transition to parenthood. These families may deal with relocation, future and past deployments (including any related trauma), inadequate support systems (e.g., being away from families of origin) and additional job stressors. Accessing mental health services may be perceived as putting the career of oneself or spouse at risk, real or not.

Fertility and perinatal counselors serve patients from diverse populations. The utilization of appropriate and inclusive language is an imperative aspect to quality patient care. Respectful inquiry into patients' preferences regarding their gender pronouns, sexual orientation and relationship status among other demographics is one step toward increasing inclusivity in fertility counseling.

LGBTQ+ Persons

Given the various ways that conception can occur (e.g., polyamorous relationships, use of gestational surrogate and reciprocal IVF), it is important for healthcare professionals to recognize the unique and complicated social, medical and legal contexts that LGBTQ+ individuals often navigate when attempting to build and/or expand their families. The LGBTQ+ community continues to face discrimination and experiences higher rates of nonperinatal mental health diagnoses than heterosexual, cisgender individuals [21]. This community may have less social support due to strained relationships with family members or friends who do not support LGBTQ+ individuals. Limited social support and history of mental illness (prior to the perinatal period) increase risk of PMADs. Protective factors against PMADs among the LGBTQ+ community include the intentionality of pregnancies and relatively equal division of child-care labor among partners [22].

Research examining the psychological experiences of pregnancy and postpartum among transgender and gender-nonconforming individuals is limited. Pregnancy and postpartum tend to be profoundly gendered life events. Transgender and gender-nonconforming individuals must navigate a heteronormative healthcare system in addition to societal rigidity and expectations regarding pregnancy and parenting.

Paternal Postpartum Adjustment

Men's mental health can be overlooked, particularly during infertility treatments, pregnancy and the first year postpartum. Fathers and noncarrying parents may feel marginalized by fertility and perinatal health services. The carrying partner is the focus of treatment and the noncarrying partner often does not need to be present for appointments.

Social practices associated with pregnancy and postpartum are, also, typically focused on maternal and infant well-being. For example, mothers and carrying parents are screened for depression at Ob/Gyn and pediatrician visits. There is no systematic mental health screening in place for fathers and noncarrying parents. More research is needed to better understand the development and course of paternal PMADs, as the current data is limited and focused on the experiences of heterosexual men.

Maternal depression is the strongest predictor of paternal postpartum depression or anxiety [23]. Mothers suffering with PMADs may not be able to engage in adequate self-care and/or feel limited in their ability to care for their infant. Fathers can then be left with levels of responsibility that they perceive to be overwhelming. Other factors that may increase risk of paternal depression and anxiety include history of depression, relationship discord, limited sexual intimacy with partner, brief paternity leave and fewer opportunities to bond with their infant. The quality and sensitivity of parenting provided to children during the first year of life can have persistent and long-lasting effects on child development [23].

In order to manage maternal PMADs, it is critical to include fathers and noncarrying parents in mental health treatments for PMADs. The focus of postpartum couple's psychotherapy is often on the optimization of the child's development via development of better communication skills between partners. Loving and supporting one another will have a positive impact on the baby. Having concrete and useable tools can help to aid this communication.

Evidence-based Treatments

Given the biopsychosocial dimensions of PMADs, multidisciplinary management of symptoms is recommended [3]. Consistent communication between obstetrics specialists and perinatal mental health professionals is imperative given the bidirectional relationship between PMADs and obstetrical complications. In addition, building professional relationships with and providing referrals to allied health professionals can optimize perinatal mental health outcomes.

Psychiatrists and psychiatric nurse mental health practitioners often play an important, sometimes vital, role in the treatment of PMADs. Nonprescribing mental health clinicians should discuss the availability of evidence-based, pharmacological mental health treatments with perinatal patients. A consult to psychiatry is particularly important when nonprescribing counselors are treating patients with moderate to severe or refractory perinatal mental illness [3]. An emerging treatment for moderately severe or severe postpartum depression is an IV-infused metabolite of progesterone named allopregnanolone [24]. This treatment is FDA-approved for postpartum depression but currently not covered by health insurance companies. Thus, it may not be an affordable treatment option for most patients.

In addition to incorporating allied professionals in the treatment plans of perinatal individuals, it is often helpful to invite the perinatal patient's loved ones to psychotherapy sessions (pending patient approval). Psychological distress experienced by perinatal individuals impacts the entire family unit [2]. As a result, perinatal psychotherapists must feel comfortable addressing the needs of several stakeholders during the perinatal period.

Providing education regarding the importance of sleep preservation is another hallmark of perinatal psychotherapy. After controlling for other risk factors, sleep deprivation increases depression and suicidal ideation among postpartum individuals [9]. Mental health clinicians frequently discuss nonpharmacological ways to maximize sleep continuity and improve sleep quality. Mothers are encouraged to take naps while their baby is sleeping. If the infant is agreeable to being bottle-fed, mothers are asked to alternate night feedings and diaper changes with their partner(s) and/or support person. When working with single parents, mental health professionals assess whether a trusted family member or, if financial resources allow, a night doula may be able to relieve the parent from some aspects of overnight infant care.

The United States Preventive Services Task Force recommends the use of evidence-based psychotherapies for the prevention and treatment of perinatal depression. The vast majority of perinatal women prefer psychotherapy as first-line treatment of their psychological symptoms, as they perceive it to be a safer treatment option that psychotropic medications during pregnancy and lactation [6,25].

With respect to evidence-based psychotherapies studied among the perinatal population, interpersonal psychotherapy (IPT) has been found to be effective in preventing and treating perinatal depression and anxiety

disorders [25]. Focusing on interpersonal functioning during the perinatal period is particularly important given that low social support and marital discord are associated with depression and anxiety among pregnant and postpartum women [2,3]. Improved interpersonal skills can help perinatal individuals mobilize their support system in a more effective manner.

The emphasis on role transitions and grief in IPT is also relevant, considering the identity and lifestyle modifications that occur during the transition to parenthood. Perinatal women treated with IPT report increased relationship satisfaction, improved social adjustment and decreased worrying [25]. It is also effective in treating perinatal depression among mothers from low socio-economic and ethnic minority backgrounds [26].

Cognitive–behavioral therapy (CBT) is another well-researched, evidence-based treatment for perinatal depression and anxiety disorders [27]. The focus of CBT on generating practical solutions to current issues is helpful for the acute psychotherapeutic needs of the perinatal population. Relaxation training aspects of CBT, such as diaphragmatic breathing and progressive muscle relation, can be utilized to reduce autonomic arousal and improve sleep patterns among parents with anxiety and depression. Cognitive restructuring is also a powerful therapeutic technique when working with the perinatal population. Common cognitive distortions experienced by perinatal individuals, including those who have undergone assisted reproduction, are listed in Table 23.4.

Regardless of the specific modality of psychotherapy utilized to care for individuals with PMADs, treatment is administered in a compassionate and flexible manner. Perinatal patients are typically not penalized for occasionally arriving late to their psychotherapy sessions or providing short-term cancellations. Parents may be tardy or cancel psychotherapy due to, for example, an ultrasound appointment running long, parents wanting to speak with certain NICU professionals and difficulties estimating the amount of time it takes to get an infant ready for an outing. Perinatal patients may also not be able to engage in or complete psychotherapy home practice assignments due to the time-consuming stressors associated with being pregnant and having a child. Postpartum, the infant is invited to join the perinatal person's psychotherapy sessions and can be very helpful in the transition to parenthood by facilitating interventions which assist in bonding and attachment. Pumping and feeding are also welcomed.

Table 23.4 Perinatal cognitive distortions

Cognitive distortion	Example
Fortune telling: Predicting that something negative/unwanted will certainly happen (without concrete evidence).	"I will miscarry again." "I will not have a healthy pregnancy."
All-or-nothing thinking: Seeing things as only right or wrong, good or bad, perfect or terrible.	"Unless I do every single thing that the pediatrician suggests, I'm a bad mom." "Only breastfed babies are healthy."
Filtering: Focusing only on the negative aspects of a situation and ignoring anything positive or good.	"My baby cries all of the time." "My doctor says that everything is going well, but my belly is measuring on the small side of normal. Something must be wrong with my baby."
Overgeneralization: Thinking that a negative situation is part of a constant cycle of bad things that will always happen. One negative event is seen as a never-ending pattern of defeat.	"The gestational carrier didn't call me back right away. She's not taking care of our pregnancy." "I didn't enjoy the first few days of motherhood so I likely won't enjoy being a mom for the rest of my life."
Catastrophizing: Believing that the worst-case scenario is the inevitable outcome of a situation and that you will not be able to cope.	"My baby will grow up to hate me because we used an egg donor. She won't love me." "The pain of childbirth is going to be unbearable. I won't be able to manage it."
Personalization: Seeing yourself as the cause of some negative external event	"My baby cries when I hold her because we used a donated embryo." "My baby has colic because I forgot to take my prenatal vitamin a few times."
Should statements: Telling yourself how you should, ought or need to act and/or feel.	"I worked really hard and paid a lot of money to have a baby. I should be really happy."

Conclusion

The therapeutic reach and influence of fertility counselors can extend well into their patients' pregnancy and postpartum experiences. Fertility counselors can help reduce the prevalence or severity of PMADs by providing evidence-based care to their patients prior to pregnancy. After reaching reproductive success, patients may benefit from exploring their expectations of pregnancy, labor/delivery and postpartum with their fertility counselors. Brief education about PMADs and referral sources (reproductive psychiatry, PSI, support groups, perinatal psychotherapists) can be disseminated to psychotherapy and nonpsychotherapy patients, such as those undergoing third-party reproduction consults and gestational surrogacy psychological screenings. While it takes a village to raise a child, it can also take a village of healthcare professionals to treat PMADs. Fertility counselors serve an important role in that village and the greater efforts to improve maternal mental health.

References

1. Long MM, Cramer RJ, Jenkins J, Bennington L, Paulson JF. A systematic review of interventions for healthcare professionals to improve screening and referral for perinatal mood and anxiety disorders. *Arch Womens Ment Health* 2019;22(1):25–36.

2. Accortt EE, Wong MS. It is time for routine screening for perinatal mood and anxiety disorders in obstetrics and gynecology settings. *Obstet Gynecol Survey* 2017;72 (9):553–568.

3. Paschetta E, Berrisford G, Coccia F, Whitmore J, Wood AG, Pretlove S, Ismail KM. Perinatal psychiatric disorders: an overview. *Am J Obstet Gynecol* 2014;210(6):501–509.

4. Mott SL, Schiller CE, Richards JG, O'Hara MW, Stuart S. Depression and anxiety among postpartum and adoptive mothers. *Arch Womens Ment Health* 2011;14(4):335–343.

5. Leach LS, Poyser C, Fairweather-Schmidt K. Maternal perinatal anxiety: a review of prevalence and correlates. *Clin Psychol* 2017;21(1):4–19.

6. Goodman JH, Watson GR, Stubbs B. Anxiety disorders in postpartum women: a systematic review and meta-analysis. *J Affect Disord* 2016;203:292–331.

7. Field T, Diego M, Hernandez-Reif M, et al. Comorbid depression and anxiety effects on pregnancy and neonatal outcome. *Infant Behav Dev* 2010;33(1):23–29.

8. Cirino NH, Knapp JM. Perinatal posttraumatic stress disorder: a review of risk factors, diagnosis, and treatment. *Obstet Gynecol Survey* 2019;74(6):369–376.

9. Orsolini L, Valchera A, Vecchiotti R, et al. Suicide during perinatal period: epidemiology, risk factors, and clinical correlates. *Front Psychiatry* 2016;7:138.

10. MGH Center for Women's Health. Can Women Suffer from Postpartum Depression after Miscarriage? Published 2006.

Available at: https://womensmentalhealth.org/posts/postpartum-depression-miscarriage [last accessed June 22, 2022].

11. Capuzzi E, Caldiroli A, Ciscato V, et al. Is in vitro fertilization (IVF) associated with perinatal affective disorders? *J Affect Disord* 2020;**277**:271–278.

12. Gressier F, Letranchant A, Cazas O, Sutter-Dallay AL, Falissard B, Hardy P. Post-partum depressive symptoms and medically assisted conception: a systematic review and meta-analysis. *Hum Reprod* 2015;**30**(11):2575–2586.

13. Barber GA, Steinberg JR. Examining the association between infertility, pregnancy intention, and postpartum depression. *Fertil Steril* 2020;**114**(3):e447–448.

14. Barnes M, Roiko A, Reed R, Williams C, Willcocks K. Outcomes for women and infants following assisted conception: implications for perinatal education, care, and support. *J Perinat Educ* 2012;**21**(1):18–23.

15. Blake L, Jadva V, Golombok S. Parent psychological adjustment, donor conception and disclosure: a follow-up over 10 years. *Hum Reprod* 2014;**29**(11):2487–2496.

16. Bouzaglou A, Aubenas I, Abbou H, et al. Pregnancy at 40 years old and above: obstetrical, fetal, and neonatal outcomes. Is age an independent risk factor for those complications? *Front Med* 2020;7:208.

17. Pope CJ, Mazmanian D. Breastfeeding and postpartum depression: an overview and methodological recommendations for future research. *Depress Res Treat* 2016;**2016**:4765310.

18. Borra C, Iacovou M, Sevilla A. New evidence on breastfeeding and postpartum depression: the importance of understanding women's intentions. *Matern Child Health J* 2015;**19**(4):897–907.

19. Ystrom E. Breastfeeding cessation and symptoms of anxiety and depression: a longitudinal cohort study. *BMC Pregnancy Childbirth* 2012;**12**(1):36.

20. Tandon SD, Cluxton-Keller F, Leis J, Le HN, Perry DF. A comparison of three screening tools to identify perinatal depression among low-income African American women. *J Affect Disord* 2012;**136**(1–2):155–162.

21. Williams AJ, Jones C, Arcelus J, Townsend E, Lazaridou A, Michail M. A systematic review and meta-analysis of victimisation and mental health prevalence among LGBTQ+ young people with experiences of self-harm and suicide. *PLoS One* 2021;**16**(1):e0245268.

22. Ross LE. Perinatal mental health in lesbian mothers: a review of potential risk and protective factors. *Women Health* 2005;**41**(3):113–128.

23. Howard LM, Khalifeh H. Perinatal mental health: a review of progress and challenges. *World Psychiatry* 2020;**19**(3):313–327.

24. Scarff JR. Use of brexanolone for postpartum depression. *Innov Clin Neurosci* 2019;**16**(11–12):32–35.

25. Sockol LE. A systematic review and meta-analysis of interpersonal psychotherapy for perinatal women. *J Affect Disord* 2018;**232**:316–328.

26. Nillni YI, Mehralizade A, Mayer L, Milanovic S. Treatment of depression, anxiety, and trauma-related disorders during the perinatal period: a systematic review. *Clin Psychol Rev* 2018;**66**:136–148.

27. Marchesi C, Ossola P, Amerio A, Daniel BD, Tonna M, De Panfilis C. Clinical management of perinatal anxiety disorders: a systematic review. *J Affect Disord* 2016;**190**:543–550.

Chapter 24

Walking the Tightrope: The Pregnant Fertility Counselor

Laura Covington and Janet Jaffe

Introduction

We've all been there. A patient asks *the* loaded question: *Do you have any kids?* This deceptively simple question is complicated for the fertility counselor; in the therapy room, we are addressing not just the patient's reproductive story, but our own as well [1]. Where we are in our own fertility journey, and how much, if, or when to disclose, is at the forefront of this chapter. Regardless of one's theoretical orientation or philosophy, self-disclosure (or not) has consequences in the therapeutic alliance, and is an essential element of psychotherapy and counseling.

This chapter delves into the unique situation of the pregnant fertility counselor and her work with reproductive patients.[1] If the counselor is or becomes pregnant during the course of treatment, it necessitates some sort of disclosure; each patient will react in his or her own unique way. For a patient who is struggling with infertility, has had a pregnancy loss or may be pregnant herself, knowing that the therapist is pregnant can trigger intense reactions. Although responses may be different, underlying themes of competition, jealousy and abandonment can emerge. Similarly, feelings about a pregnant therapist may unlock a history of trauma or previous unresolved relationships in the patient, typically arising from the family of origin. Complicated dynamics and emotions are likely to unfold, and what may look seemingly benign on the surface may tap into deep areas of pain and loss. Assessing the feelings that disclosure arouses in the client (transference), and likewise what it evokes in the therapist (countertransference) is the work we do. Complicating matters even further are the unexpected events that can occur during pregnancy: mandatory bed rest or an early

delivery, for example. These unforeseen circumstances may rob the therapist of being able to thoroughly process their patient's emotional response. How we, as fertility counselors, help our patients manage their feelings, as well as how we manage our own, can enhance, deepen and intensify the therapeutic experience [2].

This chapter is not a "how-to" lesson in self-disclosure, but rather an exploration of the potential gains and/or pitfalls that a shared experience can have on therapy. We investigate reactions from the patient's point of view, as well as that of the therapist, and analyze both the positive and negative implications that pregnancy and/or pregnancy loss can have on treatment. For example, should the fertility counselor disclose to her patient that she too is trying? Should a fertility counselor who is in the midst of her own treatment even see reproductive patients? What if one or the other becomes pregnant, or has a pregnancy loss? What if they are both working with the same doctor or clinic? These questions must be thoughtfully and compassionately addressed. Additionally, we will look at the postpartum period, including the fourth (the first 3 months postpartum) and fifth (returning back to work) trimesters, addressing the unique vulnerability of the therapist leaving for and returning from parental leave, and its impact on therapy. The transference/countertransference that is evoked when the therapist returns to work can bring challenging, but oftentimes rich, material to the therapeutic setting.

The Patient's Point of View

When reproductive patients enter therapy, most are traumatized and grief-stricken, having spent months if not years working to create a family. Their individual stories, circumstances and emotional reactions will differ, but the underlying need for understanding and support is universal. Knowing that the counselor they have sought out specializes in reproductive therapy may feel like a relief: *I have finally found someone who gets it.* It is also natural for patients to be curious about their fertility counselor's

---

[1] The chapter may use feminine terms such as "she" and "her" to describe the fertility counselor and a person trying to achieve pregnancy for purposes of simplicity, but we recognize that gender is a continuum and not all who are pregnant identify as female. Also, it should be noted that while this chapter focuses on the pregnant therapist, the issues raised pertain to all pregnant reproductive medical staff treating infertility patients.

personal life: *Why have they have chosen this particular specialty?* While patients are expected to reveal everything about their lives and inner emotions, by nature of the relationship, therapists reveal little to nothing about themselves, that is, until the therapist becomes pregnant. What the patient might think about the fertility counselor prior to her pregnancy may completely shift; the unconscious arousal of feelings toward the therapist may be fraught with enormous chaos and internal disorder.

Transference

Simply put, transference entails the shifting of patients' unconscious feelings, usually about important people (i.e., their parents), onto the counselor. The patient's beliefs of who the therapist is and how she feels are projected onto her from the patient's inner world. For example, the patient may need to see the counselor as all-knowing or perfect, because of his/her own feelings of inadequacy. Although originally seen as a component of psychoanalytic theory and practice, the idea of transference occurs across the board regardless of theoretical orientation [1].

Patients' perceptions of the clinician vary, depending on how curious they are about the therapist's personal life, and how "real" the therapist is. Living in a time of easy access to online information makes privacy nearly impossible, and many patients may know more about us than we realize. At the same time, many patients don't want to know information about their therapist. Too much knowledge of the therapist's personal life can feel overwhelming; it can flood the patient with multiple reactions and feelings. It can disrupt treatment by introducing unwanted elements into the therapy and disturb the patient's transference [3]. The therapist's pregnancy, impossible to keep hidden, is such a case. How the patient views the counselor's pregnancy may be a cause for a great deal of emotional confusion and internal disarray. While this is true for the general therapy client, it is magnified for patients who are dealing with reproductive issues.

Pregnancy Disclosure: Who, What, Where, When, Why and How?

Ideally when disclosing personal information, the therapeutic purpose and how the patient might interpret the information should be analyzed [4]. Will the information be useful to treatment, or will it be disruptive? With a pregnancy, however, disclosure is clearly necessary.

Patients will observe the growing belly and/or the clinician will go on parental leave, directly impacting the treatment. Whether or not a patient has discussed their reproductive story, when considering the disclosure of a pregnancy, the patient's reproductive journey may become more pronounced, and the therapist's reproductive story consequently becomes a part of clinical work. No matter the therapist's theoretical orientation, the patient–therapist relationship is affected with pregnancy disclosure [5].

Both the fertility counselor and the patient may feel off balance with this disclosure, and it may be difficult to deal with the disruption to treatment. Not only does the fertility counselor need to cope with the patient's reaction to the disclosure, she must manage her own feelings as well. Positive and negative impact can come from the therapist's pregnancy. It may allow an opportunity for growth as the patient can engage in a deeper understanding of his/her own reproductive story, the grief and the trauma they have experienced. Alternatively, patients may feel the clinician no longer understands them, or they may feel like a burden to the therapist. Because the therapist becomes more real in the self-disclosure, she may experience her own worries around bringing a piece of her life into the room.

Many considerations go into sharing the pregnancy with the patient: when to tell during the pregnancy; what words to use; how much to share; when to tell during the session; how will the patient react; what to do if the patient asks about the pregnancy before the counselor is ready to disclose, etc. How is pregnancy disclosure different in individual therapy versus couple's therapy, or in a group therapy setting? What is the difference in impact when doing in-person work versus telemedicine? There is not a one size fits all model, and it will vary from patient-to-patient based on his/her clinical needs. Table 24.1 offers a summary of questions and suggestions as to how to deal with the unavoidable disclosure of the pregnant counselor.

There may be contexts where a patient may not be able to observe a therapist's growing belly: in telehealth where only the shoulders and head are shown; a father or noncarrying partner; use of a gestational carrier; or adoption. This may make the therapist wonder if disclosure is actually necessary and change the timeline of when to disclose. The question becomes though, if the pregnancy is not disclosed, how does the therapist handle explaining leave? Some level of self-disclosure will become relevant, and a "medical" leave versus "parental" leave may continue to make a patient wonder and worry about the therapist.

Table 24.1 The who, what, where, when, why and how of pregnancy disclosure

Who?	Who should I tell? Which patients should I share with first?	You may consider sharing with a patient with a harder journey early on, as a way to allow them to process their feelings. It may be clinically more risky if they find out from someone else. On the flip side, you may feel more secure with other patients who may take the news positively; it can give you the opportunity to get comfortable with the words. The bottom line: treat each disclosure individually; each patient will have different needs.
What?	What information do I share? Should I share my journey to becoming pregnant? Should I share when I am due?	Does the client need to know this piece of information to make informed consent about his or her treatment? You may choose to share more broad information than specific. Make sure to share information that is clinically relevant (if you know when you will be on parental leave and for how long; who will be covering for you). However, you also don't need to have everything figured out (i.e., parental leave) when you share.
Where?	Where in the session do I share? Should I tell the patient at the beginning of the session to get it out of the way? Should I postpone it until the end so they can process it on their own? Do I wait for an opportunity to bring it up based on what the patient is sharing during the session?	Generally, it can be helpful to give some time for the patient to respond within the session and acknowledge that it will continue to be addressed in future meetings.
When?	When do I tell the patient during the pregnancy? Should I tell them in the first trimester? Should I wait until a certain point in the pregnancy? Should I wait until I am showing? Should I wait until the patient asks?	Doing telemedicine versus in-person therapy may influence this timing. Generally, between 16–22 weeks is standard, but there may be various needs for the patient and the clinician that necessitate disclosing earlier or later.
Why?	Why does the patient need to know? What value does this bring to the work we are doing?	This question is key. Always ask oneself what is helpful for this particular patient and what is not. Use this as a guide for making decisions around disclosure.
How?	How do I tell my patient? What words should I use? What information do they need to know? What do I say if someone asks before I have shared?	Honesty is best. Be brief and to the point. Use simple, direct and empathetic language. Acknowledge that feelings may arise for the patient, and offer a space to explore those feelings. You may also share that this is hard to share knowing the patient's journey. Address a plan of how this will impact the patient (i.e., parental leave).

How Patients React to the News

When the fertility counselor announces her pregnancy, the therapeutic alliance will change. For some patients, feelings may overtly intensify, for others they may be less obvious. Some patients may act out in atypical ways. The fertility counselor needs to be aware of her patients' heightened affect, while contending with her own feelings of having her personal life exposed. The clothing worn may make the pregnancy and growing belly more or less visible in the room. The patient may ask more when the baby's presence is more noticed and the belly becomes bigger. With a pregnancy disclosure, a patient may be more likely to ask personal questions, a fertility counselor may be quicker to respond or a patient may offer gifts which the fertility counselor accepts [6].

The psychological issues that get triggered for a reproductive patient are numerous and significant. Their initial reasons for entering therapy (needing support, working through grief, managing relationships) can suddenly feel threatened. What had been a safe place for the patient to share their thoughts and feelings may turn into a landscape pocked with potential landmines. There can occur a split in the shared intimacy of the therapeutic alliance, with the patient feeling isolated and alone. Resentment and betrayal may overpower therapeutic gains. While patients may be able to avoid stroller parades at the mall, or going to baby showers, they find themselves in yet another setting where they can't avoid a pregnancy. This is not what they had signed up for!

Patients may express their rage, but often they find themselves tiptoeing around feelings of anger and loss: *Will the counselor abandon me because she has someone else to care for? Will she continue to understand and have empathy for my situation? Is it still okay to talk about how alone I feel because everyone around me is pregnant or has a baby? Has my therapist "gone to the dark side"?* Patients may wonder how long the therapist has been holding onto the knowledge of her pregnancy, how long it's been kept secret, and feel deceived. Feelings of jealousy (*Why isn't it me?*), feelings of competition (*The counselor is perfect; I am not*) and feelings of aloneness (*I really don't belong anywhere*) can haunt the patient. To top it off, she may feel that she's not allowed to bring any of this up in therapy.

The amount of resentment a patient may harbor toward her counselor may not always be conscious. She may regress in ways that simulate issues of abandonment from her family of origin. Not only jealous of the baby, she may want to *be* the baby. In other words, the patient may fear the therapist will no longer be available as a source of comfort and care, and a kind of sibling rivalry between the patient and the therapist's baby may emerge. There may be deep sorrow and grief for having to share the therapist with the baby. The patient may also hold such intense bitterness that she entertains a hope for the pregnancy to fail; consequently, she may feel overwhelmingly guilty for having these thoughts. These emotions are so painful and taboo that there may be a collusion of sorts by both therapist and patient to avoid exploring them.

The patient may suddenly present as more needy (telephoning more, asking for additional appointments) in an effort to stay special or important to the therapist. The pregnancy not only represents psychological issues of abandonment, but a real disruption to the therapeutic alliance during parental leave [7]. While the therapist may attempt to bring up this hostility, it could overwhelm the patient and backfire. If the dynamics between the patient and therapist cannot be identified and processed, the patient may act out in anger by spacing out sessions, delaying payment, arriving late to sessions, missing appointments or quitting therapy completely [8].

It goes without saying that each therapeutic dyad will differ, with reactions as diverse as clients. While some patients may react negatively, others may express their need to take care of the pregnant therapist or bring her gifts. For example, if the patient has had issues of pregnancy loss, she may want to protect her therapist by avoiding the very topic she needs to address. Another patient may want to offer advice, especially if she is already a parent, relating to the therapist more as a friend or advisor. Roles may feel like they are shifting. Normal therapeutic boundaries may loosen as both therapist and client explore new, unfamiliar territory. The exposure of the therapist's private life may elicit more personal questions (i.e., what is her marital status, sexual orientation, difficulty with conception, etc.). How much the therapist decides to share should be determined based on the needs of the client and the transference material that is evoked. In other words, while questions may seem straightforward, what patients are really asking may be deeper than immediately meets the eye [7]. For example, if a patient asks when the baby is due, she may be really wondering at what point the therapist's focus will change from the patient to the baby, bringing up feelings of jealousy or abandonment. What is critical to remember is that the disequilibrium caused by the shifting of roles not only affects the patient but, as will be addressed in the next section, can be quite uncomfortable for the fertility counselor as well.

The Fertility Counselor's Perspective

Therapists want to help others on their emotional journeys and provide a healing space. Fertility counselors in particular want to help people grow their family, and deeply understand the emotional struggle when this path is marked by trauma and loss. Many of us specialize in this field because of our own fertility experiences. We are acutely aware that sharing our own pregnancy may bring up hurt, anger, sadness and jealousy for the very patient we are trying to help manage these feelings. Sensitive to our client's feelings, we might feel fear, guilt and anxiety in sharing our pregnancy. Knowing that this will likely cause pain to our clients (we have now become one of *those* women), our successful pregnancy brings us joy, setting the stage for our own internal conflict and vulnerability.

Countertransference

Countertransference is a counselor's reactions and feelings towards the patient. Countertransference is inevitable; it can be problematic when ignored, unnoticed and unexamined. When unattended to, countertransference can lead to excessive and/or inappropriate self-disclosure in treatment [9]: *Am I finding more of a need to share information with the patient?* Once realized, self-awareness of the countertransference can address the influence of the counselor's internal experience: *Where are these feelings coming from? What feelings are about my own issues? What might be highlighting something the patient is feeling? How might these feelings be influencing the therapeutic process, and how can I utilize them for the benefit of the patient?*

The pregnant fertility counselor needs to be acutely aware not only of the patient's reactions but also to how she is feeling as well. She will likely experience anxiety about sharing her news and wonder how the patient is going to react: *Will the patient want to leave therapy? What if the patient thinks I no longer understand? Will this be triggering for my patient? Should I share my journey with the patient?* There may be a desire to convince the patient that the fertility counselor does, in fact, understand and empathize with her even though she is pregnant. In an effort to try to protect the patient, the fertility counselor may have been holding onto her information for some time, trying to assess just the right time to discuss her pregnancy. It can be emotionally draining to share something so private with patient after patient.

Disclosure of the pregnancy may elicit other questions about the clinician, such as her relationship status and/or sexual orientation. Feeling imposed upon, the fertility counselor may begin to feel some resentment. For example, the reproductive patient may become more needy, phoning more or requesting additional sessions, while the therapist may feel less tolerant and more easily fatigued by the patient's struggles or feel a need to overly accommodate the patient's behaviors. As will be discussed later, patients may act out their transference, arriving late or cancelling altogether, instilling anger in the counselor. The constant tug of war between guilt for having a pregnancy while the patient is struggling to conceive, and wanting to help the patient while experiencing her own joy of becoming a mother, is mentally exhausting.

Because physical and psychological changes occur for the fertility counselor throughout the course of her pregnancy, she may become distracted and need to focus on herself rather than solely on the patient. With the third entity (the pregnant belly and baby) now fully acknowledged in the room, the ability to compartmentalize this part of her personal life is no longer possible. Feeling more vulnerable and less present, her pregnancy may cause decreased ability to empathize with the patient as a way of protecting herself. Feelings of "pregnancy brain" muddled with the countertransference related to the self-disclosure may also cause the clinician to feel "less with it" and capable. The reality of needing to schedule doctor's appointments for herself may cause further disruption, straining the therapeutic alliance even more.

The reality is that every patient will have a different reaction; there is no one right way to disclose or cope with the fertility counselor's pregnancy. Sometimes those patients we worry about the most do the best with it, and those we think will be okay have a deeper reaction than anticipated. Because it can be an acutely draining process, this is a time for knowing one's own boundaries and obtaining regular consultation. For example, it may be best to say "no" to a new fertility patient or to someone who has had a recent pregnancy loss, not only for the interest of the patient, but also for one's own well-being. Self-care is always called for, but especially during a pregnancy.

Different therapeutic contexts may also bring up various reactions and necessitate individual ways of disclosing. Addressing the needs of someone seeking a one-time consultation will be very different than patients in ongoing or long-term therapy, where the therapeutic relationship will be impacted by the therapist's pregnancy. When a pregnancy is visible, it may be helpful to share with a patient on the phone prior to meeting for the first time so they can make a decision about whether to see the fertility counselor and won't be surprised upon meeting. Challenges arise in telehealth, where there is less intimacy and more ability to hide behind a screen for both a clinician and a client. This requires less "real life" interactions and is easier for a patient to conceal feelings or disappear. When working with couples, the therapist may be dealing with managing two different responses. Similarly, group therapy, particularly support groups where people might be dropping in and out, might be a harder place to process individuals' feelings. With a group, there may be reasons to let members know prior to the group meeting, or it may be better addressed in the group. There are many unique considerations without one perfect answer.

The Fourth Trimester: Parental Leave

The pregnant counselor must assess and contemplate her and her family's needs for when the baby arrives and what the "fourth trimester" and beyond will look like. This concept of the "fourth trimester" is considered to be approximately the first 3 months postpartum, as a new parent continues to care for the baby who requires around the clock care and feedings. The postpartum body continues to go through significant and real hormonal, biological and psychological changes. The adjustment to being a new mother continues as there begins to be separation from the baby.

Considerations to determine the appropriate parental leave are multiple, and individual circumstances will influence this. The therapist needs to address self-care versus patient care, financial consideration and redefining roles (professional versus parent): *What do I need to do to care for patients? What do I need to do to care for myself, my baby, and my family? How much time can I take off from a financial perspective? How do I see my role as a professional after having a baby?*

Parental leave is a time when the fertility counselor needs to take care of herself and relinquish patient care to others. Putting in the needed supports for the patient while on leave is crucial, yet may bring up various feelings for the therapist: *But we have a long history of working together, so this other therapist won't be able to help my patient. My patient needs me and won't see someone else. What if my patient likes this other counselor more than me? I have already let my patient down by being pregnant so I need to be there for her.* Letting go can be difficult and the feelings it evokes need to be examined; supervision can help.

Boundaries are important when considering the length of parental leave and attending to the countertransference that might be occurring. The fertility counselor might feel guilt over leaving her patients behind, especially those who may be in the middle of treatment or have had a recent loss. Thus, the counselor may decide to shorten her parental leave to address the needs of her patient.

There is a need to weigh patient care but also consider the self in this scenario. This discussion around leave may also be an opportunity to model helpful boundaries of self-care and frame it with the patient in such a way. Consulting a colleague and supervision can help with working through these thoughts and worries to also be able to care for one's self.

Implications for Therapy

Pregnancy, in general, is a time of enormous physical and emotional growth. Indeed, it has been referred to as the third-individuation phase, akin to the psychological development of separation and individuation in infancy and adolescence [10]. It has been seen as a definitive transition to adult status [11], and described as a time in which a woman "… renegotiates her personal and professional identity, adjusts relationships and develops a new relation with her baby …" [8, p. 51]. The pregnant fertility counselor can no longer maintain her professional stance of neutrality as her private life is exposed.

She may be distracted by her own needs and want to focus her attention on herself and her newborn. It is no wonder then that a pregnant therapist may feel off-balance as she negotiates her new role, both inside and outside of the office.

At the same time, the therapeutic guidelines for the reproductive patient are also disrupted. While a counselor's pregnancy will have an impact on the general therapy population, for reproductive patients her pregnancy can feel devastating. Is this still a safe place to address the pain and trauma of infertility if the therapist is so obviously fertile? Is it okay for a patient to address her stillbirth, or will she feel the need to protect her therapist from worry? While there is a risk that therapy will be thrown off course with patients' newfound feelings of resentment, betrayal or competition, there is also the possibility that the fertility counselor's pregnancy will introduce an element of true human vulnerability, and the potential for deeper connection and understanding [3]. What is clear is that both members of the therapeutic dyad are simultaneously experiencing complex psychological changes, some that may augment therapy, and some that may not.

In a study exploring the client–therapist relationship with pregnant therapists, Wolfe noted a continuum of therapist responses to their clients' boundary violations [6]. Depending on the client and their particular issues, therapist reactions ranged from needing to firmly reassert boundaries to finding that their pregnancy provided an opportunity for an enhanced therapeutic alliance. There was a shared susceptibility: the times when the therapist opened up about her personal life allowed clients to be more willing to do so as well. Pregnant therapists should maintain sensitivity to their patient's needs on a case-by-case basis, while simultaneously paying attention to their own needs [6].

Dynamics in the therapeutic dyad can get even more complicated, however, if the fertility counselor and patient are both trying to conceive at the same time; it's a perfect set-up for issues of competition. Assuming that the *fertility counselor wins the race*, the patient, who likely did not even know the fertility counselor was trying, may feel a sense of loss and betrayal. The pregnant fertility counselor may feel guarded and self-protective, and not able to cope with her patient's negativity. On the other hand, if the *patient wins*, how does the fertility counselor feel? Can she manage her own internal struggles while remaining present for the joy the patient is experiencing? What if one or the other has a pregnancy loss? Or what if the practitioner and patient differ in their moral or ethical views? For example, if a patient adamantly dismisses use of donor technology, how does the clinician cope if she has arrived at egg donation as the best option for herself? The fertility counselor, having the patient's insights, knows about *the race* before the patient, and this unequal playing field may make it harder for the fertility counselor, particularly if the patient *wins*. Even if the patient and the fertility counselor *tie*, there are other competition dynamics that can continue to arise throughout the pregnancy, birth and postpartum.

Unfortunately, there is no formula for handling these complex situations, except for the clinician to monitor her own emotions and respond with sensitivity to the patient. The rule of thumb for practitioners is always to promote what is best for the patient (beneficence) and to do no harm (nonmaleficence) [12]. This may mean the clinician does not see reproductive patients while in the midst of her own reproductive situation, refers an established patient to someone else or seeks consultation to maintain a clear view of the patient's needs.

While the related chapter in the *Case Studies* volume will highlight many of these dilemmas, having an illustration of how the therapeutic alliance can be enhanced is worth noting. For example, the patient who has sought therapy to help with infertility may be able to work through feelings of isolation with the pregnant fertility counselor. With compassion, the clinician may decide to disclose her pregnancy early on to this patient rather than wait until it becomes obvious. Knowing how hard it might be to receive this news, the fertility counselor can model her own anxiety in divulging her pregnancy, and recognize that this will not be easy – for either of them. Acknowledging the pain, the fertility counselor can encourage and accept the range of her patient's feelings. Many times, new transference issues emerge as the patient may see the fertility counselor in a different light. When considering having children, it is normal for instance, to reflect on one's own upbringing and the evolution of one's own reproductive story [1]. Both therapist and patient are likely thinking about their childhood and relationships with parents. Here again, the shared experience can improve the therapeutic bond. With the therapist focused on her own growth and development, she can encourage the patient to process and learn from interpersonal relationships in her life as well. Being able to manage these intense interactions in the confines and safety of the therapeutic space enables the patient to cope better within a child-centric world.

The Fifth Trimester: Returning Back to Work

While most of what we have discussed has focused on the pregnancy, the "fifth trimester," [13] or the return to work by the fertility counselor, now also Mom, is less talked about but has equally important clinical value to consider [7]. First, the relationship of the patient and clinician after a hiatus needs to be addressed with the added concerns of what the pregnancy, absence and return means for the patient. Second, the fertility counselor is going through her own changes and trying to figure out her professional identity as a new mom. The "return to normal" working life takes time and becomes a new and different kind of normal. The plan for establishing work–parenting balance may need to be continually renegotiated with the lived-experience of being back in the office, and it may not be how originally envisioned.

If the fertility counselor is breastfeeding, this can add an additional strain on the return. The fertility counselor will need to schedule around the pumping sessions and finding a place to store the pump supplies and milk. Pumping can add a layer of stress, making the workday longer, and serve as a reminder of separation from the baby. Even if the fertility counselor is working remotely, she will have to schedule around the baby's feeding schedule. Patients and therapist alike may react to hearing a baby cry, even while working in another room.

While pregnancy is a hard experience for the reproductive patient, especially as the pregnant belly is visible, when the fertility counselor returns from parental leave, no longer pregnant, there is an awareness that it is now back to just the patient and the fertility counselor in the room. During parental leave, reproductive patients may experience abandonment issues, feeling that another person is leaving them behind and moving onto another phase of life. So many feelings may come up for the patient; in some ways it may be more difficult to address them when there is less visibility around the issue at hand. Yet, for others, they may now feel more comfortable discussing their feelings around the pregnancy, feeling less worry about the fertility counselor's well-being. The patient may have questions or curiosities about the baby, having been a part of this more personal piece of the therapist's journey, which may make her "more real."

While things may have been on hold for the patient–therapist relationship, the patient and the therapist's lives continued separately, and the reuniting may need to jump into whatever may be going on for the patient. The patient might be in the middle of a treatment cycle or had a recent loss. The crisis can make it harder to revisit and discuss what the leave meant for the patient. This processing of the pregnancy and leave is something that may come up right away or take some time to establish normalcy before the patient is willing and able to discuss.

Patients may also have beliefs and feelings about the fertility counselor's parental leave, whether the fertility counselor is taking off "too much time" or judgments around her return to work and not staying home with her baby. Managing what comes up for the patient after returning to work can cause countertransference. Maybe the fertility counselor wants to take off more time but financially is unable to, or wants to return back to work sooner but doesn't have the supports at home or in the community to do so.

The postpartum fertility counselor may return back to work before she fully feels back to herself, dealing with fluctuating hormones leveling out, sleepless nights and nursing a baby. This transition back to the office may bring up various feelings: *What if the patient asks about the baby? What if the patient doesn't ask about the baby?* In some ways, it may feel like a relief to no longer have to discuss (or not discuss, i.e., the elephant in the room) the pregnancy, as the baby is no longer in the room. On the other side, the patient *knows* the therapist had a baby, so how much does she continue to share about the baby, if a patient asks or doesn't ask.

The fertility counselor's focus and energies will have shifted when she returns from parental leave. The arrival of a baby, and the role of new parenting provide novel insights and perspective [7]. The fertility counselor now has experienced and knows pregnancy, pregnancy symptoms, birth, the hormonal shifts after delivery and parenting. These topics may have been discussed with patients pre-pregnancy but now knowing and experiencing them may allow the fertility counselor to explore ideas about pregnancy and parenting in a different way. There is lived empathy of the days after a baby is born, where the baby is feeding every couple of hours, and now wonders where the adage "sleeping like a baby" derived. Yet, this new parenting perspective may also keep the fertility counselor less neutral, as her own experience guides and informs the work.

This shift of parent–therapist role (good parent versus good professional) can be draining. The therapist may be tired, distracted and struggling with guilt of leaving a baby behind. She may still be in a "fog" similar to "pregnancy brain," making her feel ineffective both as a therapist and parent.

If a patient asks about the baby, the fertility counselor may once again feel vulnerable, crossing a boundary into her personal life. While she may be happy when the patient expresses interest, she may also wonder: *Why does she want to know?* This ongoing self-disclosure can be challenging: *When do I just answer my patient's question, and when do I explore where the question is coming from?*

The fertility counselor's reproductive story now is a part of the therapy. She is perceived as "more real" and a sexual being. There may be important themes to discuss about the fertility counselor's reproductive story in relationship to the patient's reproductive story. Countertransference is again important to consider in the return back to work, as one considers how much to share about the baby. Because this piece of information, that would otherwise be unknown to a patient, is out in the open, it can become a more delicate line to dance in the sharing of information.

Summary

Pregnancy disclosure for the fertility counselor adds a complex dynamic to the therapy process and makes for more present transference and countertransference interactions. There is no one-size-fits-all model for sharing. This disclosure will depend on the patient, the fertility counselor and the clinical setting. It is hard to predict how a patient will react to the news and what it will mean for the ongoing therapy relationship. Having support and a place to process the disclosure is useful for managing and understanding both the patient's transference and the therapist's countertransference.

References

1. Jaffe J, Diamond MO. *Reproductive Trauma: Psychotherapy with Infertility and Pregnancy Loss Clients.* Washington, DC: American Psychological Association, 2011.

2. Hayes JA, Gelso CJ, Hummel AM. Managing countertransference. *Psychother* 2011;**48**;88–97.

3. Ulman KH. Unwitting exposure of the therapist: transferential and countertransferential dilemmas. *J Psychother Pract Res* 2001;**10**:14–22.

4. Derlaga VJ, Berg JH, Eds. *Self-disclosure: Theory, Research, and Therapy.* New York, NY: Kluwer Academic/ Plenum, 1987.

5. Fallon AE, Brabender V. *Awaiting the Therapist's Baby: A Guide for Expectant Parent-practitioners.* New York, NY: Psychology Press, 2003.

6. Wolfe E. The therapist's pregnancy and the client–therapist relationship: an exploratory study. Doctoral Dissertation, Smith College School for Social Work, 2013.

7. Waldman J. New mother/old therapist: transference and countertransference challenges in the return to work. *Am J Psychother* 2003;**57**(1):52–63.

8. Schmidt FMD, Fiorini GP, Ramires VRR. Psychoanalytic psychotherapy and the pregnant therapist: a literature review. *Res Psychother* 2015;**18**(2):50–61.

9. Redlinger-Grosse K. Countertransference: making the unconscious conscious. In Veach PM, LeRoy BS, Callanan NP, Eds. *Genetic Counseling Practice*. Hoboken, NJ: Wiley Blackwell, 2020, 153–175.

10. Colarusso CA. The third individuation: the effect of biological parenthood on separation-individuation processes in adulthood. *Psyc Study Child* 1990;**45**:179–194.

11. Arnett JJ. Emerging Adulthood. *Amer Psych* 2000;**55**:469–480.

12. Peterson ZD. More than a mirror: the ethics of therapist self-disclosure. *Psychother* 2002;**39**:21–31.

13. Brody LS. The fifth trimester: the working mom's guide to style, sanity, and big success after baby. Broadway, NY: Doubleday Books, 2017.

Chapter 25

Telemental Health in Fertility Counseling

Lauren Magalnick Berman and Carrie Eichberg

March 13, 2020: Two days after the World Health Organization declared COVID-19 a pandemic, the United States (US) declared COVID-19 a national emergency. Countries all over the world were similarly affected. Life as we once knew it changed. Within short shrift of that announcement, many businesses shuttered their doors and most fertility practices went into hiatus. No one knew whether it was safe to work from office buildings and many mental health professionals experimented for the first time with telemental health (TMH).

The COVID-19 pandemic temporarily shifted the way we practice fertility counseling and many of these changes are likely to be permanent. How many of our clients will prefer to continue taking 1 hour out of their day to meet with us via videoconference rather than fighting traffic, finding parking and making excuses to their employers? How many more clients will be able to access us remotely from small towns 2 or 3 hours from large fertility centers rather than blocking off an entire day to drive into a large, metropolitan area? Or to see an expert reproductive mental health professional rather than a local professional who has little or no training in this highly specialized field? How many couples or individuals will prefer to use TMH rather than make expensive travel plans to conduct preliminary meetings of multiparty, gestational carrier or donor arrangements?

The COVID-19 pandemic brought grief, tragedy, business failures, mental health crises, economic hardship, loneliness, loss and long-term illness among other challenging and unfathomable consequences. But is also brought creative approaches to the practice of reproductive mental health along with greater access to care. This is a powerful and positive outcome of those terrible times. It behooves us to examine these remote approaches and to incorporate whatever we can to benefit clients and the field as a whole.

Telemental health via videoconference came to fruition coincident with technological advances which made it relatively simple to deliver video access to personal computers and devices. However, other forms of TMH have been available and practiced since the advent of the telephone. Zara Greenbaum, in a 2020 article, shares research in TMH dating back to 1960 [1]. TMH includes all types of remote administration of client/professional interface including, but not limited to, telephone, text, email, chat, fax and artificial intelligence platforms.

Modern video technologies have been studied since as early as 2008 with forays into delivering mental health services into prisons and military outposts [2]. The central question posed by many of these studies and the question that hovers to this day is whether TMH delivery of services is equivalent to or as effective as in-person delivery of services.

Advantages and Disadvantages

We learned so many lessons during the very challenging pandemic years. We have, hands down, discovered many of the benefits of TMH. For patients and clients, TMH has been a major vehicle for access to care. During the pandemic years and beyond, clients were able to meet with their fertility counselors in a physically safe manner without increasing their risk of COVID-19. At the same time, clients no longer have to juggle taking 2 hours away from work for their mental health appointment. In cities like New York, Atlanta, Los Angeles, London and San Francisco, traffic can be miserable and drive times unpredictable. In many cities, parking arrangements are complicated and expensive. TMH has taken the burden of commuting off the shoulders of the client. Additionally, for people who live in rural communities, TMH reduces the need to travel 2 or 3 hours to a major metropolitan center in order to access the highly specialized care that we offer. For clients with social anxiety, disabilities or other conditions that may create barriers to physical presence in a professional office, TMH opens access to care. For clients who have small children or school-age children, TMH provides the benefit of reducing the need for added childcare hours or making it less worrisome

The addenda referred to in this chapter are available for download at www.cambridge.org/covington-clinical-guide

about being home in time to meet the bus. TMH makes it possible to maintain crucial continuity of care, even during the most trying of times, like a pandemic.

For fertility counselors, TMH has had its advantages as well. TMH makes it possible to provide services when it is inconvenient, untenable or impossible to work from one's professional office. The COVID-19 pandemic provides a case study in TMH advantages. Except for during the beginning of the pandemic, when most of the fertility clinics were closed, TMH allowed fertility counselors to continue practicing without interruption during a true national emergency. It offers the ability to provide services from flexible locations and enables clients to access services in locations that are convenient to them. During the pandemic, many fertility counselors moved further than commuting distance away from their physical offices or gave up offices altogether. These changes improved counselors' quality of life and potentially reduced expenses.

Furthermore, TMH "invites" us into our clients' homes and offices. We might meet our clients' pets, spouses or children, giving us a more contextual portrait of our clients' lives and personalities. For fertility counselors, TMH provides potential solutions for the challenges of multiparty, multilocation, third-party arrangements such as known donors and gestational surrogacy arrangements.

There are also pitfalls and challenges to the adoption of TMH in clinical practice. In fact, studies show that while clients find TMH to be just as helpful or satisfying as in-person meetings, practitioners tend to find it less so [3].

Prior to the pandemic, most mental health professionals lacked specific training in TMH and its requisite technology [4]. Training opportunities in TMH began to expand in the 2010s and multiplied in 2020. A great many are now offered directly through mental health professional associations. However, it is unclear as to how many practitioners have taken any training in TMH. Furthermore, many practitioners report that the technology itself remains a significant challenge. Internet connections are sometimes interrupted or pixilated. Mental health professionals (MHP) have some control over their own Internet quality. However, the quality of both the technological and the human connection in TMH might also depend on the patient's Internet connection quality. Sometimes the onus is on mental health professionals to be technology problem-solvers; for many, this is uncomfortable. Additionally, clients might join their TMH appointments from a smartphone rather than a computer

screen. Does a smaller screen size or poor-quality Internet connection change the nature of the relationship between counselor and client? We are still uncertain about what impact the quality of the "picture" might have on the therapeutic meeting and, surely, this will be studied in the future. For MHPs, who rely on nonverbal cues and body language to learn more about their clients, video meetings might obscure the ability to access this information.

Another disadvantage of providing services through TMH is the intensity of "face-to-face" connections made through videoconferencing. A 2021 study of psychotherapists who adopted TMH practice during the COVID-19 pandemic found that 70% of professionals surveyed reported that they found remote work to be more draining than the in-person contact they were accustomed to pre-pandemic [5]. Indeed, "Zoom fatigue" has become a validated phenomenon, most recently studied by Jeremy Bailenson and his colleagues at the Stanford Virtual Human Interaction Laboratory [6]. Bailenson isolated four factors which seem to underlie Zoom fatigue. First, is the unnatural way that people make eye contact when engaged in teleconferences. Viewing faces in a larger than normal size can invade one's natural personal space meter and create an internal stress response. Another factor is having one's own face in view staring back. Bailenson describes this as like having someone follow you around all day with a mirror. For many people, this contributes to fatigue. A third factor is that videoconferencing is a sedentary activity. Therapists are accustomed to sitting for long periods of time but also shifting positions and getting up between sessions. TMH demands that we do not move or shift positions and this can make us more fatigued at the end of the day. The final factor is that videoconferencing demands that we learn new ways to project and interpret nonverbal cues: this can stress us.

Clearly, there are advantages and disadvantages to the TMH format. TMH is here to stay and it is likely that most MHPs will work within a hybrid format in the future [5].

Definitions

Telemental health includes a wide range of service modalities beyond videoconferencing and it is likely that these services will only expand as technology progresses. Telephone therapy predates videoconferencing by many years. Texting or emailing with clients is also considered to be TMH. Furthermore, Internet platforms and technology startups are now offering therapy by chat or text. There are also many apps which provide psychoeducation and features of cognitive-behavioral therapy in an asynchronous fashion to assist clients with anxiety management and coping skills between therapy sessions. There are even technology companies that are experimenting with artificial intelligence responses to common questions that arise in therapy. For the purposes of this chapter, the focus will be on TMH via videoconferencing.

Applicability of Telemental Health to Fertility and Implications Counseling

Telemental health lends itself well to many aspects of fertility counseling. The fertility journey is a physically taxing and an emotionally challenging process. Patients describe treatment as an emotional roller coaster, one in which periods of hope can be followed by periods of despair. The longer treatment persists, the more draining and depleting it becomes. Access to care during waiting periods is recommended [7].

Fertility patients are often required to take considerable time off from work for multiple visits to their physician's office. One of the primary goals of fertility counseling is to reduce the suffering of the patient. TMH can reduce the burden on patients by offering services with minimal need to carve out additional time-off from work, school and home responsibilities. Recent studies have found that psychotherapists and patients notice few barriers to forming and maintaining therapeutic relationships in TMH [8,9]. Patients and therapists surveyed in these studies also report their TMH treatment to be effective.

In many ways, teletherapy is no different from in-person psychotherapy or counseling. Teletherapy involves a connection or relationship between the therapist and the client or clients.

The therapist comes to the relationship with the promise of expertise, privacy, confidentiality and an empathic presence. Expertise and an empathic presence are easily achieved through remote technologies [3]. However, privacy and confidentiality are wholly dependent on where the client and therapist are sitting during the session. A typical therapy office provides a safe, comforting and quiet place. Many therapists build out their office space with added soundproofing in order to ensure clients that their private musings will not be overheard. There are no interruptions in a typical, in-person therapy hour. Phones are turned off and, often "Do Not Disturb" signs are posted. For in-person sessions, clients

are often comforted by returning to a familiar space week after week. Because this familiar space creates a sense of security, clients may be jarred by changes in the therapy setting. Some clients even report feeling discomforted by changes in decor or the therapist's hair style. The "sacred" therapy space can be lost in teletherapy. Therefore, teletherapy requires therapists to re-create as much of this sacred space as possible.

When TMH sessions are conducted from the therapist's home to the client's home, therapists must consider the background of their images and try to create the impression of a therapy office. Some therapists have thoughtfully designed home offices and some videoconferencing platforms allow the background to be manipulated. Conducting TMH sessions from a therapist's bathroom or bedroom may project too much of a sense of familiarity and might detract from professionalism. With TMH, a therapist can travel or go to a vacation home but still continue practicing. Similar to changes in décor, changes in location/video background can have an impact on a client's sense of safety and security. They may impact the therapy. Further, when practicing from home, there are often interruptions which might include pets, family members and merchandise deliveries. These interruptions can also impact the client's sense of safety, privacy and confidentiality as well as the perception of therapeutic boundaries [10].

To some extent, the therapist can control Internet connection quality, background image and the creation of a quiet space on one side of the videoconference. However, the therapist has little or no control of where the client sits. Although the client is watching the therapist, who can sit in a thoughtfully designed environment, the client may be sitting in a space that is ill-suited to psychotherapy or counseling. Anecdotal reports from therapists find TMH clients sitting in restrooms, bedrooms, public buildings, automobiles and even coffee shops. There are also considerations about clients using office computer equipment and networks. Some companies monitor their employees' computers and their Internet use. A client's discovery of employer monitoring of a therapy session can create problems and issues beyond what is brought to therapy. Furthermore, office spaces are often not soundproofed and considerations must be made about coworkers overhearing the conversation. Counselors need to consider what effect this potential loss of confidentiality and privacy might have on the client and on the therapeutic relationship.

Telemental health also requires different processes for informed consent. Informed consent is not simply a document that clients sign, but a process for informing clients of the potential risks of engaging in a certain treatment. For in-person therapy, informed consent occurs within the first visit. Information about the purpose of the session, limitations of confidentiality and releases are explained. Informed consent for TMH is more complicated and additional consents are recommended. The American Psychological Association ([11], p. 795) recommends that:

Psychologists strive to obtain and document informed consent that specifically addresses the unique concerns related to the telepsychology services they provide. When doing so, psychologists are cognizant of the applicable laws and regulations, as well as organizational requirements that govern informed consent in this area.

One of the complications of TMH consent is that, as soon as clients join the videoconference, they are vulnerable to certain risks. Videoconferencing platforms can be hacked. Clients must be informed of the risks of TMH before joining the call [12]. Table 25.1 describes issues that need to be addressed in a TMH informed consent document. These issues include an authorization for electronic transmission, qualitative differences in the interaction, information about technology failures and an alert to security concerns.

One additional precaution should be noted. TMH gives therapists the opportunity to reach clients who are situated far from the therapist's home community. Therapists are typically familiar with hospitals, psychiatrists and emergency services within their home

Table 25.1 Checklist for telemental health informed consent

Authorization of electronic transmission of mental health information.

Agreement to use own equipment, not an employer's.

Agreement not to video record, take photographs or screenshots.

Statement that there are interpersonal and emotional differences from in-person services, including distortion.

Statement that technology can fail, transmission can be unclear and platforms can be hacked.

Information about local emergency options and request for emergency support numbers.

Statement that there is a greater risk of confidentiality, security risks and data security breaches.

Notification that billing (and reports) reflect that session was conducted via videoconference.

Notification that failure of technology has potential to impact the relationship

communities. Remote TMH, particularly for clients who suffer from personality disorders or who are in crisis, may require therapists to have knowledge of these resources.

Evaluating Donors and Gestational Carriers

Telemental health can be used to evaluate donors and gestational carriers but it carries certain risks. MHPs are trained to attend to both the content of clients' verbalizations as well as their nonverbal behaviors. Videoconferencing reveals only the client's face. Therefore, we can observe a client's facial expressions but no other body language. We cannot see whether the client has an anxious leg bounce or whether she is picking at her nails. We miss the way a client strides into the office and we cannot see her posture. We cannot smell alcohol or cigarettes on the client's breath. We do not see tattoos or injuries. We cannot observe the condition or style of her clothing. Because a couple must artificially squeeze into the frame by sitting close together, we cannot detect whether a couple would naturally sit in close proximity to each other or further apart. We cannot note whether the client's spouse reaches out for her hand or elbows her under the table. When a client is physically present in our offices, we collect a plethora of significant information that enables us to better interpret content from the clinical interview and results of psychological testing. Videoconference assessments deprive the clinician of this valuable information.

On the other hand, TMH reduces the burden of travel for the gestational carrier or donor candidate as well as the financial burden on intended parents. Additionally, videoconferencing offers opportunities to observe the gestational carrier or donor within their own home. With videoconferencing, the clinician has the opportunity to observe housekeeping standards, décor, pets and living conditions. While in-person assessment is considered best practice for donors and carrier evaluation, there are extenuating circumstances under which in-person interviews are not possible. Where videoconference is deemed to be the best option for a particular donor or carrier, the rationale for this should be noted in the report and measures should be taken to gather additional information about the client's living circumstances.

Special Considerations in Psychological Testing

American Society for Reproductive Medicine (ASRM) Guidelines strongly recommend that psychological testing is used for evaluation of gestational carriers, gamete donors and, where appropriate, intended parents [13]. The standardized, psychological testing instruments that are most often used in these evaluations are the Personality Assessment Inventory (PAI) and versions of the Minnesota Multiphasic Personality Inventory (MMPI-2, MMPI-2-RF or MMPI-3). Fertility counselors and other MHPs rely on standardized testing because these instruments have norms which enable professionals to compare the testing subject to others. Considerable data is collected to create these norms for precise interpretation and tests have undergone rigorous construct validation. Some clinicians also use projective testing such as the Thematic Apperception Test or the Rorschach [14]. The administration and interpretation of psychological testing instruments requires specialized training, including graduate level courses on psychological assessment and training specific to the test being administered [15]. These assessment instruments have been developed, normed and validated using in-person administration with a standardized protocol and standardized procedures. Since validation of these tests is based on statistical analyses and standardized instructions and procedures, the validity of these instruments under nonstandard procedures (i.e., remotely) has not been firmly established. We do not currently know whether a divergence from standard administration will be defensible in a court of law.

Psychological testing includes the development of some type of rapport prior to administration. It is unclear whether meeting via videoconference rather than in-person impacts rapport. Tests are interpreted through the lens of the clinical interview. When we are missing behavioral cues we may also be missing the texture for interpretation. Further, testing may also be sensitive to camera angle, screen size, setting and technology glitches [16]. A 2005 study by Grady and Melcer found that socially anxious people tend to underreport anxiety during remote assessments [17]. This study suggests that setting can skew the results of the administration. Other issues that might impact testing results are distractions, technology glitches, computer notifications and accessibility to Internet searches during testing.

Test security is another significant issue for remote administration. Testing validity is partially related to the confidentiality of test content. If testing items were somehow shared, this might compromise the power and validity of the test. In a remotely administered psychological assessment, the possibility exists for the client to take screen shots of test items or share them via email. This

is one reason for the recommendation that remote administrations be monitored by the MHP or a trained proctor. Virtual monitoring should include identity verification and, where possible, multiple screens.

American Psychological Association guidelines for TMH [11] suggest that psychologists must fully consider these issues when contemplating the remote use of instruments that were validated for in-person assessment. Until such time as research establishes that assessment instruments demonstrate sufficient validity in remote assessment, in-person assessment will remain as best practice. Luxton, Pruitt and Osenbach ([16], p. 30) conclude:

> ... it would be inappropriate practice to select, develop, or modify assessment instruments or alter procedures for remote administration without evidence of sufficient scientific validation or the appropriate disclosure of limitations. It is therefore necessary for practitioners to be familiar with what measures or techniques are supported by the scientific literature before using them.

If the clinician concludes that remote testing is necessary, the clinician must account for, explain and document the reasons. When the test is administered remotely, the report must reflect this and include an explanation for divergence from standard (that is, in-person) administration. Remote assessment should be monitored.

Legal Considerations and Ethical Issues in Telemental Health

All MHP associations have their own sets of ethical codes and within the past 10 years, these associations have included codes specific to TMH. The codes from the different professions are quite similar to one another but all ethical codes address issues of informed consent, access to care, cultural competency, confidentiality and best interests of clients.

It is important to note that TMH is not always the best modality for all clients. The most important question to ask for ethical practice is *Whom does it serve?* That is, does remote administration simply convenience the clinician or does it also benefit the client? Clearly, safety issues supersede all other concerns. During such extraordinary times as the COVID-19 pandemic, it was clearly in the best interest of clients to use TMH in order to minimize risks of disease transmission. But, in normal times, clinicians need to continually ask themselves this question before choosing TMH for any client: *Whom does the modality benefit?* And *Why use this technology with this patient?* Eric Harris and Jeffrey Younggren ([18], p. 416) offer this advice:

> It is important to remember that if there is no advantage to providing remote services over in-person services, the risk-managing psychologist will choose in-person services, even if it means referring the prospective client to someone else.

It is valuable for each clinician to have an established process for ethical decision-making in TMH. All ethical decision-making begins with the ethical guidelines offered by MHP associations. Clinicians should be familiar with their own profession's guidelines.

Ethical guidelines in all MHPs require that professionals practice only within their spheres of expertise. While fertility counselors typically have undergone rigorous training in infertility, third-party reproduction and counseling techniques, most have not received specialized training in TMH. In order to develop competence in TMH required for ethical practice, specific TMH training should be taken.

Another ethical consideration highlighted in these documents is the importance of maintaining confidentiality of both client information and data. Ethical practice must include careful consideration about maintaining the client's privacy and data security. Using a videoconferencing platform that does not offer Health Insurance Portability and Accountability Act (HIPAA)-compliance might constitute an ethical violation. HIPAA-compliance is a process that includes not only, a secure videoconferencing platform, but also a Business Associate Agreement, a signed contract that specifies how private information (PHI) must be treated.

In the US, professional guidelines for the various MHPs include cautions about interjurisdictional practice. MHPs are typically licensed in the state where they reside. Some are also licensed in contiguous states or states where they once lived. It is important to understand that licensing laws also apply to the state where the client sits during the TMH session. If the fertility counselor is licensed in New York state and the client is sitting in New Jersey, then the counselor is actually practicing in New Jersey – even if the client is a resident of New York state. Unfortunately, professional licensing laws are like a patchwork quilt. One state's laws often do not align with laws from other states. For example, temporary psychology practice in Alabama requires that a psychologist register with the state, send proof of licensure in the home state and complete a form. Mississippi, a neighboring state, requires a Temporary Practice Certificate which is accompanied by a $100 fee and necessitates passing a test on Mississippi state law. Some states do not permit out-of-state telepractice at all. Other countries may differ in laws about privacy, confidentiality, licensing and informed consent.

In US-based cross-jurisdictional TMH, it is incumbent on fertility counselors to research the laws of the state where the client will be sitting prior to engaging in interjurisdictional practice. These include a familiarity with reporting requirements in the remote state. Federal HIPAA laws also need to be observed. Even if a fertility counselor is permitted to practice in another state, liability insurance may limit the professional from practicing. Additionally, the client's healthcare insurance may restrict the use of interstate TMH.

Nurses and psychologists in the US have the advantage of having multistate "compacts" to practice in multiple states. The nursing pact is called the Enhanced Nursing Licensure Compact (eNLC) and the Psychology compact is called PSYPACT. These compacts are agreements between state licensing boards to permit professionals licensed in states that are member of the compact to practice temporarily in other states that have joined the compact. Professionals who reside in eNLC or PSYPACT states can apply to participate in these programs: once accepted, these professionals can practice interjurisdictionally in member states without additional research or permissions. The Association of Social Work Boards is in process of developing an interstate compact and the American Counseling Association is currently in the exploration phase. These compacts will facilitate greater use of interjurisdictional TMH.

Ethical practice of TMH also requires that TMH is documented in the medical record, billing documents and any reports. The reasoning for using TMH in the particular case should also be noted. As already stated, informed consent should be specific to TMH and should include a discussion of the security risks.

The "How-Tos" and "How-Not-Tos" of Telemental Health

This chapter has outlined definitions of TMH and the advantages and risks of using it. This section is primer for setting up a TMH practice. The most important starting point is securing a HIPAA-compliant videoconferencing platform. In the US, deciding which platform to use will include queries on data security, potential for hacking and the existence of a Business Associate Agreement. In the United Kingdom (UK), the National Health Service publishes its own security standards for telehealth. Having a reliable Internet connection is crucial. Technology glitches can be disruptive to the session, rapport and the therapeutic relationship. An ethernet connection is the most reliable technology for videoconferencing. Size matters – at least when it comes to screens. Behavioral observations are more accurate when a computer monitor is used rather than a phone screen. Sound quality is also critical. Most computers have built-in microphones but these microphones may be insufficient unless the practitioner is quite close to the screen. Bluetooth headsets are useful as are external, conference-style microphones.

In order to ensure a professional presentation and for concern about client privacy and confidentiality, it is important for the fertility counselor to create a private, quiet place without external noise or distractions for the TMH session. Background programs, email applications and cell phones should be closed before the session. These programs can interfere with the Internet connection and create noise or distractions.

Having some kind of professional backdrop is very helpful. This means sitting in a place which projects "office" to your patient. A garage or bedroom backdrop might be quiet but unsettling. Some videoconferencing platforms allow the insertion of a professional-looking background.

Telemental health demands a close attention to facial and upper body appearance that in-person sessions do not. MHPs are not typically trained for televised appearances. There are also some helpful tricks tools. It is helpful to prop the computer up on a stack of books or platforms so that the camera lens is just above eye level. Tilting the camera lens down to eye level gives the counselor the ability to see the screen while making eye contact. Also, lighting has a significant impact on how the client sees and perceives the MHP. Using a lamp placed slightly behind and slightly to the side of the computer creates a professional image. Some practitioners are now using a studio light called a ring lamp (see Addendum 25.1).

Addressing certain administrative issues in advance of the session enables the flow of a TMH session. It is critical to gather information about where the client will be sitting during the session. Fertility patients often travel significant distances from remote states in order to consult with a particular physician or clinic. Physicians, in turn, refer to local fertility counselors with whom they are accustomed to working. Interjurisdictional restrictions and state licensing laws make it risky for fertility counselors who do not inquire about the client's locale prior to

the session. Informed consent documents specific to TMH should also be gathered prior to the session. TMH requires that the client's identity is confirmed through the presentation of a driver's license or other form of photo ID. This should be documented in the client record.

It is often helpful to provide TMH clients with an instruction sheet prior to the session (see Addendum 25.2). The instruction sheet can outline the following:

- The importance of having the session in a private location.
- Instructions for facilitating the highest quality connection.
- A request that clients make every effort to have adequate lighting so that they can be seen.
- Preparation for presenting photo identification.
- A request to not record the session or take screenshots.
- A notice that insurance may not cover the TMH session.
- A warning about using an employer's device or unsecured (nonprivate) networks.
- A notification that technology might fail or might distort the interaction.

Once the first call begins, it is helpful to create a plan with the client about what to do in case of a technology issue. It is sometimes helpful to have a client telephone number in the event of technology glitches. The telephone can be used, instead of the computer microphone, for continued conversation if the videoconference stops and starts. Table 25.2 provides a checklist for TMH practice.

Reflection and Summary

Telemental health is an exciting modality which offers significant benefits to clients and practitioners. It is convenient, inexpensive, easily accessible and effective. Without TMH, most clients would not have been able to access critical mental health care and fertility counseling during the COVID-19 pandemic. During those dark times, TMH bolstered the ability of fertility counselors to continue practicing without having to choose between the risk of a potentially fatal illness and the ability to provide necessary care. TMH enables clients who live far from fertility counselors to utilize these specialized services. It offers timesaving care for clients who are saddled with multiple physician appointments.

Telemental health requires significant changes from in-person practice and entails some risks and cautions. Licensing laws, insurance issues, technology failures,

Table 25.2 Checklist for provision of telemental health services

What service(s) do you plan to deliver? Psychotherapy, support, psychoeducation, supervision, evaluation?

In which state(s) are you licensed and in which state will the client sit during the session?

What are the state laws about TMH in the state where you are licensed *and* in the state where the client is sitting?

Have you reviewed your profession's ethical guidelines about TMH? If so, what do they say about the ethics of the service you want to offer?

Does your professional liability insurance cover your TMH practice? If so, under what conditions?

If you are planning to bill the insurance company, does your client's insurance plan cover remote or TMH treatment?

What videoconferencing platform are you using for TMH and does it qualify for HIPAA-compliance? What additional legwork do you need to do in order to be HIPAA-compliant when using this platform?

Have you received specialized training in TMH?

How competent are you with the technology platform you are using and with TMH, in general?

What is the quality of your Internet connection and how secure is it?

Have you assessed your client's competence with videoconferencing technology and his/her/their Internet quality?

What is your Plan B if the technology fails or freezes?

What advance instructions have you given your client in order to help him/her/them mimic the therapy office and maintain privacy?

Where will your client be sitting – Home? Work? An automobile?

What device will your client use – smartphone? tablet? laptop? – and how might this impact the session?

Are you in your office? If not, what precautions are you taking to ensure the client's privacy?

Have you created an informed consent addendum to specifically address TMH? If so, what is your process for advance notice of informed consent?

Have you explained the differences of receiving services via TMH versus in-person to your client?

Have you researched emergency resources in your client's locale and has your client provided you with emergency contacts?

Have you received specialized training in TMH?

Have you reviewed the pertinent literature/research that might justify your use of this modality?

Have you assessed the risks and benefits of providing TMH services for this particular client?

Have you informed the client that identity will need to be validated with photo ID?

privacy concerns and distortions in transmission all impact the quality and utility of TMH. There is a significant learning curve for fertility counselors to become proficient in TMH and its particular requirements and procedures. Specific training in TMH facilitates this learning and enables fertility counselors to practice effectively and ethically.

Telemental health is particularly useful for fertility counseling. It is of great utility for implications counseling for intended parents in gestational surrogacy gamete donation cases. It eases the scheduling burden on these clients in complicated, third-party reproduction counseling. TMH offers substantial convenience for evaluating gestational carriers and gamete donors. However, considerable caution is recommended when using TMH and teleassessment in these evaluations.

Telemental health is best used by professionals who approach this modality thoughtfully and who are knowledgeable about the practice, the ethics and the laws pertaining to it.

References

1. Greenbaum Z. How well is telepsychology working? Researchers are pinpointing what we know – and what we need to learn – about these treatment options. *Monit Psychol* 2020;**51**(5):46.

2. Morgan RD, Patrick AR, Magaletta PR. Does the use of telemental health alter the treatment experience? Inmates' perceptions of telemental health versus face-to-face treatment modalities. *J Consult Clin Psychol* 2008;**76** (1):158–162.

3. Jenkins-Guarnieri MA, Pruitt LD, Luxton DD, Johnson K. Patient perceptions of telemental health: systematic review of direct comparisons to in-person psychotherapeutic treatments. *Telemedicine and e-Health* 2015;**21**(8):652–660.

4. Topooco N, Riper H, Araya R, et al. Attitudes towards digital treatment for depression: a European stakeholder survey. *Internet Interventions* 2017;**8**:1–9.

5. Shklarski L, Abrams A, Bakst E. Navigating changes in the physical and psychological spaces of psychotherapists during Covid-19: when home becomes the office. *Pract Innov* 2021;**6**(1):55–56.

6. Bailenson JN. Nonverbal overload: a theoretical argument for the causes of Zoom fatigue. *Technology, Mind and Behavior* 2021;**2**(1) (online). https://doi.org/10.1037 /tmb0000030

7. Domar AD, Gross J, Rooney K, Boivin J. Exploratory randomized trial on the effect of a brief psychological intervention on emotions, quality of life, discontinuation, and pregnancy rates in in vitro fertilization patients. *Fertil Steril* 2015;**104**(7):440–451e7.

8. Aafes van Doorn K, Békés V, Prout TA. Grappling with our therapeutic relationship and professional self-doubt during COVID-19: will we use video therapy again?

Counselling Psychology Quarterly 2020 (online). https://doi.org/10.1080/09515070.2020.1773404

9. Békés V, Aafes-van Doorn K. Psychotherapists' attitudes toward online therapy during the COVID-19 pandemic. *J Psychother Integr* 2020;**30**(2):238–247. https://doi.org/10.1037/int0000214

10. Drum KB, Littleton HL. Therapeutic boundaries in telepsychology: unique issues and best practice recommendations. *Prof Psychol Res* 2014;**45**(5):309–315.

11. American Psychological Association. Guidelines for the practice of telepsychology. *Am Psychologist* 2013;**60**(9):791–800.

12. Barrett JE, Kolmes K. The practice of tele-mental health: ethical, legal and clinical issues. *Pract Innov* 2016;**1**(1):53–66.

13. American Society for Reproductive Medicine. Recommendations for practices utilizing gestational carriers: a committee opinion. *Fertil Steril* 2017;**107**(2): e3–e10.

14. Riddle MP. Psychological assessment of gestational carrier candidates: current approaches, challenges and future considerations. *Fertil Steril* 2020;**13**(5):897–902.

15. American Society for Reproductive Medicine. Guidance on qualifications for fertility counselors: a committee opinion. *Fertil Steril* 2021;**115**(6):1411–1415.

16. Luxton DD, Pruitt LD, Osenbach JE. Best practices for remote psychological assessment via telehealth technologies. *Prof Psychol Res Pract* 2014;**45**(1):27–35. https://doi.org/10.1037/a0034547

17. Grady BJ, Melcer T. A retrospective evaluation of telemental health care services for remote military populations. *Telemedicine and e-Health* 2005;**11**:551–558. https://doi.org/10.1089/tmj.2005.11.551

18. Harris E, Younggren J. Risk management in the digital world. *Prof Psychol Res Pract* 2011;**42**(6):412–418.

Chapter 26

Nuts and Bolts of Fertility Counseling
Legal Issues and Practice Management

Margaret Swain and William Petok

Introduction

Family building is seldom a straight-line march to the finish, even for those fortunate individuals who avoid a detour into the ethical and legal minefield of assisted reproductive technology (ART). The landscape has become ever more rugged, notably complicated by, among other issues, third-party reproductive collaboration, accessibility to care, protections against exploitation of women, and concerns for the safety and well-being of children. The client is influenced by cultural mores and religious beliefs, as well as by general societal pressure, but also by more practical concerns such as affordability of and access to medical care, feasible aspects of participating in these arrangements and the like. Further, the client selects courses of action based not only on personal choice, but also upon the integrated influences of the surrounding local community, and in some sense, through the input of the larger global society. Most importantly, intended parents and their third-party helpers often lack fundamental information about the parties' status to any child created – who is a parent, what rights the respective parties possess, and how those rights are protected. Unless appropriately addressed, these issues may contribute to misunderstandings, misperceptions and confusion, all of which may be laid at the feet of the fertility counselor.

Additionally, few other areas of clinical counseling are so intimately aligned with the law. The two disciplines grew in parallel tracks as the needs within ART developed. Sometimes, the intertwining provides for affirmative action and clear resolutions. Other times, the lack of qualified assistance from one or both fields is glaring, or simply, the "perfect storm" of circumstances arises and the need becomes excruciatingly apparent. This chapter will guide the fertility counselor in recognizing risky situations; analyzing them with a critical eye; practicing within the parameters of competence, ethics and legal sound stricture; and applying best practice principles.

The addenda referred to in this chapter are available for download at www.cambridge.org/covington-clinical-guide

In a previous edition we discussed a case where a legally blind woman sued several physicians and their practices for discriminating against her by refusing to provide infertility services, allegedly because of her blindness. Further, she claimed discrimination because she was required to provide proof she was fit to be a mother after the defendant had provided those services previously without these assurances. Ultimately, evidence established that the plaintiff's blindness was not a motivating factor in the decision to defer treatment until medically appropriate concerns about her ability to care for the child were resolved. The patient also had a history of clinical depression, was emotionally abused as a child, and subsequently demonstrated problems interacting with others. The defendants were able to show that the patient consistently perceived that people were always trying to prevent her from following her plans and making her own choices. She admitted to jumping to conclusions about others' desires to interfere with her wishes and that she had a hard time understanding people's true intentions. She also dealt inappropriately with authority figures. A psychiatrist who examined her testified that she had traits of borderline personality disorder as well as major depressive disorder and narcissistic personality disorder [1].

The case is illustrative of a few of the myriad legal issues that a fertility counselor might consider in working with a patient who is seeking treatment for infertility. It highlighted the impact of the law on the delivery of mental health services attached to reproductive medicine clinics. While most cases the fertility counselor will face are not nearly as complex, it points out the multilevel nature of our work and the need for collaboration between knowledgeable professionals on both sides of the law–mental health axis.

A Multidisciplinary Approach to Crisis Management: The Fertility Counselor's Role

Inherent in the previously mentioned case, but also typical for many situations in fertility counseling, are medical, psychological, nursing and legal issues, all of which influence the final outcome. Collaboration among the various professionals is the best plan to address the interests of the medical practice, the concerns of the professionals involved, and the safety, well-being and equitable treatment of the patient. Assigning possible resolutions and treatments according to the scrutiny suggested below should provide some protection to all the stakeholders. In the development of a team approach, the following guideposts should be in the forefront.

Professional Standards of Practice for Counselors

Professional competency provides the basic theoretical approach of fertility counseling in the context of the law. Competency involves a collection of skills, abilities, habits, character traits and knowledge a person must have to perform a specific job well. An individual performs effectively within the professional construct when s/he possesses the skills, abilities and knowledge that constitute competence. Competency is based upon knowledge, training and standards that a profession has identified as necessary to perform a job effectively. These standards, with some variations, provide the bedrock for licensing, credentialing and discipline-specific regulations, both in the United States (US) and abroad. Each fertility counselor is responsible for compliance with the requirements in their jurisdiction of practice.

Credentialing and Licensure

In the US, psychiatrists, psychologists, social workers, psychiatric nurses, licensed professional counselors and marriage and family therapists are credentialed separately, typically under distinct legislative titles. State statutes provide for a licensing entity that specifies licensing and certification requirements and enumerates prohibited actions, as well as penalties, for violations of the code. Standards of practice and ethical guidelines are typically promulgated by professional associations, and in some countries, are the basis for licensure. Once adopted by the organization, these guidelines may be viewed as the legal standards against which practitioners in each category may be judged. Of interest in the US are the American Psychological Association's (APA) Ethical Principles of Psychologists and Code of Conduct [2] the National Association of Social Workers (NASW) Code of Ethics [3] and the National Board for Certified Counselors (NBCC) Code of Ethics [4]. Also pertinent may be: the American Association for Marriage and Family Therapy (AAMFT) Code of Ethics [5]; the American Psychiatric Association (the APA), The Principles of Medical Ethics with Annotations Especially Applicable to Psychiatry [6]; and the American Psychiatric Nurses' Association (APNA), Scope and Standards of Psychiatric and Mental Health Nursing [7].

In countries other than the US, psychiatrists and psychologists are regulated separately from other MHPs, and systems for regulating social workers and other types of counselors are not uniform. The majority of registration systems operate in tandem with a competency evaluation and a disciplinary procedure, and registration is defined by statute. For example, in the United Kingdom (UK), credentialing of fertility counselors is available through the British Infertility Counselling Association (BICA) and the British Fertility Society (BFS) [8].

The UK's Human Fertilisation and Embrology Authority (HFEA) requires that fertility counselors hold a recognized clinical psychology, counseling psychology or psychotherapy qualification to a minimal level of diploma of higher education, and be accredited under the British Infertility Counselling Association (or actively working towards the accreditation) [9]. Australia requires that working psychologists comply with registration requirements of the State and Territory Psychologists Registration Boards. Generally, all states or territories require completion of a 4-year course of undergraduate study in psychology, and 2 full-time, additional years of postgraduate work or supervised fieldwork as a probationary/conditional registered psychologist. Social workers are expected to comply with the ethical requirements of state regulatory bodies, such as the South Australian Council on Reproductive Technology, established as a function of the Reproductive Act of 1998 [10].

Professional Guidelines for the Area of Practice

The American Society for Reproductive Medicine (ASRM) Practice Guidelines are mostly applicable to medical healthcare professionals. However, where the substantive content relates to mental health and legal issues, the guidelines are at least arguably applicable to fertility counselors and attorneys, as practitioners in both professions are accepted as members of the organization and both maintain separate professional groups within ASRM. In the absence of other established guidelines, these recommendations may be legitimately viewed as standards of care against which professional behavior in this field is evaluated and judged. Also, ASRM has recently published updated practice guidelines regarding qualifications for fertility counselors [11].

The specific national standards of practice for each particular discipline of fertility counselors, as well as the bylaws and guidelines of pertinent professional groups within parent organizations for reproductive medicine are critical (e.g., the Mental Health Professional Group [MHPG] of ASRM). Since MHPs have a separate professional group within ASRM, the guidelines established through this body do speak specifically to fertility counselors, as do those within ESHRE and its Psychology and Counseling Special Interest Group. Another similar organization is the International Infertility Counseling Organization (IICO). One of the goals of IICO is " … to establish professional standards and guidelines for the psychosocial care and treatment of infertile patients" [12]. The guidelines established by these professional groups fall short of enforceable rules, but nevertheless provide the framework for professional standards, competency, and possibly credentialing for fertility counselors.

Scope of Practice

ASRM recommends that fertility counselors should be qualified to provide the following services or appropriately refer clients if the individual MHP cannot offer an enumerated particular service [11]. Table 26.1 describes the types of service a fertility counselor may provide.

Other Professional Pronouncements

Both ASRM and ESHRE Ethics Committee Opinions are available to members and are printed in the respective society's journals and, for both members and nonmembers, on their websites (ASRM.org and ESHRE.eu) These types of considered and thoughtfully written opinions provide justification for professional decisions and, should a dispute arise, may provide a basis for defense of those actions.

Laws Affecting Outcomes for Reproductive Technology Patients

While the fertility counselor is not expected to know and provide information about state, federal, or international law, it is important to recognize that clients may be considering arrangements that are restricted or prohibited in their state or country. Acting in contravention to those laws can lead to unintended and highly problematic situations. Advising clients that such laws may exist and apply to their situations and that a consultation with an experienced reproductive law attorney as indicated is helpful and appropriate. Additionally, international

Table 26.1 Fertility counselor services

Diagnosis and treatment of mental disorders
Grief counseling
Supportive counseling
Crisis intervention
Education/information counseling
Decision-making counseling
Third-party evaluation and implications counseling
Psychometric test administration/interpretation
Sexual counseling
Support group counseling
Psychotherapy
Couples and family therapy
Referral/resource counseling
Reproductive endocrinology and infertility (REI) staff education and consultation

clients should be told that a consultation with an immigration attorney may be necessary. International clients may not be aware that in order to return home with a child born abroad through a surrogacy arrangement, they will need a passport or other border pass documents for their child. Proper counseling may involve asking clients if they know what is necessary for them to accomplish their goal of returning home with their baby.

General Principles of Sound Business Practice

These drive institutional policy and procedure and should be part of the decision-making matrix. It is best practice to develop uniform and consistently applied formal policies for all parts of the fertility counseling practice: financial, process and practical. While counselors who are employed by institutions will be expected to adhere to institutional policies, independent practitioners should employ the same practices as may pertain to their individual businesses. For example, providers in the US who are in solo practice must still adhere to the guidelines promulgated by the Health Insurance Portability and Accountability Act (HIPAA) [13], and provide policy statements to clients. In addition, anyone who uses a credit card processing machine to collect fees is required to complete a Payment Card Industry (PCI) compliance evaluation every year, adhere to the guidelines developed by the Security Standards Council and document such adherence [14]. As a general statement, informal policies invite misunderstanding and are typically indefensible in a lawsuit. To protect itself and, if part of a larger group, then to make certain that all members of the team are reliably following clear standards in a predictable manner, the practice should ensure that:

- Well-defined, unambiguous written policy and procedures are maintained.
- Such policies are applied uniformly, and exceptions are not entertained without substantial and compelling reason and further review, preferably by an outside entity.
- Any evaluation is a customary and usual part of a standard protocol.
- Patients are informed at the outset that interviews may be conducted with an eye toward evaluating the intended parent's ability to safely participate.

Collaboration with Other Disciplines

Including members of all the related professions in an orchestrated manner provides for safeguards and protections, not just for the client, but for members of the treatment team, including the independent practitioner. Typically, the group might include physicians, nurses, geneticists, embryologists, office managers and practice coordinators, matching program directors and coordinators, fertility counselors and attorneys. When team members all practice within the same group, the various members should all meet periodically to review cases and patient information, update policy and assess the overall success of the team. Input of other professionals not part of the practice, such as independent fertility counselors and lawyers, should be solicited as needed. For problematic and more complex arrangements, it is wise to have access to an Ethics Review Board. If this is not part of a usual protocol within a facility, such a board could be convened on an ad hoc basis. If practicing as an independent healthcare professional, it is useful for the fertility counselor to have a "team" of trusted professionals from other disciplines who can be consulted when difficult issues arise. At a minimum, this team should include an experienced reproductive law attorney and another fertility counselor with comparable or greater experience. Additional consults with knowledgeable physicians and nursing professionals can be useful as well.

A Primer for Practice

The following are offered as minimal guidelines and suggestions for establishing oneself as a competent provider of fertility counseling services and carrying out those services.

Evidence of Competency as a Fertility Counselor

Proper licensure to practice in the field as a psychologist, social worker, marriage and family therapist or other state sanctioned mental healthcare professional.

This would include proof of a degree in the field, the necessary supervised experience to become licensed and evidence of licensure from the state in which one practices. Membership in other professional certifying organizations, such as the National Register of Health Service Psychologists or status as a Certified Social Worker in Health Care (C-SWHC), provide further evidence of competency. Adherence to the minimum standards for training, such as those provided by the MHPG of ASRM or the Psychology and Counseling Special Interest Group of ESHRE, also offer skill-building and aptitude in this specialized field.

For those not licensed in both states and utilizing telehealth across state lines, participation with PSYPACT or comparable organizations is essential and is discussed in greater detail in Chapter 25 on telemental health in fertility counseling.

Membership in professional organizations devoted to the provision of mental health services to fertility patients.

This would include the above mentioned: these organizations offer continuing education opportunities not often found in other continuing education programs. In addition, access to current thought and practice in the medical aspects of infertility is available via membership in these organizations. Mentoring programs and the opportunity to consult with thought leaders in the field is available through membership in many of these organizations. Finally, ethical and practice guidelines for the profession are found within their publications.

Building Blocks of Contemporary Business Practice

Forms play an important role in documenting the professional relationship that exists between the fertility counselor and clients. They are equally important in authorizing and facilitating conversation with clients' attorneys or medical practices conducting ART. Carefully worded, intentional documentation is the key to avoiding misunderstanding and legal mishaps. This would include but not be limited to written statements about policies on confidentiality, privacy (HIPAA) and fees. In the case of evaluations, forms should clearly delineate who is the client, the clinic, the agency, the individual being considered as a gestational carrier or the intended parents. Retainers establish the fertility counselor's role and limitations. The nature of the services to be provided and the compensation for those services are also contained here. These documents are useful in the general practice of providing therapy services and in the more specialized practice of evaluations and psychosocial educational consultations. Also, with the increasing popularity of telemental health counseling, consents particular to these sessions must be in the practitioner's arsenal. Further, choosing a secure and professionally acceptable video-conferencing service is critical to conducting remote counseling.

Documentation of therapy sessions is essential. The oft-repeated concept that, if something wasn't documented in writing, it never happened, is still applicable. While it is impossible to write down everything that takes place in a session, it is possible to document many aspects of one. At a minimum the following information should be contained in a note following a session:

- date, time and length of session
- diagnosis code (if appropriate)
- procedure code (ICD–10, DSM-V or whatever standard is dictated by law and practice guidelines)
- session behavior
- level of functioning and stressor levels
- treatment goals
- homework or recommendations
- signature of counselor.

Documentation becomes quite important should a problem develop. In the great majority of cases no problems do develop and the work goes smoothly. However, in the rare circumstance when something does go awry, having a well-documented record is invaluable to the counselor's professional and mental health! It will also provide valuable assistance for legal counsel, should you need it, and will substantiate your adherence to standards and policies.

Informed consent in psychotherapy grew out of a 1985 case, Osheroff v. Chestnut Lodge Inc., in which a client alleged that he was not given access to all available treatments and would have improved dramatically had he been prescribed medication sooner [15]. ASRM practice guidelines address informed consent when conducting psychological screening for ART, as well as when counseling clients about the ART process [16]. A good informed consent will outline the fertility counselor's role with the client during the process, what process and procedures might take place with the context of the interactions, and what the client can expect from the counselor. It will also describe the limits of confidentiality that the counselor must adhere to by law and ethics.

Conflict of interest waivers can ameliorate the difficulty of one fertility counselor representing two parties in an ART arrangement. These documents make it clear that conflicts may exist and a fertility counselor may give advice that is contrary to the wishes of one of the parties. Clients should be given the option of accepting this arrangement, or opting out of treatment or evaluation by the same fertility counselor as is involved with the other party. Professional liability, however, cannot be waived within such documents.

Retainers are often employed by attorneys for similar purposes and will be well understood by the legal professionals with whom you work. A good retainer will outline what action will take place in the event of a dispute, as well as describe the specific services to be performed.

Reports and evaluations are a necessary part of an integrated team approach that includes evaluating and counseling participants in third-party arrangements. They are equally present when the counselor is part of a team or an independent practitioner. In either case, the fertility counselor should be certain to document the client's understanding of the nature of the consultation, what information will be contained in any report and that he or she may be disqualified from participation in fertility treatments by the evaluation.

The question of how and by whom those reports may be used, and to whom they may be released, is an irksome one and, among other things, turns on the intent and language in the fertility counselor's consents and releases. Generally speaking, the records belong to the person whose private health information they contain. The client is entitled to those records. If an appropriate, HIPAA-compliant release has been voluntarily and knowingly signed by the client, then the records (or whatever portion of them is designated) may be shared with whomever the client designates. However, the fertility counselor may have an agreement with a referral source that limits release of the report to the fertility center and/or matching program, and, as a consequence, limits the client's access to the report. In cases where there is this type of restrictive agreement, the counselor must carefully review the restriction with the participant and be sure the limitation is clearly disclosed in the signed informed consent document. Regarding psychological testing, raw test data from the report is not released to clients, clinics or other practitioners in the same way test materials themselves are not to be released in accordance with the APA's ethics guidelines.

Evaluations, as well as other written or electronically generated reports or notes, should be stored in compliance with HIPAA, state law and professional guidelines. In many cases that means these records are to be maintained, securely, for 7 years after the end of therapy or, in the case of a minor, 3 years after the minor reaches the age of majority. Many counselors maintain records in perpetuity as a matter of course. However, it is easy to see how a busy practice could generate significant paper or electronic data and have a need for off-site storage that is HIPAA compliant. While the APA has not provided "official" guidance regarding online/off-site storage, recent publications have addressed its significance, at least one noting that, "... the implementation of these advancements in mental healthcare involves consequences to digital privacy and might increase clients' risk to unintended breaches of confidentiality" [17]. Additional resources for practitioners can be found at the U.S. Department of Health and Human Services, Office for Civil Rights website [18] and in documents prepared by the APA Practice Organization [19].

One suspects that as time and technology go forward, most if not all of these records will be converted to electronic or digital format, thereby reducing the amount of space they require for maintenance. Accordingly, secure cloud storage or other protected storage options have become increasingly important considerations. Electronic health record (EHR) systems offer this style of data storage, not without risk. As noted, any number of safeguards have been implemented, to "... enhance the governance of healthcare data"; however, e-health data has been frequently breached. In addition, as the accessibility and usability of e-health data increase, its security attack vectors have also been widening. Over the last decade, 1.5 million medical devices have been compromised due to software vulnerabilities and their wireless connection" [20]. Data storage companies are in the process of creating highly secure systems that are intended to offer the necessary security for these very reasons. The APA offers guidelines for every type of data storage (www.apa.org/practice/guidelines/record-keeping) and special emphasis on electronic record storage is outlined in Guideline 9 [21]. NASW guidelines and instruction may be found at: www.socialworkers.org/includes/newIncludes/homepage/PRA-BRO-33617.TechStandards_FINAL_POSTING.pdf.

Disclaimers: Wise or Waste of Time?

A disclaimer is a statement limiting or providing specifics about a scope of responsibility in a legally recognized relationship. Examples of those relationships might be landlord–tenant, host–guest, common carrier–passenger, or parties to a contract. Typically, disclaimers are introduced when there is a risk inherent in the relationship.

Disclaimers may or may not be enforceable. Their enforceability turns on the nature of the disclaimer, the laws of the particular jurisdiction, and whether the aggrieved party consented to the risk or uncertainty addressed in the disclaimer. For instance, if the language of the disclaimer is not clear and unambiguous or if it is not visible or apparent to the concerned party, a court may decide that the party suffering harm never consented to that risk. Additionally, a party seeking the protection of a disclaimer should be certain that the statement includes the specifics of the matter, as opposed to a blanket statement of no liability. Further, if the party is seeking protection from misrepresentation of omission within a contract and it is demonstrated that the party knew that certain facts were misrepresented or omitted, the disclaimer is likely to be set aside.

Fee Agreements and Similar Documents

That said, a careful, unambiguous and specific disclaimer may provide a measure of protection in a contract or other document, but, in the event of a dispute, it does not guarantee recognition and enforceability of its terms. Overly general, boilerplate statements, tacked onto an agreement or other document may potentially be viewed as a mechanism to escape any responsibility whatsoever by the author. These are not useful and may place the writer in a more vulnerable position of scrutiny by a court.

A disclaimer is not likely to protect a professional from a claim of professional malpractice. For example, in many states, a clause in an attorney's fee agreement that attempts to limit his liability or exculpate him for his own negligence, thereby avoiding a claim for legal malpractice, is prohibited. However, laws do vary from state to state. The fertility counselor should be aware of the laws governing the mental health profession and particular licensure regulations or rules.

Reports of Evaluations and Testing

The fertility counselor should include a particular disclaimer in anticipation of the following situation: an evaluation is conducted and a report issued for a gestational carrier and a set of, or an individual, intended parent(s). For some reason, the arrangement does not move forward, or is indefinitely postponed. The agency or participant requests that (or simply uses without asking) the report, specifically issued and pertaining only to the gestational carrier and a particular set of intended parents, be recycled for use in a new match, or even for a subsequent arrangement with the same parties. This is concerning because, of course, the relationship between the gestational carrier and the intended parents, at that specific point in time, is a critical component. To address this concern, and to protect the fertility counselor, the report should include, in bold writing, the following or similar language:

> The evaluation documented in this report was conducted for the specific purpose and intent of (name of gestational carrier) acting as a gestational carrier for (name of intended parent/s), in an arrangement to proceed within a reasonable time period from the date of this report. The writer makes no recommendation as to any other circumstance or arrangement that may arise in the future, including the parties entering into a similar situation with another gestational carrier or intended parent. Further, circumstances may change among the parties, which may make this recommendation inappropriate and void as to any future arrangement, even between the same parties. The following comments, opinions and recommendation are limited to the parties evaluated at this time and are only applicable for a reasonable time period within which to complete the presently contemplated arrangement.

In summary, it may be wise, and in some circumstances very important, to include disclaimers in certain client documents, such as fee agreements, retainers and reports. If doing so:

- Ensure the language is bold and conspicuous.
- Explain the risks that the disclosure addresses.
- Ask the clients to initial the disclaimer section.
- Use specific and unambiguous language when writing a disclaimer.

Legal Consultation

Attorneys and counselors are necessarily involved in third-party ART arrangements and working collaboratively with fertility counselors (and, not incidentally, with the fertility centers) serves the best interests of the clients. It is helpful to the legal professionals to understand the mental health evaluation process, the time involved, the timeline for the evaluation to be completed, the cost and

the nature of the reports that the fertility counselor provides. The fertility counselor will need an authorization from the client to share the report or other communications.

The legal consultation is generally comprised of the following discussions and topics: laws of the relevant jurisdiction; overall legal process; rationale for a written agreement; independent representation of the parties; terms of that agreement; implications of those provisions; risks involved in these arrangements; remedies available for breach; acknowledgment that the surrogate/carrier is the medical manager of the pregnancy; and, that ultimately, a surrogate's refusal to undergo or deciding to undergo any type of medical procedure in contravention of contract terms is not amenable to remedy by "specific performance" or by injunctive relief. We also describe how parentage will be obtained and will review timelines involved in every step. Finally, a written retainer agreement is presented to the client for review and approval, including a reference that the surrogate's fee is paid by the intended parent(s), but that the attorney representing the surrogate has a singular duty and responsibility to the surrogate, regardless of who pays the fee. A conflict waiver statement is also included. Each attorney should present to the client, whether the client is the intended parent or the surrogate/gamete/embryo donor, a written retainer specific to the type of client, as it includes a description of the attorney's services and for the intended parent, the fee structure.

Fertility counselors may be surprised to learn that many ART agreements, especially gestational surrogacy contracts, require the parties to meet with a counselor if a dispute arises during the term of the agreement, or may require that a party seek counseling if the other party requests it. Should such a consultation be requested, it benefits everyone if the fertility counselor and the attorneys involved discuss the situation, if for no reason other than the fertility counselor being forewarned that the client(s) will likely be unsettled and perhaps angry. The fertility counselor should ask the client which attorneys are representing the parties in the contract drafting review and finalization phase, and should feel free to request the relevant language pertaining to any dispute resolution.

In the course of preparing consent forms for the fertility counseling practice, it makes good sense to consult with a qualified and experienced legal professional. There are 14 examples of consent forms for reference contained in Addendum 26, but state-specific requirements should be reviewed with your practice attorney.

Table 26.2 How to avoid a lawsuit

Do	Do not
Practice within the scope of your competence	Make exceptions
Follow professional Code of Ethics	Skip steps
Obtain adequate consents	Fail to document phone calls and other communications
Consult when you have a question	Be afraid to turn down a questionable referral
Be aware of the law and legal implications	Answer legal questions or give legal advice
Establish policies and follow them	Fail to clarify your role to all parties
Follow ASRM/ESHRE practice guidelines	
Refer clients for legal consultation with a qualified attorney in third-party cases	

Table 26.2 provides helpful guidance on what fertility counselors need to consider regarding how to avoid legal conflicts.

Dilemmas in Policy Implementation

Inevitably, a time will come in a fertility counselor's practice where a request is made to "bend the rules," thereby challenging one's policies and procedures. The two examples that follow demonstrate how many of the above points can place one in a sticky situation.

Many fertility counselors have faced a call from a clinic coordinator, or an attorney representing a gestational carrier (GC) or intended parent (IP), requesting an evaluation "quickly." Often these calls indicate that a cycle is about to happen and the psychological evaluation is the only thing holding up the process. The individuals involved are likely under a great deal of stress to complete the process and their urgency is obvious. What do you do under these circumstances? Do you feel compelled to assist the process to move rapidly or do you take a more reasoned approach?

Working in this field requires not only an understanding of the psychological problems and issues inherent in the overall process, but also insight into the medical considerations. Accommodating both types of concerns, within boundaries, is appropriate. Rush situations have unnecessary stress attached to them and undermine the goals associated with the evaluation (i.e., making sure all parties understand the long-range implications of assisted reproduction, are making an informed decision and are at the best place possible to move forward treatment). Are you going to point this out to the parties when you decline the evaluation? Will it have a negative impact on your practice if you do decline or will the parties gain respect for your concern for a best-case outcome and want to work with you in the future? If you accept the case, will you include a disclaimer indicating there is no guarantee that your work will be concluded within the posited time frame? Attorneys also face this pressure, with the same consequences and issues. Your consideration of these types of requests should include a review of the previously stated business practice guidelines, particularly those addressing exceptions. While circumstances vary from case to case, it is almost always better to adhere to your own internal policies and procedures when addressing these requests.

While this kind of situation provides an opportunity for a "teaching moment," the coordinator, the legal professional or other parties involved may not be open to learn! You may decide that on a one-time basis you'll take the evaluation, turn it around quickly and have a subsequent conversation with the professionals explaining why you can't do it again under future, similar circumstances. Fertility counselors early in their careers who are eager for work may be willing to take the evaluation regardless and worry that to not take the case would not only impact their future reputation but might as well constitute an improper refusal to provide services. Does your state law require that you provide service to anyone who requests it or do you have the ability to refuse a case? In all likelihood you have the right to be selective. It would be unreasonable to expect that every professional has a schedule that permits taking every case opportunity. Furthermore, borrowing from the medical code of "do no harm," you may be colluding to increase stress and reduce positive outcomes. Would it be better for the recipients to have their treatment team plan thoroughly for these situations, so no one is subjected to undue pressure and encouraged by the timeline to do shoddy work? Most of us would answer in the affirmative!

Other, more specific issues can give rise to procedural and ethical dilemmas for the fertility counselor. A call came from a couple asking to conduct a psychological evaluation for a GC. The couple was referred by their reproductive endocrinologist (RE), who was known to the fertility counselor. The IP wife noted in her call that she had been working with the RE for 9 years and that it was clear that they needed a GC. She mentioned that the fertility counselor might want to know that there are "extenuating circumstances." It turned out that those circumstances included the fact that the GC was a single woman who had never given birth. The couple had identified her via an Internet advertisement and the physician thought she might make a good candidate because she had a cranial abnormality and would likely never marry or have children.

The fertility counselor not only saw a "red flag" but also heard sirens wailing! This IP couple was most likely very frustrated by their long treatment without a successful birth. Furthermore, the physician sounded like he was equally frustrated and desperately wanted to help the couple. On questioning, the fertility counselor ascertained that the couple had not yet retained an attorney but were "looking into it." The fertility counselor explained that an evaluation would be impossible because it violated the practice guidelines of ASRM. The absence of a pregnancy carried to term was a "rule out" for GCs and the counselor adhered to those guidelines. The guideline existed to ensure that the GC could give informed consent and the lack of a prior birth precluded her ability to give it. The explanation went further to include the rationale that, particularly in this case where the GC was unlikely to marry or have a child of her own, she was even more vulnerable to develop an attachment to the fetus and have a difficult time following through with her intention to place the baby with the intended parents. The potential long-term psychological consequences for her were too significant. In fact, what appeared to be a reason to the couple and the physician to work with her was a glaring reason to exclude her. The physician clearly felt that the proposed GC's physical problem was more cosmetic and that created a mitigating circumstance for not observing the ASRM practice guideline that all GCs have given birth before acceptance as a carrier. Finally, the fertility counselor advised that the couple seek legal advice sooner rather than later as they pursued a suitable GC. The wife said she understood the fertility counselor's position and thanked the counselor for being frank with her.

Knowing and adhering to the practice guidelines and the possibility of legal complications averted a potential disaster for at least three and possibly four individuals: the GC, the couple and the potential child.

Conclusion

As practices in this area have developed, and science continues to push the limits of the possible, the problematic issues have become even more multifaceted and complex. Our responses must be reasoned, measured and frequently crafted after the science has leapt forward. It seems that the interface of law and mental health with regard to reproductive medicine is always playing catch up! Fertility counselors who pay attention to the issues outlined in this chapter will have tools to reduce their own stress and potential liability, and presumably provide a better service not only to their clients but also to the professionals in other disciplines who refer to them.

References

1. Swain M, Petok WD. Legal issues for fertility counselors. In Covington SN. Ed. *Fertility Counseling Clinical Guide and Case Studies.* Cambridge: Cambridge University Press, 2015, 296–307.

2. American Psychological Association. *Ethical Principles of Psychologists and Code of Conduct.* Washington, DC: The American Psychological Association, 2016. Available at: www.apa.org/ethics/code [last accessed June 16, 2022].

3. National Association of Social Workers. Code of Ethics [pamphlet]. Washington, DC: National Association of Social Workers, 2021. Available at: www.socialworkers.org/about/ethics/code-of-ethics [last accessed June 16, 2022].

4. National Board for Certified Counselors (NBCC). Code of Ethics. Washington, DC. Published 2016. Available at: www.counselorprep.com/nbcc-revised-code-of-ethics/#:~:text=The%20National%20Board%20for%20Certified%20Counselors%20%28NBCC%29%20published,counselors%20certified%20by%20NBCC%20or%20applicants%20for%20certification [last accessed June 16, 2022].

5. American Association of Marriage and Family Counselors. Code of Ethics. Available at: www.aamft.org/Legal_Ethics/Code_of_Ethics.aspx [last accessed June 16, 2022].

6. American Psychiatric Association. Ethical Code. The Principles of Medical Ethics with Annotations Especially Applicable to Psychiatry. Published 2013. Available at: www.psychiatry.org/psychiatrists/practice/ethics [last accessed June 16, 2022].

7. Code of Ethical Practice for Psychiatric Nursing and Foundations of Psychiatric Nursing Practice. Available at: http://54.65.62.192/english/pdf/ethicalandfoundations.pdf. See also: and www.slideshare.net/guylamunyon/ana-psychiatric-mental-health-scope-and-standards-of-practice [last accessed June 16, 2022].

8. British Infertility Counseling Association. Available at: www.bica.net.

9. Human Fertilisation Embryology Authority. Code of Practice, 9th ed., with 2019 updates. Available at: https://portal.hfea.gov.uk/knowledge-base/read-the-code-of-practice/ [last accessed June 16, 2022].

10. ANZICA. Guidelines on Professional Standards of Practice: Infertility Counseling. Published August 2018. Available at: www.fertilitysociety.com.au/professional-groups-anzica-australia-new-zealand/ [last accessed June 16, 2022].

11. Guidance on Qualifications for Fertility Counselors: A Committee Opinion. *Fertil Steril* 2021;**115**(6):1411–1415.

12. International Infertility Counseling Association. Compendium of Fertility Counseling Organizations Across the Globe. Available at: www.iico-infertilitycounseling.org [last accessed June 16, 2022].

13. Health Insurance Portability and Accountability Act of 1996, Public Law 104–191, 110 Stat. 1936. Washington, DC: The United States Senate, 1996.

14. PCISSD. Data Security Standards Overview [Internet]. [Cited May 29, 2014] Available at: www.pcisecuritystandards.org/pci_security/standards_overview [last accessed June 16, 2022].

15. *Osheroff v. Chestnut Lodge, Inc.*, 490 A. 2d 720, 62 Md. App. 519 (1985).

16. Consideration of the gestational carrier: an Ethics Committee opinion. *Fertil Steril* 2018;**100**(6):1017–1021.

17. Lustgarten SD, Garrison YL, Sinnard MT, Flynn AWP. Digital privacy in mental healthcare: current issues and recommendations for technology use. *Curr Opin Psychol* 2020;**36**:25–31. https://doi.org/0.1016/j.copsyc.2020.03.012

18. Available at: www.hhs.gov/ocr/index.html [last accessed June 16, 2022].

19. 2003, 2005, 2013. Available at: www.apaservices.org/practice/business/hipaa [last accessed June 16, 2022]; solely or in collaboration with the APA Insurance Trust (APA Practice Organization & APA Insurance Trust).

20. Yaqoob T, Abbas H, Atiquzzaman M. Security vulnerabilities, attacks, countermeasures, and regulations of networked medical devices – a review. *IEEE Commun Surv Tutor* 2019;**21**:3723–3768; cited in *Int J Environ Res Public Health* 2021;**18**:9668. https://doi.org/10.3390/ijerph18189668

21. The American Psychological Association. Record-keeping guidelines, *Am Psychol* 2007;**62**:993–1004.

Chapter 27

Ethical Platform of Assisted Reproduction

Julianne Zweifel and Jeanne O'Brien

Reproductive endocrinology and infertility (REI) was officially recognized as a subspecialty of medicine in the United States (US) in 1972. The first US baby born as a result of in vitro fertilization (IVF) dates back to 1981. Since then, the field of reproductive medicine has witnessed dramatic medical and technological advances. However, the early practitioners of IVF were harshly criticized for unethical human experimentation [1]. These historical clinical experiments appear to have violated many currently accepted ethical prerequisites for responsible translational research. The human clinical research that produced the first IVF child would require extensive modifications to fulfill what we now consider to be appropriate. Swift emergence of clinically complex advances is a hallmark of reproductive medicine done in the name of meeting patient needs, yet progress often outpaces ethical deliberation, highlighting our dilemma. Examination of our dilemmas is further complicated by the fact that the determination of what constitutes good ethics and the consequent choices we make will change over time.

The initial development, continuing biomedical innovation and increasing availability of assisted reproductive technology (ART) raises a series of ethical questions, some of which have no prior references for comparison. How do we approach an ethical dilemma when there is no prior information or case study to inform decision-making? Reproductive healthcare professionals frequently face the question of, "Just because we can do it, should we do it or not?" These questions become more challenging in the context of different societal structures and rapidly changing norms of what constitutes acceptable applications of reproductive medicine. There is also an uneasy element of commercial competition in the ART field. If an ART provider thinks someone else will do it if they do not, then why not be in on it as well?

Treatment decisions in reproductive medicine involve not just the intended parent(s) but a potential future child, as well as all ART professionals participating in helping to create this child. When we make treatment decisions, we do not have any knowledge of what the future outcome will be for all the present and future participants. While we strive to avoid a horrible result in terms of the health and future well-being of all the participants, our specialty requires unique considerations. We need to appreciate the vulnerability of our patients and the extraordinary lengths that desperate patients are willing to go to in order to have a child; especially a child that is genetically related to them. These risks were presciently articulated by Kass in his 1971 *New England Journal of Medicine* article before the first successful IVF birth [1]. This innate desire to pass on our genetic identity and the competitive commercial environment of many reproductive clinics places our specialty in a precarious position. How do we remain cognizant of not over-promising with incautious and unproven medical treatments for infertility or even appropriate treatments applied to a futile clinical situation? How do we consider the future psychosocial ramifications of children and the families created through these technologies? We must remain diligent for the sake of our patients who place their trust in us to remain unbiased and act in the best interests of all involved, even if it means declining to proceed with treatment.

Basic Ethical Principles

As noted previously, the choices we face are difficult and often lack prior comparisons for guidance. A frequent phrase in the ART clinic is *I have never encountered this clinical result or considered such a treatment scenario.* Broadly speaking, ethics can be defined as a way of understanding and examining the moral life. Clinicians can be challenged with how to provide competent and ethical treatment in novel or complex situations. The consideration of the four widely accepted basic ethical principles provides a starting place to form a narrative of understanding for reproductive decision-making; a strategy to utilize when the decisions are straightforward but also unclear. While principals can be narrow, they provide a foundation that respects reproductive autonomy and choice, while minimizing potential harm. The four basic principles we are all familiar with include *autonomy, beneficence, nonmaleficence, and justice*. In isolation each principle appears clear-cut, however when choices are made the principles do not always remain aligned and might even conflict with each other.

Autonomy describes the ability for an individual to be self-determined. The individual is competent to make willing, informed decisions regarding which medical tests and treatments to undergo. Although autonomous decision-making is viewed as relevant to the individual patient, the decision-making is not occurring in a bubble. Rather, as King writes, "The patient is seen as having a responsibility to society in his or her decisions just as the physician does" ([2], p. 5). King advises that autonomy must be considered in balance with other relevant factors. She notes that, "We must guard against mistakenly acquiescing to requested interventions that go against our clinical judgment, ostensibly to honor patient autonomy" ([2], p. 6).

Reproductive autonomy represents the right of individuals to make decisions about if, when and the manner in which they become parents. If unable to conceive naturally or lacking a partner, patients make the intentional decision whether or not to utilize reproductive technologies. It also includes the utilization of an expanding array of preconception and prenatal genetic testing options driven by biotechnology and commercialism. This constitutes a new genetic autonomy. Patients now have the opportunity to do more than select against disease. The clinical practice of ART usually involves an extensive informed consent process with expanded discussions of the possible risks. Overly strict reliance on the ethical principle of autonomy risks ignoring potential confounding influences as well. One significant confounding variable is the desire to pass on one's own genetic material. We will go to extraordinary lengths to try and accomplish the passage of this unique, evolving, and inherited information that defines who we are in the world.

Beneficence is the responsibility of the healthcare professional to further the patient's welfare and interests. Healthcare professionals have an obligation to protect their patients from harm. However, it is not always clear what is best for the patient. In ART, the patient is not the only concern. In reproductive medicine, ethical issues relate to more than one person, usually a couple and beyond to include a family and future child. Advances in reproductive medicine are routinely creating new ethical questions which require weighing the intense desire to have a child against the potential future well-being of that not yet real child.

Nonmaleficence is the principle, when assessed in the aggregate, to do no harm or to leave the patient in a worse condition. Most healthcare professionals would consider it unlikely their care would result in maleficence. Reproductive care, however, encompasses a complex dynamic between medical, psychological, and economic considerations for each patient(s) and unfortunately, ART might unintentionally leave a patient in a worse position when, for example, biology fails to provide a successful pregnancy. It is one of the special nuances of reproductive medicine: How do we care for patients who fail all that medicine has to offer and yet provide them hope for the future, a future that does not involve a biologically related child or any child?

Distributive justice broadly refers to equality, fairness, and inclusion in healthcare. As applied to reproductive medicine, distributive justice calls attention to the question of who has access to ART in the general population. Finer examination of justice asks how do we define equality, fairness, and inclusion in healthcare and how do we provide equitable access and expert care? Access to reproductive healthcare is far from just and inclusive in many parts of the world. While beyond the scope of this chapter, the benefits (of having a child) and burdens (costs) of ART are unequally distributed. Legitimate application of certain eligibility criteria appropriately guides the allocation of scarce resources in a society. Those criteria may include parental age, length of infertility, diagnosis, prior parity, and ability to afford treatment, among others. When a country applies a more consistent approach to ART access using merit-based criteria, the decision for the general population tends to lose respect for the interests of the individual. For example, the system used for organ allocation in the US clearly defines the factors that prioritize one patient over the other [3]. Difficult decisions must be made to make the best use of a scarce resource. Even with objective criteria, the application to individual decision-making will not resolve all questions. To arrive at a just decision requires weighing the specific individual circumstances. Ultimately, each society through its form of governance decides what is permissible when considering ethical principles. The healthcare professional must also be aware of current societal consensus and how quickly it changes.

Again, ethics are a way of examining and considering a moral life, the lens of which can incorporate the individual, the family, community, and broad society. The basic ethical principles discussed above are a starting place for examining reproductive decisions. Considerable attention has been paid to developing and applying ethical frameworks specific to the realm of reproductive decisions. Below is an introduction to ethical frameworks influential in current reproductive care.

Procreative Liberty

John Robertson's book, *Children of Choice: Freedom and the New Reproductive Technologies* [4], has been described as, "the most important book on reproductive choice to date, and one that is required reading for philosophers, lawyers, ethicists, and anyone else interested in legal and ethical aspects of procreation" ([5], p. 3). Robertson's concept of "Procreative Liberty" (used interchangeable with the term, "Reproductive Freedom"), as discussed in the book, became the underpinning of influential ethics opinions, as well as clinical policies, and individual patient assertions. Although Robertson's arguments are contested, as will be discussed here, it is essential that professionals working in the field of assisted reproduction familiarize themselves with the main points of the Robertson argument so that they are equipped to assist in addressing and/or resolving ethical questions in assisted reproduction.

Robertson's argument is framed within a *rights-based approach*. For Robertson, the utility of a rights-based approach is that (a) rights claims and discourse are a normative part of our political, legal, and public life and thus, draw on a familiar method of reasoning; (b) many ethical concerns in the field of reproduction can be construed as deserving of rights protection, again a concept that is familiar in our society; and (c) a rights-based approach outlines a familiar and structured strategy for resolving disputes that includes identifying the competing reproductive and social interests stake. Robertson has employed this rights-based approach to argue against actual and proposed laws that could limit the use of reproductive technologies by single women, lesbians, and gay men as well as the use of gamete/embryo donation, surrogacy, and genetic testing.

The corner stone in Robertson's Procreative Liberty/ Reproductive Freedom thesis is that procreation, regardless of intent to rear the offspring, is a crucial, self-defining experience and "deserves presumptive respect because of its central importance to individual meaning,

dignity, and identity" ([4], p. 16). Simply stated, reproductive freedom is a cardinal right that is not easily constrained. Robertson asserts that denying an individual the opportunity to reproduce "denies a person's respect and dignity at the most basic level" ([4], p. 4). Procreative Liberty dictates that individuals have the freedom, or right, to decide whether or not to reproduce and the freedom to reproduce when, with whom, and by what means one chooses. Robertson suggests that, "decisions about reproductive technology should, in almost all cases, be left to the individuals directly involved" ([4], p. 4).

Robertson asserts further that individuals have the right to enact decisions regarding their reproductive plan that they feel are central to their overall decision to reproduce, including use of technology to influence the traits of their offspring. Robertson writes, "If a person thought that she would realize the benefits (of reproduction and parenting) only from a child with particular characteristics, then she should be free to select offspring to have those preferred traits. The right to procreate would thus imply the right to take actions to assure that offspring have the characteristics that make procreation desirable or meaningful for that individual" ([4], p. 152). For Robertson, objections to selecting genetic traits of offspring based on eugenics and protecting the child's welfare are "not convincing grounds" to oppose the use of technology [6]. Robertson acknowledged that the human genome project, as well as other scientific advancements, may continue to present future ethical dilemmas in reproductive care, but he asserted that, "If we are to take procreative liberty seriously, there may be no way to avoid recognizing the prebirth liberty of parents to exercise control over offspring characteristics" ([7], p. 39).

While Reproductive Freedom is held in the highest regard, the Robertsonian thesis notes that no liberties are without limits. The threshold for what constitutes a sufficient reason to constrain Reproductive Freedom, however, is set quite high. Robertson concedes that reproductive technologies may produce children who are physically or psychologically injured by the techniques in question but, in order to justify limiting procreative choice, the severity of that harm must be such that the resultant child would have preferred not to have been born at all. This argument invokes the *nonidentity problem*.

The linchpin of the *nonidentity dilemma* argument is that, in all but the worst of circumstances, it is better to exist than to not exist. In the context of adults exercising reproductive freedom, it is argued that offspring that result from deliberate reproductive decisions, even unwise or harmful decisions, enjoy the opportunity to exist and, if different decisions had been made, they would not have existed (e.g., use of a different embryo, sperm cell or oocyte would result in a different child and a choice not to reproduce would result in no child), which is deemed far worse. The argument, in a nutshell, is that we cannot "protect" children by preventing their births ([5], p. 7). This complex issue bears restating. An individual who incurs harm as a result of the reproductive decisions/plan of the parents cannot claim to have been harmed by their parents or the reproductive plan because, if a different decision or plan had been enacted, the child would not exist, and nonexistence is viewed as a more severe harm than existence with physical or psychological harm. In essence, it is a matter of degrees of harm rather than harm or no harm, and in the nonidentity dilemma construct, nonexistence is almost always considered the worst harm. The upshot of this rationale is that anything short of an offspring's claim that their life is not worth living (i.e., a claim of very severe harm that cannot be remedied or lessened), falls short of what is sufficient to curtail the parent generation's full reproductive freedom.

A final important Robertson contribution to convey here is a recommendation for a two-step process for arbitrating ethical disputes. The first step is to determine whether there is an individual with a procreative interest. For Robertson, if the individual seeking to reproduce finds significance in reproduction, then the first step has been satisfied. The second step is to consider whether the potential harm inherent in the reproductive plan is sufficient to override the presumption of procreative liberty. The burden is on the opponents of the plan to show that the potential harm justifies limiting reproductive liberty and Robertson asserts that this consideration should tilt the balance in favor of reproducing.

Critique of Procreative Liberty

While Robertson could reasonably be considered the Dean of Reproductive Ethics, it is important to understand varied perspectives as well as criticisms of Robertson's Reproductive Freedom. Criticisms begin with the foundational concept of procreative liberty/reproductive freedom. Some view procreative liberty and the associated rights that extend from it as "a moral bulldozer that crushes all competing interests" ([8], p. 5) due to its enshrinement as a cardinal right that is so wrapped in private values and personal conceptions of

meaning and dignity, that any meaningful ethical or practical debate is off limits [8,9].

Procreative liberty is bestowed cardinal status based on the importance to the individual in reproduction. It can be argued, however that it may be harmful to construe reproduction as a crucial, self-defining experience, the frustration of which is deleterious to personal meaning, dignity and identity. Such concepts set up women, and to a lesser extent men, to feel that reproductive failure is equivalent to failure as a woman (or man) and failure to be fully human [8]. Robertson's portrayal of procreative liberty is also criticized as narrow and narcissistic in that the motivation for reproduction is isolated in the desires and needs of the individual, or parent, with little regard or empathy for how others are impacted [9]. Lastly, critics have objected to Robertson's unyoking reproduction from child-rearing and have argued that the individual need to reproduce (differentiated from a need to parent) is an insufficient basis to elevate procreative liberty to the status that he appoints. Rather, to be enshrined as a cardinal right, procreative liberty needs to include not only the right to reproduce, but also the goal to rear a child in a manner that is intended to be positive [5,10].

A second, and increasingly relevant, criticism of Robertson's characterization of procreative liberty is the consequent entitlement of individuals to select their offspring's traits. Although genetic technology emerged primarily as an attempt to treat life-limiting disease or prevent profound genetic disorders, it "now beckons as an instrument of improvement and consumer choice" ([11], p. 2). Opponents of the unfettered use of genetic technology to influence the traits of children see this as chipping away at the dignity of offspring [9]. They argue that parents are stewards of the children that they bear and raise and, as such, need to see them as having dignity equal to that of their parents, rather than seeing them as "projects" or "objects of our design" [9,11]. Further criticism of prenatal selection of offspring characteristics is that, rather than allowing for the natural occurrence and development of traits, prearranging of traits is an effort to predetermine the characteristics and life experiences of the child. It has been noted that, "the more choices we have, the higher our expectations tend to become" ([10], p. 97). In this context of prenatal selection of traits, it may lead to unreasonable parental expectations of the child. This is counter to the assertion that each child has a right to "an open future;" the right to have future options open until they reach adulthood. Finally, it is argued that the attempt to have mastery over the traits of offspring and bowing to society's competitive demand to improve or perfect, misses, or may even destroy the sense of life as a gift. And the corollary that the beneficial development of individual humility is fostered by the acceptance that not everything in the world is open to what we may desire or devise [11].

A final, and perhaps pivotal criticism of Robertson's Procreative Liberty is its unreasonable reliance on the nonidentity dilemma to counter almost any objections to the potentially harmful use of reproductive technology. As Prusak states, the nonidentity problem, "appears to dissolve the worry that parents can *harm* a child in bringing him or her into being, and so absolve would-be-parents of any culpability for a child's existence in all instances but when it can be predicted that the child's life would be so terrible that it would not even be worth living" ([10], p. 8). This standard has been argued to be too low and that we owe it to potential children to not conceive them if they can be expected to have too low a quality of life [8]. While Prusak and Purdy object to the nonidentity dilemma, they do not dismantle it; however this is done effectively by Cohen. Cohen takes on the core argument of the nonidentity dilemma: that even a poor existence is better than not existing. Cohen notes that "*nonexistence before coming into being* and *nonexistence after having lived* are two distinct concepts" ([12], p. 23). She writes further that there is no harm in nonexistence unless one "assumes that children with an interest in existing are waiting in a spectral world of nonexistence where their situation is less desirable than it would be were they released into this world" ([12], p. 21).

Ethical Expansion Beyond Procreative Liberty

Beyond critiques of the Robertson position, are additional ethical frameworks including virtue ethics, feminist ethics, care-based ethics and communitarian ethics.

Virtue ethics and the moral parental obligations to a potential child factor into arbitrating ethical disputes. As discussed above, the Robertson argument is based on rights. Virtue ethics has its roots in ancient Greek philosophers, including Aristotle, and describes a goal of being a moral or virtuous person. It goes beyond simply behaving in a virtuous manner, and instead focuses on *being a person of a deep virtuous nature*. From this nature, comes a virtuous approach to decisions and actions. Virtue ethics applied to reproduction means approaching the complex aspects of having and raising a child as a virtuous parent would. This is a more down to earth and less aspirational perspective than it may appear. One

fundamental aspect of virtue ethics in having and rearing a child is parental acceptance of the child regardless of nonhealth impacting characteristics, such as the child's sex [13]. Another is that parents provide a sense of emotional security and belonging for their child. For the child, the parent is someone who is committed to their well-being, whose own well-being is tightly bound up with the child's, and being someone who can be counted on to be there for the child in a way that most others cannot [10]. It is suggested that the emotional security inherent in this type of parent–child relationship is not easily transferrable to another responsible adult. While another adult may be able to meet the practical needs of a child, it is not possible to ensure that someone else will love the child as a parent [10]. In the end, it is argued that, by bringing a child into being, a parent faces "prima facie obligations, not only to prevent harm and to prepare the child for a decent life, but to provide, *in person*, support, warmth, and affection during the child's minority and beyond" ([10], p. 37).

Feminist ethics adds to reasoning in reproductive ethics by employing a skepticism of embedded, unrecognized assumptions [14]. Primary in this is the recognition that, historically, societal beliefs and values as well as scientific study, has been founded on the male experience. This androcentric perspective takes the male experience to be the generic human experience and the female experience to be a variation [15]. This can lead to the promotion of reproductive technologies that speak more to the needs of men than the needs of women. For example, it has been suggested that IVF, rather than IUI with donor sperm, is often the primary treatment recommendation when low sperm count is causal in a couple's fertility struggle. This prioritizes and values genetic continuity for men over shielding women from unnecessary medical treatment [14]. A feminist perspective also challenges a culture of "compulsory motherhood" where a woman's identity is centralized on reproductive function and success leading to avoidable distress and subjugation of her needs. Finally, a feminist perspective demands that the consequences for children not be overlooked in reproductive discourse. In particular, as genetic technology advances, feminist ethics demands caution in the question of what type of children we should want [14].

Care-based ethics overlaps and has ties to feminist theory and virtue ethics. In contrast to an individualistic rights perspective, it prioritizes a moral responsibility of care including compassion, empathy and commitment that arises from the interdependent relationships amongst individuals. Care ethicists assert that "human beings are not best understood as individual rights bearers or property owners, but as vulnerable beings-in-relationship who rely on one another for care, concern, nurture, and identity" ([16], p. 335). The moral equality and value of care for both the one cared for and the caregiver is considered as fundamental to humanity. Care-based ethics are particularly important in considering and implementing reproductive health decisions that can be vulnerable to overlooking or discounting the value of others. For example, in the realm of gestational carrier arrangements, a set of intended parents are not just entering into a contract with the carrier; rather, they are embarking on a relationship with her that necessitates a recognition of moral equality, respect, caring and empathy [16].

Communitarian ethics look to expand ethical decision-making to not only incorporate the perspective of the individual but also the impact for the community which is increasingly global. It emerged in response to the ascension of individualist liberalism which incorporated a laissez-faire outlook [17]. The main thrust of communitarian ethics in the realm of assisted reproduction is a demand for personal autonomy be exercised with a consideration for the impact on the community. For example, an individual rights perspective may allow patients the opportunity to select the sex of their child; however, a communitarian ethics argument may resist this by asserting that, although the impact of one patient choosing the sex of their child is negligible, a global community trend towards allowing sex selection risks dramatic impact. With this in mind, it would be argued that communal values and interests sometimes trump personal autonomy [15].

Regulatory Frameworks

We have analytical frameworks for common morality to consider ethical dilemmas in reproductive medicine. What regulatory frameworks have societies enacted to consider ethical dilemmas in this field? The British model covers the regulation of ART for all citizens regardless of the type of treatment clinic (public or private). The Human Fertilisation and Embryology Act (HFEA) was originally drafted in 1990 [18]. It provides an example of the value of legal regulation as well as the drawbacks. Its strength has been in its revision over time. When originally written, fertility treatment was linked to the presence of a male partner. This was subsequently amended in 2008 to a concept of supportive parenting. Initially, HFEA had opposed many treatments which were then revised over time.

American reproductive medicine provides a stark contrast to the United Kingdom (UK). In the US, there is no federal oversight of IVF beyond a recommendation to report IVF outcomes to the Society for Assisted Reproductive Technology (SART). In 2018, 86% of IVF clinics in the US were members of SART [19]. This remains an important aspect of US reproductive care as it provides a way to fairly establish and limit positional advantage among competing clinics. Clinics provide sworn outcome data regarding all treatment cycles. Each clinic decides who to treat and which treatments to offer. The competitive environment for improved clinical outcomes and potential commercial advantages might unjustly limit access to care for patients considered less likely to succeed.

A Format to Address Reproductive Ethical Questions

How are ethical challenges in reproductive medicine best approached? In the majority of cases, there is no clear right or wrong answer. In 1975, a group of eminent scientists, legal scholars and ethicists met at the now famous Asilomar Conference to consider how to safely proceed with genetic engineering. The Nobel laureate, David Baltimore, stated, "We are here ... to balance the benefits and hazards right now and to design a strategy which will maximize the benefits and minimize the hazards for the future" ([20], p. 58). The statement is applicable to our situation in so many ways. It is not a question of *if* we proceed. It is a matter of *how* we proceed.

Ethicists have written extensively regarding strategies for proceeding with ethical deliberation and decision-making. The American College of Obstetrics and Gynecology (ACOG), in particular, has created a helpful committee opinion on ethical decision-making, much of which is incorporated below [15]. While guiding steps are outlined in this section, elemental to constructive ethical consideration is involvement of a multidisciplinary team (e.g., ethicists, physicians, mental health professionals, nurses, attorneys, chaplains and administrators) when available. It is also advised that those addressing ethical questions consider respected opinions about similar cases and utilize established ethical resources including published opinions by the American Society for Reproductive Medicine (ASRM) and the European Society of Human Reproduction and Embryology (ESHRE), as well as institutional ethics committees. A seven-step decision-making process in reproductive ethics is presented below and outlined in Table 27.1.

Table 27.1 Seven-step decision-making process in reproductive ethics

Step 1: *Identify the persons with a direct interest at stake*

Step 2: *Gather medical, psychosocial and legal information relevant to the interests of each identified stake holder*

Step 3: *Identify all medically appropriate decision options*

Step 4: *Review each potential decision option with respect to autonomy, beneficence and nonmaleficence, and justice*

Step 5: *Identify and utilize additional ethical frameworks that may be relevant*

Step 6: *Evaluate each potential resolution*

Step 7: *Reevaluate the decision*

Step 1: Identify the persons with a direct interest at stake. At a minimum, this will include an individual patient seeking reproductive care but frequently will include the interests of a spouse or partner and potentially children of either of these individuals. In third-party reproduction decisions, this can include the interests of a gamete donor or gestational carrier and potentially that individual's partner and children. Often overlooked due to their current state of nonexistence, yet important, are the interests of the prospective child. The relative standing of each individual's interests is specific to the concerns identified.

Step 2: Gather medical, psychosocial and legal information relevant to the interests of each identified stake holder with the goal of increasing understanding of their position, values and interests. As relevant, identify the personal, professional, institutional and societal values, perspectives and potential biases that are contributing to the processing of the ethical concern.

Step 3: Identify all medically appropriate decision options including those put forward by the patient and other concerned individuals as well as options suggested by relevant consultants.

Step 4: **Review each potential decision option with respect to the core ethical principles** of respect for autonomy (including procreative liberty), beneficence and nonmaleficence, and justice.

Step 5: Identify and utilize additional ethical frameworks that may be relevant to the question at hand. This may include procreative responsibility, virtue ethics, feminist ethics, care-based ethics and communitarian ethics.

Step 6: After consideration of core ethical principles and additional helpful ethical frameworks, **evaluate each**

potential resolution to identify how each option impacts the interests of the individuals who have a stake in the decision. Select the option that can be best justified.

Step 7: Reevaluate the decision as information becomes available regarding the outcome and its impact on the interested individuals with the goal of positively impacting decision-making in future ethical concerns.

Emerging Ethical Challenges and Conclusion

The ASRM chronicles the timeline of assisted reproduction and notes as a starting place the first successful pregnancy using frozen sperm, which occurred in 1953 [21]. The timeline portrays a continual emergence of reproductive technologies including the first successful IVF (1978), the first successful pregnancy with donor oocytes (1983), the first successful pregnancy by a gestational carrier (1985), the first child born following pre-implantation genetic diagnosis (1990), and the first successful pregnancy after uterine transplant (2014). Across this same timeline are legal advances including the 1965 Supreme Court ruling allowing married couples to use birth control, the 1973 Roe v Wade ruling permitting abortions, and the 2015 ruling legalizing same sex marriage. Further, across this same timeline we have witnessed increasing diversity of patients seeking care to include LGBTQ patients, single patients, fertility preservation patients, and patients of advanced age. The advancing and changing face of reproductive care has always been accompanied by varying degrees of societal pushback and the emerging and ever more complex ethical dilemmas will require rigorous societal debate.

As the rapid pace of technological innovation in reproductive medicine continues, we grapple with new ethical questions. The expanding role of genetics, beyond the prevention of severe disease through the selection of unaffected embryos into the selection of a more advantaged embryo, ushers in particularly difficult ethical challenges. The discovery of CRISPR-Cas9 in 2012 and its rapidly evolving iterations compels ethical debate including considerations that raise significant questions: What diseases qualify as sufficiently severe to warrant germline modification? How is severity evaluated? What if it were possible to remove the extra chromosome in an embryo with trisomy 21? Is it reasonable to use genetics to enhance a child's health, intelligence, skills or physical abilities?

The perspectives of procreative liberty, virtue ethics, feminist ethics, care-based ethics and communitarian ethics are all important voices as these questions are debated. The ethical challenges associated with genetics are particularly formidable. While it will always be reasonable for a parent to want a healthy child, society needs a diverse population for many reasons, not the least of which is to position ourselves to have sufficient diversity within the species to adapt to the challenges we will face from pandemics such as COVID-19, evolution, or those created by ourselves. In 1962, eminent geneticist and evolutionary biologist Theodosius Dobzhansky stated that, "genetic diversity is mankind's most precious resource, not a regrettable deviation from an ideal state of monotonous sameness" ([22], p. 112), emphasizing that a society of uniformly perfect individuals with similar characteristics is ill-positioned for future challenges. Prioritizing the hardiness of humanity over the prebirth liberty of parental control in offspring characteristics is a delicate balance and apt to be met with resistance. Undoubtedly, we will be evermore pressed to balance the reproductive liberties of the individual with the needs of society.

Technology will march on, and patients will bring increasingly complex requests to healthcare professionals. The question is not are we going to employ innovative technologies or expand reproductive care, but rather, how do we balance individual patient desires with ethics.

References

1. Kass LR. Babies by means of in vitro fertilization: unethical experiments on the unborn? *N Engl J Med* 1971;**285**(21):1174–1179.

2. King LP. Should clinicians set limits on reproductive autonomy? *Hastings Cent Rep* 2017;**47**(Suppl. 3):S50–S56.

3. University of Minnesota's Center for Bioethics. Ethics of Organ Transplantation. 2004. Available at: www.ahc.umn.edu/img/assets/26104/Organ_Transplantation.pdf [last accessed June 16, 2022].

4. Robertson JA. *Children of Choice: Freedom and the New Reproductive Technologies*. Princeton, NJ: Princeton University Press, 1994.

5. Steinbock B. Review Essay/Procreative Liberty. *Crim Justice Ethics* 1996;**15**(1):67–74.

6. Robertson JA. Ethics and the future of preimplantation genetic diagnosis. *Reprod Biomed Online* 2005;**10**(S1):97–101.

7. Robertson JA. Genetic selection of offspring characteristics. *B.U.L. Rev* 1996;**76**(3):421–482.

8. Purdy L. Children of choice: whose children? At what cost? *Wash Lee Law Rev* 1995;**52**(1):197–224.

9. Meilaender G. Products of the will: Robertson's children of choice. *Wash Lee Law Rev* 1995;**52**(1):173–195.

10. Prusak BG. *Parental Obligations and Bioethics*. New York, NY: Routledge, 2013.

11. Sandel MJ. The case against perfection: what's wrong with designer children, bionic athletes, and genetic engineering. *The Atlantic Online*. Published April 2004. Available at: www.theatlantic.com/magazine/archive/2004/04/the-case-against-perfection/302927/ [last accessed June 16, 2022].

12. Cohen CB. Give me children or I shall die! New reproductive technologies and harm to children. *Hastings Cent Rep* 1996;**40**(4):19–27.

13. McDougall R. Acting parentally: an argument against sex selection. *J Med Ethics* 2005;**31**:601–605.

14. Overall C. *Ethics and Human Reproduction: A Feminist Analysis*. London: Routledge, 1987.

15. American College of Obstetrics and Gynecology. ACOG Committee Opinion No. 390, December 2007. Ethical decision making in obstetrics and gynecology. *Obstet Gynecol* 2007;**110**(6):1479–1487. https://doi.org/10.1097/01.AOG.0000291573.09193.36

16. Parks JA. Care ethics and the global practice of commercial surrogacy. *Bioethics* 2010;**24**(7):333–340.

17. Tam H. Communitarianism, Sociology of. In: Wright JD (editor-in-chief), *International Encyclopedia of the Social & Behavioral Sciences*, 2nd ed., vol. **4**. Oxford: Elsevier, 2015, 311–316.

18. Doyle P. The U.K. Human Fertilisation and Embryology Authority. How it has contributed to the evaluation of assisted reproduction technology. *Int J Technol Assess Health Care* 1999;**15**(1):3–10.

19. What is SART? Available at: www.sart.org/patients/what-is-sart/ [last accessed June 16, 2022].

20. Weiner C. Social responsibility in genetic engineering: historical perspectives. In: Nordgren A. *Gene Therapy and Ethics: Studies in Bioethics and Research Ethics*, 4th ed. Uppsala, Sweden: Uppsala University Press, 1999, 51–64.

21. Timeline of Advances in the Field of Reproductive Medicine. Available at: www.asrm.org/about-us/history-of-asrm/ [last accessed June 16, 2022].

22. Dobzhansky T. Genetics and equality. *Science* 1962;**137**(3524):112–115.

The International Glossary on Infertility and Fertility Care, 2017[*]

Term	Consensus definition
Acrosome	A membrane-bound structure covering the anterior of the sperm head that contains enzymes necessary to penetrate the zona pellucida of the oocyte.
Adenomyosis	A form of endometriosis marked by the presence of endometrium-like epithelium and stroma outside the endometrium in the myometrium.
Adhesions	Bands of fibrous scar tissue that may bind the abdominal and pelvic organs, including the intestines and peritoneum, to each other. They can be dense and thick or filmy and thin.
Age-specific fertility rate (ASFR)	The number of live births per woman in a particular age group in a specific calendar year expressed per 1,000 women in that age group.
Agglutination	Clumping of spermatozoa in the ejaculate.
Andrology	The medical practice dealing with the health of the male reproductive system.
Aneuploidy	An abnormal number of chromosomes in a cell. The majority of embryos with aneuploidies are not compatible with life.
Anti-sperm antibodies	Antibodies that recognize and bind to antigens on the surface of the spermatozoon.
Aspermia	Lack of external ejaculation.
Assisted hatching	An ART procedure in which the zona pellucida of an embryo is either thinned or perforated by chemical, mechanical or laser methods.
Assisted reproductive technology (ART)	All interventions that include the *in vitro* handling of both human oocytes and sperm or of embryos for the purpose of reproduction. This includes, but is not limited to, IVF and embryo transfer (ET), intracytoplasmic sperm injection (ICSI), embryo biopsy, preimplantation genetic testing (PGT), assisted hatching, gamete intrafallopian transfer (GIFT), zygote intrafallopian transfer, gamete and embryo cryopreservation, semen, oocyte and embryo donation, and gestational carrier cycles. Thus, ART does not, and ART-only registries do not, include assisted insemination using sperm from either a woman's partner or a sperm donor. (See broader term, medically assisted reproduction, (MAR).)

* With permission: Zegers FZ, Adamson GD, Dyer S, et al. The International Glossary on Infertility and Fertility Care: Led by ICMART in Partnership with ASRM, ESHRE, IFFS, March of Dimes, AFS, GIERAF, ASPIRE, MEFS, REDLARA, FIGO. *Fertil Steril* 2017;108(3):393–406.

Asthenoteratozoospermia	Reduced percentages of motile and morphologically normal sperm in the ejaculate below the lower reference limit. When reporting results, the reference criteria should be specified.
Asthenozoospermia	Reduced percentage of motile sperm in the ejaculate below the lower reference limit. When reporting results, the reference criteria should be specified.
Azoospermia	The absence of spermatozoa in the ejaculate.
Binucleation	The presence of two nuclei in a blastomere (cell).
Biochemical pregnancy	A pregnancy diagnosed only by the detection of beta hCG in serum or urine.
Birth (single)	The complete expulsion or extraction from a woman of a fetus after 22 completed weeks of gestational age, irrespective of whether it is a live birth or stillbirth, or, if gestational age is unknown, a birth weight more than 500 grams. A single birth refers to an individual newborn; and a delivery of multiple births, such as a twin delivery, would be registered as two births.
Blastocele	Fluid-filled central region of the blastocyst.
Blastocyst	The stage of preimplantation embryo development that occurs around day 5–6 after insemination or ICSI. The blastocyst contains a fluid-filled central cavity (blastocele), an outer layer of cells (trophectoderm) and an inner group of cells (inner cell mass).
Blastomere	A cell in a cleavage stage embryo.
Blastomere symmetry	The extent to which all blastomeres are even in size and shape.
Bleeding after oocyte aspiration	Significant bleeding, internal or external, after oocyte aspiration retrieval requiring hospitalization for blood transfusion, surgical intervention, clinical observation or other medical procedure.
Canceled ART cycle	An ART cycle in which ovarian stimulation or monitoring has been initiated with the intention to treat, but which did not proceed to follicular aspiration or in the case of a thawed or warmed embryo did not proceed to embryo transfer.
Childlessness	A condition in which a person, voluntarily or involuntarily, is not a legal or societally recognized parent to a child, or has had all children die.
Chimerism	Presence in a single individual of two or more cell lines, each derived from different individuals.
Cleavage stage embryos	Embryos beginning with the 2-cell stage and up to, but not including, the morula stage.
Clinical fertility	The capacity to establish a clinical pregnancy.
Clinical pregnancy	A pregnancy diagnosed by ultrasonographic visualization of one or more gestational sacs or definitive clinical signs of pregnancy. In addition to intra-uterine pregnancy, it includes a clinically documented ectopic pregnancy.
Clinical pregnancy rate	The number of clinical pregnancies expressed per 100 initiated cycles, aspiration cycles or embryo transfer cycles. When clinical pregnancy rates are recorded, the denominator (initiated, aspirated or embryo transfer cycles) must be specified.

Clinical pregnancy with fetal heart beat

A pregnancy diagnosed by ultrasonographic or clinical documentation of at least one fetus with a discernible heartbeat.

Cohort total fertility rate (CTFR)

The observed average number of live born children per woman applied to a birth cohort of women as they age through time. This is obtained from data on women after completing their reproductive years.

Compaction

The process during which tight junctions form between juxtaposed blastomeres resulting in a solid mass of cells with indistinguishable cell membranes.

Complex aneuploidies

Two or more aneuploidies involving different chromosomes in the embryo. When autosomes are involved, this condition is not compatible with human life.

Congenital anomalies

Structural or functional disorders that occur during intra-uterine life and can be identified prenatally, at birth or later in life. Congenital anomalies can be caused by single gene defects, chromosomal disorders, multifactorial inheritance, environmental teratogens and micronutrient deficiencies. The time of identification should be reported.

Congenital anomaly birth rate

The number of births exhibiting signs of congenital anomalies per 10,000 births. The time of identification should have been reported.

Congenital bilateral absence of the vasa deferentia (CBAVD)

The absence, at birth, of both duct systems (vas deferentia) that connect the testes to the urethra and may be associated with cystic fibrosis transmembrane conductance regulator (CTFR) gene mutation. Although the testes usually develop and function normally, men present with azoospermia.

Conventional in vitro insemination

The co-incubation of oocytes with sperm in vitro with the goal of resulting in extracorporeal fertilization.

Corona radiata cells

The innermost cells of the cumulus oophorus.

Cross-border reproductive care

The provision of reproductive health services in a different jurisdiction or outside of a recognized national border within which the person or persons legally reside.

Cryopreservation

The process of slow freezing or vitrification to preserve biological material (e.g. gametes, zygotes, cleavage-stage embryos, blastocysts or gonadal tissue) at extreme low temperature.

Cryptorchidism

Testis not in scrotal position within the neonatal period and, up to but not limited to, 1 year post birth. If the testis has not descended into the scrotum, this condition can cause primary testicular failure and increased risk of testicular cancer development.

Cumulative delivery rate per aspiration/ initiated cycle with at least one live birth

The number of deliveries with at least one live birth resulting from one initiated or aspirated ART cycle, including all cycles in which fresh and/or frozen embryos are transferred, until one delivery with a live birth occurs or until all embryos are used, whichever occurs first. The delivery of a singleton, twin, or other multiples is registered as one delivery. In the absence of complete data, the cumulative delivery rate is often estimated.

Cumulus oophorus

The multi-layered mass of granulosa cells surrounding the oocyte.

Cytoplasmic maturation

The process during which the oocyte acquires the capacity to support nuclear maturation, fertilization, pronuclei formation, syngamy and subsequent early cleavage divisions until activation of the embryonic genome.

Cytoplasmic transfer	A procedure that can be performed at different stages of an oocyte's development to add to or replace various amounts of cytoplasm from a donor egg.
Decreased spermatogenesis	A histological finding in which spermatogenesis is present with few cells in the seminiferous tubules, resulting in a decreased number or absence of sperm in the ejaculate.
Delayed ejaculation	A condition in which it takes a man an extended period of time to reach orgasm and ejaculation.
Delayed embryo transfer	A procedure in which embryo transfer is not performed within the time frame of the oocyte aspiration cycle but at a later time.
Delivery	The complete expulsion or extraction from a woman of one or more fetuses, after at least 22 completed weeks of gestational age, irrespective of whether they are live births or stillbirths. A delivery of either a single or multiple newborn is considered as one delivery. If more than one newborn is delivered, it is often recognized as a delivery with multiple births.
Delivery rate	The number of deliveries expressed per 100 initiated cycles, aspiration cycles, or embryo transfer cycles. When delivery rates are recorded, the denominator (initiated, aspirated or embryo transfer cycles) must be specified. It includes deliveries that resulted in the birth of one or more live births and/or stillbirths. The delivery of a singleton, twin or other multiple pregnancy is registered as one delivery. If more than one newborn is delivered, it is often recognized as a delivery with multiple births.
Delivery rate after fertility treatment per patient	The number of deliveries with at least one live birth or stillbirth, expressed per 100 patients, after a specified time and following all treatments.
Delivery with multiple births after fertility treatments	A single delivery with more than one newborn, following all fertility treatments.
Diandric oocytes	An oocyte with an extra set of haploid chromosomes of paternal origin.
Digynic oocytes	An oocyte with an extra set of haploid chromosomes of maternal origin.
Diminished ovarian reserve	A term generally used to indicate a reduced number and/or reduced quality of oocytes, such that the ability to reproduce is decreased. (See ovarian reserve.)
Diploidy/euploidy	The condition in which a cell has two haploid sets of chromosomes. Each chromosome in one set is paired with its counterpart in the other set. A diploid embryo has 22 pairs of autosomes and two sex chromosomes, the normal condition.
Disomy	The normal number of chromosomes characterized by 22 pairs of autosomal chromosomes and one pair of sex chromosomes (XX or XY). The chromosome number in human cells is normally 46.
Donor insemination	The process of placing laboratory processed sperm or semen from a man into the reproductive tract of a woman who is not his intimate sexual partner, for the purpose of initiating a pregnancy.
Double embryo transfer (DET)	The transfer of two embryos in an ART procedure. This may be elective (eDET) when more than two embryos of sufficient quality for transfer are available.
Early neonatal death/mortality	Death of a newborn within 7 days of birth.

Ectopic pregnancy	A pregnancy outside the uterine cavity, diagnosed by ultrasound, surgical visualization or histopathology.
Ejaculation	Co-ordinated contractions of the genitourinary tract leading to the ejection of spermatozoa and seminal fluid.
Ejaculation retardata	A condition resulting in an inability to ejaculate during vaginal intercourse.
Ejaculatory duct	The canal that passes through the prostate just lateral to the verumontanum where the vas deferens and the duct from the seminal vesicle coalesce.
Elective embryo transfer	The transfer of one or more embryos, selected from a larger cohort of available embryos.
Elective single embryo transfer (eSET)	The transfer of one (a single) embryo selected from a larger cohort of available embryos.
Embryo	The biological organism resulting from the development of the zygote, until 8 completed weeks after fertilization, equivalent to 10 weeks of gestational age.
Embryo bank	Repository of cryopreserved embryos stored for future use.
Embryo donation (for reproduction)	An ART cycle, which consists of the transfer of an embryo to the uterus or Fallopian tube of a female recipient, resulting from gametes that did not originate from the female recipient or from her male partner, if present.
Embryo fragmentation	The process during which one or more blastomeres shed membrane vesicles containing cytoplasm and occasionally whole chromosomes or chromatin.
Embryo recipient cycle	An ART cycle in which a woman's uterus is prepared to receive one or more cleavage stage embryos/blastocysts, resulting from gametes that did not originate from her or from her male partner, if present.
Embryo transfer (ET)	Placement into the uterus of an embryo at any embryonic stage from day 1 to day 7 after IVF or ICSI. Embryos from day 1 to day 3 can also be transferred into the Fallopian tube.
Embryo transfer cycle	An ART cycle in which one or more fresh or frozen/thawed embryos at cleavage or blastocyst stage are transferred into the uterus or Fallopian tube.
Emission (semen)	Co-ordinated contractions of the vas deferentia, seminal vesicles, and ejaculatory ducts leading to deposition of semen into the urethral meatus prior to ejaculation.
Endometriosis	A disease characterized by the presence of endometrium-like epithelium and stroma outside the endometrium and myometrium. Intrapelvic endometriosis can be located superficially on the peritoneum (peritoneal endometriosis), can extend 5 mm or more beneath the peritoneum (deep endometriosis) or can be present as an ovarian endometriotic cyst (endometrioma).
Epididymis	A convoluted, highly coiled duct that transports the spermatozoa from the testis via the efferent ducts to the vas deferens.
Erectile dysfunction	Inability to have and/or sustain an erection sufficient for intercourse.
Euploidy	The condition in which a cell has chromosomes in an exact multiple of the haploid number; in the human this multiple is normally two. Thus, a normal embryo that is euploid is also diploid.

Excessive ovarian response	An exaggerated response to ovarian stimulation characterized by the presence of more follicles than intended. Generally, more than 20 follicles >12 mm in size and/or more than 20 oocytes collected following ovarian stimulation are considered excessive, but these numbers are adaptable according to ethnic and other variables.
Expectant fertility management	Management of fertility problems including infertility without any specific active clinical or therapeutic interventions other than fertility information and advice, to improve natural fertility, based upon the probability of becoming pregnant.
Extremely low birth weight	Birth weight less than 1000 g.
Extremely preterm birth	A birth that takes place after 22 but before 28 completed weeks of gestational age.
Fecundability	The probability of a pregnancy, during a single menstrual cycle in a woman with adequate exposure to sperm and no contraception, culminating in a live birth. In population-based studies, fecundability is frequently measured as the monthly probability.
Fecundity	Clinically defined as the capacity to have a live birth.
Female infertility	Infertility caused primarily by female factors encompassing: ovulatory disturbances; diminished ovarian reserve; anatomical, endocrine, genetic, functional or immunological abnormalities of the reproductive system; chronic illness; and sexual conditions incompatible with coitus.
Fertility	The capacity to establish a clinical pregnancy.
Fertility awareness	The understanding of reproduction, fecundity, fecundability, and related individual risk factors (e.g. advanced age, sexual health factors such as sexually transmitted infections, and life-style factors such as smoking, obesity) and nonindividual risk factors (e.g. environmental and work place factors); including the awareness of societal and cultural factors affecting options to meet reproductive family planning, as well as family building needs.
Fertility care	Interventions that include fertility awareness, support and fertility management with an intention to assist individuals and couples to realize their desires associated with reproduction and/or to build a family.
Fertility preservation	Various interventions, procedures and technologies, including cryopreservation of gametes, embryos or ovarian and testicular tissue to preserve reproductive capacity.
Fertilization	A sequence of biological processes initiated by entry of a spermatozoon into a mature oocyte followed by formation of the pronuclei.
Fetal loss	Death of a fetus. It is referred to as early fetal loss when death takes place between 10 and 22 weeks of gestational age; late fetal loss, when death takes place between 22 and 28 weeks of gestational age; and stillbirth when death takes place after 28 weeks of gestational age.
Fetus	The stages of development of an organism from 8 completed weeks of fertilization (equivalent to 10 weeks of gestational age) until the end of pregnancy.
Freeze-all cycle	An ART cycle in which, after oocyte aspiration, all oocytes and/or embryos are cryopreserved and no oocytes and/or embryos are transferred to a woman in that cycle.

Frozen-thawed embryo transfer (FET) cycle	An ART procedure in which cycle monitoring is carried out with the intention of transferring to a woman, frozen/thawed or vitrified/warmed embryo(s)/blastocyst(s). Note: a FET cycle is initiated when specific medication is provided or cycle monitoring is started in the female recipient with the intention to transfer an embryo.
Frozen-thawed oocyte cycle	An ART procedure in which cycle monitoring is carried out with the intention of fertilizing thawed/warmed oocytes and performing an embryo transfer.
Full-term birth	A birth that takes place between 37 and 42 completed weeks of gestational age.
Gamete intrafallopian transfer (GIFT)	An ART procedure in which both gametes (oocytes and spermatozoa) are transferred into a Fallopian tube(s).
Germinal vesicle (GV)	The nucleus in an oocyte at prophase I.
Gestational age	The age of an embryo or fetus calculated by the best obstetric estimate determined by assessments which may include early ultrasound and the date of the last menstrual period and/or perinatal details. In the case of ART, it is calculated by adding 2 weeks (14 days) to the number of completed weeks since fertilization. Note: for frozen-thawed embryo transfer (FET) cycles, an estimated date of fertilization is computed by subtracting the combined number of days an embryo was in culture pre-cryopreservation and post-thaw/-warm, from the transfer date of the FET cycle.
Gestational carrier	A woman who carries a pregnancy with an agreement that she will give the offspring to the intended parent(s). Gametes can originate from the intended parent(s) and/or a third party (or parties). This replaces the term "surrogate."
Gestational sac	A fluid-filled structure associated with early pregnancy, which may be located inside or, in the case of an ectopic pregnancy, outside the uterus.
Globozoospermia	Describes spermatozoa with a reduced or absent acrosome.
Haploidy	The condition in which a cell has one set of each of the 23 single chromosomes. Mature human gametes are haploid, each having 23 single chromosomes.
Hatching	The process by which an embryo at the blastocyst stage extrudes out of, and ultimately separates from, the zona pellucida.
Heterotopic pregnancy	Concurrent pregnancy involving at least one embryo implanted in the uterine cavity and at least one implanted outside of the uterine cavity.
High-order multiple births	The complete expulsion or extraction from their mother of three or more fetuses, after 22 completed weeks of gestational age, irrespective of whether they are live births or stillbirths.
High-order multiple gestation	A pregnancy with three or more embryos or fetuses.
Hydrosalpinx	A distally occluded, dilated, fluid-filled Fallopian tube.
Hypergonadotropic hypogonadism	Gonadal failure associated with reduced gametogenesis, reduced gonadal steroid production and elevated gonadotropin production.
Hyperspermia	High volume of ejaculate above the upper reference limit. When reporting results, the reference criteria should be specified.

Hypogonadotropic hypogonadism	Gonadal failure associated with reduced gametogenesis and reduced gonadal steroid production due to reduced gonadotropin production or action.
Hypospermatogenesis	Histopathologic description of reduced production of spermatozoa in the testes.
Hypospermia	Low volume of ejaculate below the lower reference limit. When reporting results, the reference criteria should be specified.
Iatrogenic testicular failure	Damage to testicular function after radiation, chemotherapy or hormone treatment; or devascularization as a consequence of hernia surgery.
Immature oocyte	An oocyte at prophase of meiosis I, (i.e. an oocyte at the germinal vesicle (GV)-stage.)
Implantation	The attachment and subsequent penetration by a zona-free blastocyst into the endometrium, but when it relates to an ectopic pregnancy, into tissue outside the uterine cavity. This process starts 5 to 7 days after fertilization of the oocyte, usually resulting in the formation of a gestation sac.
Implantation rate	The number of gestational sacs observed divided by the number of embryos transferred (usually expressed as a percentage, %).
In vitro fertilization (IVF)	A sequence of procedures that involves extracorporeal fertilization of gametes. It includes conventional *in vitro* insemination and ICSI.
In vitro maturation (IVM)	A sequence of laboratory procedures that enable extracorporeal maturation of immature oocytes into fully mature oocytes that are capable of being fertilized with potential to develop into embryos.
Induced abortion	Intentional loss of an intrauterine pregnancy, through intervention by medical, surgical or unspecified means. (See induced embryo/fetal reduction.)
Induced embryo/fetal reduction	An intervention intended to reduce the number of gestational sacs or embryos/fetuses in a multiple gestation.
Infertility	A disease characterized by the failure to establish a clinical pregnancy after 12 months of regular, unprotected sexual intercourse or due to an impairment of a person's capacity to reproduce either as an individual or with his/her partner. Fertility interventions may be initiated in less than 1 year based on medical, sexual and reproductive history, age, physical findings and diagnostic testing. Infertility is a disease, which generates disability as an impairment of function.
Infertility counseling	A professional intervention with the intention to mitigate the physical, emotional and psychosocial consequences of infertility.
Initiated medically assisted reproduction cycle (iMAR)	A cycle in which the woman receives specific medication for ovarian stimulation or in which cycle monitoring is carried out with the intention to treat, irrespective of whether or not insemination is performed, follicular aspiration is attempted in an ovarian stimulation cycle or whether egg(s) or embryo(s) are thawed or transferred in a frozen embryo transfer (FET) cycle.
Inner cell mass	A group of cells attached to the polar trophectoderm consisting of embryonic stem cells, which have the potential to develop into cells and tissues in the human body, except the placenta or amniotic membranes.

Intended parent(s)	A couple or person who seek(s) to reproduce with the assistance of a gestational carrier or traditional gestational carrier.
Intra-cervical insemination	A procedure in which laboratory-processed sperm are placed in the cervix to attempt a pregnancy.
Intracytoplasmic sperm injection (ICSI)	A procedure in which a single spermatozoon is injected into the oocyte cytoplasm.
Intra-uterine insemination	A procedure in which laboratory-processed sperm are placed in the uterus to attempt a pregnancy.
Intra-uterine pregnancy	A state of reproduction in which an embryo has implanted in the uterus.
Laparoscopic ovarian drilling	A surgical method for inducing ovulation in females with anovulatory or oligo-ovulatory polycystic ovarian syndrome, utilizing either laser or electrosurgery.
Large for gestational age	A birth weight greater than the 90th centile of the sex-specific birth weight for a given gestational age reference. When reporting outcomes, the reference criteria should be specified. If gestational age is unknown, then the birth weight should be registered.
Leukospermia	A high number of white blood cells in semen above the upper reference limit. When reporting results, the reference criteria should be specified.
Leydig cell	Type of testicular cell located in the interstitial space between the seminiferous tubules, that secretes testosterone.
Live birth	The complete expulsion or extraction from a woman of a product of fertilization, after 22 completed weeks of gestational age; which, after such separation, breathes or shows any other evidence of life, such as heart beat, umbilical cord pulsation or definite movement of voluntary muscles, irrespective of whether the umbilical cord has been cut or the placenta is attached. A birth weight of 500 grams or more can be used if gestational age is unknown. Live births refer to the individual newborn; for example, a twin delivery represents two live births.
Live birth delivery rate	The number of deliveries that resulted in at least one live birth, expressed per 100 cycle attempts. In the case of ART/MAR interventions, they can be initiated cycles, insemination, aspiration cycles or embryo transfer cycles. When delivery rates are given, the denominator (initiated, inseminated, aspirated or embryo transfer cycles) must be specified.
Low birth weight	Birth weight less than 2,500 g.
Luteal phase defect	A poorly defined abnormality of the endometrium presumably due to abnormally low progesterone secretion or action on the endometrium.
Luteal phase support	Hormonal supplementation in the luteal phase, usually progesterone.
Major congenital anomaly	A congenital anomaly that requires surgical repair of a defect, is a visually evident or life-threatening structural or functional defect, or causes death.
Male infertility	Infertility caused primarily by male factors encompassing: abnormal semen parameters or function; anatomical, endocrine, genetic, functional or immunological abnormalities of the reproductive system; chronic illness; and sexual conditions incompatible with the ability to deposit semen in the vagina.
Maternal spindle transfer	Transfer of the maternal spindle (including maternal chromosomes) from a patient's oocyte into a donated oocyte in which the maternal spindle with chromosomes has been removed.

Mature oocyte	An oocyte at metaphase of meiosis II, exhibiting the first polar body and with the ability to become fertilized.
Maturing oocyte	An oocyte that has progressed from prophase I but has not completed telophase I, thus does not exhibit the first polar body.
Medically assisted reproduction (MAR)	Reproduction brought about through various interventions, procedures, surgeries and technologies to treat different forms of fertility impairment and infertility. These include ovulation induction, ovarian stimulation, ovulation triggering, all ART procedures, uterine transplantation and intra-uterine, intracervical and intravaginal insemination with semen of husband/partner or donor.
Microdissection testicular sperm extraction (MicroTESE)	A surgical procedure using an operating microscope to identify seminiferous tubules that may contain sperm to be extracted for IVF and/or ICSI.
Micromanipulation in ART	A micro-operative ART procedure performed on sperm, egg or embryo; the most common ART micromanipulation procedures are ICSI, assisted hatching and gamete or embryo biopsy for PGT.
Microsurgical epididymal sperm aspiration/ extraction (MESA/MESE)	A surgical procedure performed with the assistance of an operating microscope to retrieve sperm from the epididymis of men with obstructive azoospermia. In the absence of optical magnification, any surgical procedure to retrieve sperm from the epididymis should also be registered as MESE.
Mild ovarian stimulation for IVF	A protocol in which the ovaries are stimulated with gonadotropins, and/or other pharmacological compounds, with the intention of limiting the number of oocytes following stimulation for IVF.
Missed spontaneous abortion/missed miscarriage	Spontaneous loss of a clinical pregnancy before 22 completed weeks of gestational age, in which the embryo(s) or fetus(es) is/are nonviable and is/are not spontaneously absorbed or expelled from the uterus.
Modified natural cycle	An ART procedure in which one or more oocytes are collected from the ovaries during a spontaneous menstrual cycle. Pharmacological compounds are administered with the sole purpose of blocking the spontaneous LH surge and/or inducing final oocyte maturation.
Monosomy	The absence of one of the two homologous chromosomes in embryos. Autosomal monosomies in embryos are not compatible with life. Embryos with sex chromosome monosomies are rarely compatible with life.
Morula	An embryo formed after completion of compaction, typically 4 days after insemination or ICSI.
Mosaicism	A state in which there is more than one karyotypically distinct cell population arising from a single embryo.
Multinucleation	The presence of more than one nucleus in a cell.
Multiple birth	The complete expulsion or extraction from a woman of more than one fetus, after 22 completed weeks of gestational age, irrespective of whether it is a live birth or stillbirth. Births refer to the individual newborn; for example, a twin delivery represents two births.
Multiple gestation	A pregnancy with more than one embryo or fetus.
Natural cycle ART	An ART procedure in which one or more oocytes are collected from the ovaries during a menstrual cycle without the use of any pharmacological compound.

Necrozoospermia	The description of an ejaculate in which no live spermatozoa can be found.
Neonatal death/mortality	Death of a live born baby within 28 days of birth. This can be sub-divided into (a) early, if death occurs in the first 7 days after birth; and (b) late, if death occurs between 8 and 28 days after birth.
Neonatal mortality rate	Number of neonatal deaths (up to 28 days) per 1,000 live births.
Neonatal period	The period which commences at birth and ends at 28 completed days after birth.
Non-obstructive azoospermia	Absence of spermatozoa in the ejaculate due to lack of production of mature spermatozoa.
Nuclear maturation	The process during which the oocyte resumes meiosis and progresses from prophase I to metaphase II.
Obstructive azoospermia	Absence of spermatozoa in the ejaculate due to occlusion of the ductal system.
Oligospermia	A term for low semen volume now replaced by hypospermia to avoid confusion with oligozoospermia.
Oligozoospermia	Low concentration of spermatozoa in the ejaculate below the lower reference limit. When reporting results, the reference criteria should be specified.
Oocyte	The female gamete (egg).
Oocyte aspiration	Ovarian follicular aspiration performed with the aim of retrieving oocytes.
Oocyte bank	Repository of cryopreserved oocytes stored for future use.
Oocyte donation	The use of oocytes from an egg donor for reproductive purposes or research.
Oocyte donation cycle	An ART cycle in which oocytes are collected from an egg donor for reproductive purposes or research.
Oocyte cryopreservation	The freezing or vitrification of oocytes for future use.
Oocyte maturation triggering	An intervention intended to induce an oocyte *in vitro* or *in vivo* to resume meiosis to reach maturity (i.e. to reach metaphase II).
Oocyte recipient cycle	An ART cycle in which a woman receives oocytes from a donor, or her partner if in a same sex relationship, to be used for reproductive purposes.
Oolemma	The cytoplasmic membrane enclosing the oocyte.
Ooplasm	The cytoplasm of the oocyte.
Ovarian hyperstimulation syndrome (OHSS)	An exaggerated systemic response to ovarian stimulation characterized by a wide spectrum of clinical and laboratory manifestations. It may be classified as mild, moderate or severe according to the degree of abdominal distention, ovarian enlargement and respiratory, hemodynamic and metabolic complications.
Ovarian reserve	A term generally used to indicate the number and/or quality of oocytes, reflecting the ability to reproduce. Ovarian reserve can be assessed by any of several means. They include: female age; number of antral follicles on ultrasound; anti-Mullerian hormone levels; follicle stimulating hormone and estradiol levels; clomiphene citrate challenge test; response to gonadotropin stimulation, and oocyte and/or embryo assessment during

an ART procedure, based on number, morphology or genetic assessment of the oocytes and/or embryos.

Ovarian stimulation (OS)
Pharmacological treatment with the intention of inducing the development of ovarian follicles. It can be used for two purposes: (1) for timed intercourse or insemination; (2) in ART, to obtain multiple oocytes at follicular aspiration.

Ovarian tissue cryopreservation
The process of slow-freezing or vitrification of tissue surgically excised from the ovary with the intention of preserving reproductive capacity.

Ovarian torsion
Partial or complete rotation of the ovarian vascular pedicle that causes obstruction to ovarian blood flow, potentially leading to necrosis of ovarian tissue.

Ovulation
The natural process of expulsion of a mature egg from its ovarian follicle.

Ovulation induction (OI)
Pharmacological treatment of women with anovulation or oligo-ovulation with the intention of inducing normal ovulatory cycles.

Parthenogenetic activation
The process by which an oocyte is activated to undergo development in the absence of fertilization.

Parthenote
The product of an oocyte that has undergone activation in the absence of the paternal genome, with (induced) or without (spontaneous) a purposeful intervention.

Percutaneous epididymal sperm aspiration (PESA)
A surgical procedure in which a needle is introduced percutaneously into the epididymis with the intention of obtaining sperm.

Perinatal death/mortality
Fetal or neonatal death occurring during late pregnancy (at 22 completed weeks of gestational age and later), during childbirth, or up to 7 completed days after birth.

Perinatal mortality rate
The number of perinatal deaths per 1,000 total births (stillbirths plus live births).

Period total fertility rate (PTFR)
The estimated average number of live born children per woman that would be born to a cohort of women throughout their reproductive years, if the fertility rates by age in a given period remained constant at the current age-specific fertility rate.

Perivitelline space
The space between the cytoplasmic membrane enclosing the oocyte and the innermost layer of the zona pellucida. (This space may contain the first and second polar bodies and extracellular fragments.)

Pituitary down-regulation
A medical or pharmacological method to prevent the release of gonadotropins (FSH, LH) from the pituitary gland.

Polar bodies
The small bodies containing chromosomes segregated from the oocyte by asymmetric division during telophase. The first polar body is extruded at telophase I and normally contains only chromosomes with duplicated chromatids (2 c); the second polar body is extruded in response to fertilization or in response to parthenogenetic activation and normally contains chromosomes comprising single chromatids (1 c).

Polycystic ovary syndrome (PCOS)
A heterogeneous condition, which requires the presence of two of the following three criteria: (1) oligo-ovulation or anovulation; (2) hyperandrogenism (clinical evidence of hirsutism, acne, alopecia and/or biochemical hyperandrogenemia); (3) polycystic ovaries, as assessed by ultrasound scan with more than 24 total antral follicles (2–9 mm in size) in both ovaries.

Polycystic ovary (PCO)	An ovary with at least 12 follicles measuring 2–9 mm in diameter in at least one ovary (Rotterdam criteria). PCO may be present in women with PCOS, but also in women with normal ovulatory function and normal fertility.
Polyploidy	The condition in which a cell has more than two haploid sets of chromosomes: e.g. a triploid embryo has three sets of chromosomes and a tetraploid embryo has four sets. Polyploidy in a human embryo is not compatible with life.
Polyspermy	The process by which an oocyte is penetrated by more than one spermatozoon.
Poor ovarian responder (POR) in assisted reproductive technology	A woman treated with ovarian stimulation for ART, in which at least two of the following features are present: (1) advanced maternal age (≥40 years); (2) a previous poor ovarian response (≤3 oocytes with a conventional stimulation protocol aimed at obtaining more than three oocytes); and, (3) an abnormal ovarian reserve test (i.e. antral follicle count 5–7 follicles or anti-Mullerian hormone 0.5–1.1 ng/ml (Bologna criteria); or other reference values obtained from a standardized reference population.)
Poor ovarian response (POR) to ovarian stimulation	A condition in which fewer than four follicles and/or oocytes are developed/obtained following ovarian stimulation with the intention of obtaining more follicles and oocytes.
Post-implantation embryo	An embryo at a stage of development beyond attachment to the endometrium to 8 completed weeks after fertilization, which is equivalent to 10 weeks of gestational age.
Post-term birth	A live birth or stillbirth that takes place after 42 completed weeks of gestational age.
Posthumous reproduction	A process utilizing gametes and/or embryos from a deceased person or persons with the intention of producing offspring.
Pregnancy	A state of reproduction beginning with implantation of an embryo in a woman and ending with the complete expulsion and/or extraction of all products of implantation.
Pregnancy loss	The outcome of any pregnancy that does not result in at least one live birth. When reporting pregnancy loss, the estimated gestational age at the end of pregnancy should be recorded.
Pregnancy of unknown location (PUL)	A pregnancy documented by a positive human chorionic gonadotropin (hCG) test without visualization of pregnancy by ultrasound. This condition exists only after circulating hCG concentration is compatible with ultrasound visualization of a gestational sac.
Pre-implantation embryo	An embryo at a stage of development beginning with division of the zygote into two cells and ending just prior to implantation into a uterus.
Preimplantation genetic testing (PGT)	A test performed to analyze the DNA from oocytes (polar bodies) or embryos (cleavage stage or blastocyst) for HLA-typing or for determining genetic abnormalities. These include: PGT for aneuploidies (PGT-A); PGT for monogenic/single gene defects (PGT-M); and PGT for chromosomal structural rearrangements (PGT-SR).
Preimplantation genetic diagnosis (PGD) and screening (PGS)	These terms have now been replaced by preimplantation genetic testing PGT. (See term PGT and its definitions.)
Premature ejaculation	A condition in which semen is released sooner than desired.

Premature ovarian insufficiency	A condition characterized by hypergonadotropic hypogonadism in women younger than age 40 years (also known as premature or primary ovarian failure). It includes women with premature menopause.
Preterm birth	A birth that takes place after 22 weeks and before 37 completed weeks of gestational age.
Primary childlessness	A condition in which a person has never delivered a live child, or has never been a legal or societally recognized parent to a child.
Primary female infertility	A woman who has never been diagnosed with a clinical pregnancy and meets the criteria of being classified as having infertility.
Primary involuntary childlessness	A condition in a person with a child wish, who has never delivered a live child, or has never been a legal or societally recognized parent to a child. A major cause of primary involuntary childlessness is infertility.
Primary male infertility	A man who has never initiated a clinical pregnancy and meets the criteria of being classified as infertile.
Pronuclei transfer	Transfer of the pronuclei from a patient's zygote to an enucleated donated zygote.
Pronucleus	A round structure in the oocyte surrounded by a membrane containing chromatin. Normally, two pronuclei are seen after fertilization, each containing a haploid set of chromosomes, one set from the oocyte and one from the sperm, before zygote formation.
Recipient (ART)	A person or couple who receives donated eggs, sperm or embryos for the purposes of initiating a pregnancy with the intention of becoming a legally recognized parent.
Recipient ART cycle	An ART cycle in which a woman receives zygote(s) or embryo(s) from donor(s) or a partner.
Recurrent spontaneous abortion/ miscarriage	The spontaneous loss of two or more clinical pregnancies prior to 22 completed weeks of gestational age.
Reproductive surgery	Surgical procedures performed to diagnose, conserve, correct and/or improve reproductive function in either men or women. Surgery for contraceptive purposes, such as tubal ligation and vasectomy, are also included within this term.
Retrograde ejaculation	A condition that causes the semen to be forced backward from the ejaculatory ducts into the bladder during ejaculation.
Salpingectomy	The surgical removal of an entire Fallopian tube.
Salpingitis isthmica nodosa (SIN)	A nodular thickening of the proximal Fallopian tube (where the tubes join the uterus), which can distort or occlude the tubes and increase the risk of ectopic pregnancy and infertility.
Salpingostomy	A surgical procedure in which an opening is made in the Fallopian tube either to remove an ectopic pregnancy or open a blocked, fluid-filled tube (hydrosalpinx).
Secondary female infertility	A woman unable to establish a clinical pregnancy but who has previously been diagnosed with a clinical pregnancy.
Secondary involuntary childlessness	A condition in a person with a child wish, who has previously delivered a live child, or is or has been a legal or societally recognized parent to a child. A major cause of secondary involuntary childlessness is infertility.

Secondary male infertility	A man who is unable to initiate a clinical pregnancy, but who had previously initiated a clinical pregnancy.
Semen analysis	A description of the ejaculate to assess function of the male reproductive tract. Characteristic parameters include volume, pH, concentration, motility, vitality, morphology of spermatozoa and presence of other cells.
Semen liquefaction	The process whereby proteolytic enzymes degrade proteins causing seminal plasma to liquefy.
Semen viscosity	The description of the relative fluidity of seminal plasma.
Semen volume	The amount of fluid in an ejaculate.
Semen/ejaculate	The fluid at ejaculation that contains the cells and secretions originating from the testes and sex accessory glands.
Seminal plasma	The fluids of the ejaculate.
Sertoli cell	The nongerminal cell type in the seminiferous tubule that mediates the actions of testosterone and FSH in the testis, provides nutrients and proteins to the developing spermatogenic cells, creates the blood–testis barrier, and secretes Mullerian-inhibiting hormone.
Sertoli cell-only syndrome	A condition in which only Sertoli cells line the seminiferous tubules with usually a complete absence of germ cells; also referred to as germ cell aplasia. Spermatogenesis in isolated foci can be observed in rare cases.
Severe ovarian hyperstimulation syndrome (OHSS)	A systemic response as a result of ovarian stimulation interventions that is characterized by severe abdominal discomfort and/or other symptoms of ascites, hemoconcentration (Hct > 45) and/or other serious biochemical abnormalities requiring hospitalization for observation and/or for medical intervention (paracentesis, other).
Single embryo transfer (SET)	The transfer of one embryo in an ART procedure. Defined as elective (eSET) when more than one embryo of sufficient quality for transfer is available.
Slow-freezing	A cryopreservation procedure in which the temperature of the cell(s) is lowered in a step-wise fashion, typically using a computer-controlled rate, from physiological (or room) temperature to extreme low temperature.
Small for gestational age	A birth weight less than the 10th centile for gestational age. When reporting results, the reference criteria should be specified. If gestational age is unknown, the birth weight should be registered.
Sperm bank	Repository of cryopreserved sperm stored for future use.
Sperm concentration	The (measure of the) number of spermatozoa in millions per 1 ml of semen.
Sperm density	A measure of the mass/volume ratio (specific gravity) for spermatozoa.
Sperm isolation	A procedure that involves the separation of sperm through centrifugation and resuspension in culture media. It can be used to remove seminal plasma and infectious agents before IUI and ART procedures. This procedure has been shown to be effective in the removal of HIV. It may also be effective in removing other infectious particles but clinical safety and efficacy have to be established for each particular infection. This term is sometimes referred to as "sperm washing."
Sperm motility	The percentage of moving spermatozoa relative to the total number of spermatozoa.

Sperm recipient cycle	A MAR cycle in which a woman receives spermatozoa from a person who is not her sexually intimate partner. In the case of ART registry data, a sperm recipient cycle would only include data from cycles using ART procedures.
Sperm vitality	The percentage of live spermatozoa relative to the total number of spermatozoa.
Spermatogenic arrest	Failure of germ cells to progress through specific stages of spermatogenesis at onset or during meiosis.
Spermatozoon	The mature male reproductive cell produced in the testis that has the capacity to fertilize an oocyte. A head carries genetic material, a midpiece produces energy for movement, and a long, thin tail propels the sperm.
Spontaneous abortion/miscarriage	The spontaneous loss of an intra-uterine pregnancy prior to 22 completed weeks of gestational age.
Spontaneous reduction/vanishing sac(s)	The spontaneous disappearance of one or more gestational sacs with or without an embryo or fetus in a multiple pregnancy documented by ultrasound.
Sterility	A permanent state of infertility.
Stillbirth	The death of a fetus prior to the complete expulsion or extraction from its mother after 28 completed weeks of gestational age. The death is determined by the fact that, after such separation, the fetus does not breathe or show any other evidence of life, such as heartbeat, umbilical cord pulsation, or definite movement of voluntary muscles. Note: it includes deaths occurring during labor.
Stillbirth rate	The number of stillbirths per 1,000 total births (stillbirths plus live births).
Subfertility	A term that should be used interchangeably with infertility.
Syngamy	The process during which the female and male pronuclei fuse.
Teratozoospermia	A reduced percentage of morphologically normal sperm in the ejaculate below the lower reference limits. When reporting results, the reference criteria should be specified.
Testicular sperm aspiration/extraction (TESA/TESE)	A surgical procedure involving one or more testicular biopsies or needle aspirations to obtain sperm for use in IVF and/or ICSI.
Thawing	The process of raising the temperature of slow-frozen cell(s) from the storage temperature to room/physiological temperature.
Time to pregnancy (TTP)	The time taken to establish a pregnancy, measured in months or in numbers of menstrual cycles.
Time-lapse imaging	The photographic recording of microscope image sequences at regular intervals in ART, referring to gametes, zygotes, cleavage-stage embryos or blastocysts.
Total delivery rate with at least one live birth	The total number of deliveries with at least one live birth resulting from one initiated or aspirated ART cycle, including all cycles in which fresh and/or frozen embryos are transferred, including more than one delivery from one initiated or aspirated cycle if that occurs, until all embryos are used. Note: the delivery of a singleton, twin or other multiple pregnancy is registered as one delivery. In the absence of complete data, the total delivery rate is often estimated.

Total fertility rate (TFR)	The average number of live births per woman. It may be determined in retrospect, observed data (Cohort Total Fertility Rate, (CTFR)) or as an estimated average number (Period Total Fertility Rate, (PTFR)).
Total sperm count	The calculated total number of sperm in the ejaculate (semen volume multiplied by the sperm concentration determined from an aliquot of semen).
Traditional gestational carrier	A woman who donates her oocytes and is the gestational carrier for a pregnancy resulting from fertilization of her oocytes either through an ART procedure or insemination. This replaces the term "traditional surrogate."
Trisomy	An abnormal number of chromosome copies in a cell characterized by the presence of three homologous chromosomes rather than the normal two. The majority of human embryos with trisomies are incompatible with life.
Trophectoderm	Cells forming the outer layer of a blastocyst that have the potential to develop into the placenta and amniotic membranes.
Tubal pathology	Tubal abnormality resulting in dysfunction of the Fallopian tube, including partial or total obstruction of one or both tubes (proximally, distally or combined), hydrosalpinx and/or peri-tubal and/or peri-ovarian adhesions affecting the normal ovum pick-up function. It usually occurs after pelvic inflammatory disease or pelvic surgery.
Unexplained infertility	Infertility in couples with apparently normal ovarian function, Fallopian tubes, uterus, cervix and pelvis and with adequate coital frequency; and apparently normal testicular function, genito-urinary anatomy and a normal ejaculate. The potential for this diagnosis is dependent upon the methodologies used and/or those methodologies available.
Unisomy	The condition in a cell resulting from loss of a single chromosome yielding a single copy of that particular chromosome rather than the normal two. The majority of unisomies in human embryos are incompatible with life.
Vaginal insemination	A procedure whereby semen, collected from a nonlubricated condom or similar method, is deposited into the vaginal cavity of a female. An intervention that can be self-administered by a woman attempting pregnancy.
Varicocele	A venous enlargement in the testicular pampiniform plexus.
Varicocelectomy	Procedure to occlude or remove part of the internal spermatic vein in situations in which it has expanded into a varicocele.
Vasectomy	Procedure to occlude the vas deferens. It is usually carried out bilaterally in order to secure sterilization.
Very low birth weight	Birth weight less than 1,500 g.
Viscosity	The description of the relative fluidity of the semen.
Vitrification	An ultra-rapid cryopreservation procedure that prevents ice formation within a cell whose aqueous phase is converted to a glass-like solid.
Voluntary childlessness	A condition describing a person who does not have or has not had a child wish and does not have any biologically, legally or societally recognized children.
Warming (cells)	The process of raising the temperature of a vitrified cell or cells from the storage temperature to room/physiological temperature.

Y-chromosome microdeletions   Missing segments of the genetic material on the Y-chromosome that are associated with abnormal spermatogenesis.

Zona pellucida   The glycoprotein coat surrounding the oocyte.

Zygote   A single cell resulting from fertilization of a mature oocyte by a spermatozoon and before completion of the first mitotic division.

Zygote intrafallopian transfer (ZIFT)   An ART procedure in which one or more zygotes is transferred into the Fallopian tube.

Index

Printed in the United States
by Baker & Taylor Publisher Services